Contemporary Issues
in Bioethics

Contemporary Issues in Bioethics

A Catholic Perspective

James J. Walter
Thomas A. Shannon

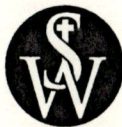

A SHEED & WARD BOOK

ROWMAN & LITTLEFIELD PUBLISHERS, INC.
Lanham • Boulder • New York • Toronto • Oxford

A SHEED & WARD BOOK

ROWMAN & LITTLEFIELD PUBLISHERS, INC.

Published in the United States of America
by Rowman & Littlefield Publishers, Inc.
A wholly owned subsidiary of The Rowman & Littlefield Publishing Group, Inc.
4501 Forbes Boulevard, Suite 200, Lanham, Maryland 20706
www.rowmanlittlefield.com

PO Box 317
Oxford
OX2 9RU, UK

British Library Cataloguing in Publication Information Available
Library of Congress Cataloging-in-Publication Data

Contemporary issues in bioethics : a Catholic perspective / by James J. Walter
and Thomas A. Shannon.
    p.   cm.
Includes bibliographical references and index.
ISBN 0-7425-5060-5 (hardcover : alk. paper)—ISBN 0-7425-5061-3
(pbk. : alk. paper)
1. Medical ethics—Religious aspects—Catholic Church. 2. Bioethics—Religious
aspects—Catholic Church. I. Walter, James J. II. Shannon, Thomas A.
[DNLM: 1. Bioethical Issues. 2. Catholicism. WB 60 C761 2005]
R725.56.C66   2005
174.2—dc22   2005016779

Printed in the United States of America

♾ ™ The paper used in this publication meets the minimum requirements of American
National Standard for Information Sciences—Permanence of Paper for Printed Library
Materials, ANSI/NISO Z39.48-1992.

To
Jennifer K. Walter
Robert J. Walter

May the love that both of you have for the art and practice of medicine and for the study of bioethics nourish and sustain you in your care of patients and the teaching of students.

To
Ashley E. Shannon
Courtney Shannon Pinto
Dino Pinto

You have wonderful gifts that you offer to your students. May you continue to find joy and fulfillment in your teaching and in your lives.

Contents

Acknowledgments

We gratefully acknowledge permission to reprint the following chapters:

Chapter 1. "Religion and Bioethics: A Value Added Discussion," by Thomas A. Shannon. In *Notes From a Narrow Ridge: Religion and Bioethics*, edited by D. S., Davis and L. Zoloth. Hagerstown, MD: University Publishing Group, 1999, 129–50.

Chapter 4. "The Communitarian Perspective: Autonomy and the Common Good," by Thomas A. Shannon. In *Meta-Medical Ethics*, edited by M. A. Grodin. The Netherlands: Kluwer Academic Publishers, © 1995, with kind permission of Springer Science and Business Media, 61–76.

Chapter 5. "Reflections on the Moral Status of the Pre-embryo," by Thomas A. Shannon and Allan B. Wolter, OFM. *Theological Studies* 51 (December 1990): 603–26.

Chapter 7. "Cloning, Uniqueness and Individuality," by Thomas A. Shannon. *Louvain Studies* 19 (1994): 283–306.

Chapter 8. "Reproductive Technologies: Ethical and Religious Issues," by Thomas A. Shannon. In *God Forbid: Religion and Sex in American Public Life*, edited by Kathleen M. Sands, copyright © 2000 by Oxford University Press, Inc. Used by permission of Oxford University Press, Inc.

Chapter 9. "Theological Parameters: Catholic Doctrine on Abortion in a Pluralist Society," by James J. Walter. In *Abortion and Public Policy: An Interdisciplinary Investigation within the Catholic Tradition*, edited by Gerard Magill and R. Randall Rainey. Omaha, NE: Creighton University Press, 1996, 91–130.

Chapter 10. "Perspectives on Medical Ethics: Biotechnology and Genetic

Medicine," by James J. Walter. In *A Call to Fidelity: On the Moral Theology of Charles E. Curran*, edited by James J. Walter, Timothy E. O'Connell & Thomas A. Shannon. Washington, DC: Georgetown University Press, 2002, 135–52. Copyright with permission of Georgetown University Press.

Chapter 12. "The Meaning and Validity of Quality of Life Judgments in Contemporary Roman Catholic Medical Ethics," by James J. Walter. *Louvain Studies* 13 (Fall, 1988): 195-208.

Chapter 13. "Terminal Sedation: A Catholic Perspective" by James J. Walter. Reprinted with permission of Loma Linda University Center for Christian Bioethics from *Update: Loma Linda University Center for Christian Bioethics* 18 (September 2002): 6–8, 12.

Chapter 14. "The PVS Patient and the Forgoing/Withdrawing of Medical Nutrition and Hydration," by Thomas A. Shannon and James J. Walter. *Theological Studies* 49 (December, 1988): 623-647.

Chapter 15. "Health Beat: Artificial Nutrition, Hydration: Assessing Papal Statement," by Thomas A. Shannon and James J. Walter. *National Catholic Reporter* 40 (April 16, 2004): 9–10.

Chapter 16. "Implications of the Papal Allocution on Feeding Tubes," by Thomas A. Shannon and James J. Walter. *Hastings Center Report* 34 (July/August 2004): 18–20.

Chapter 17. "Assisted Nutrition and Hydration and the Catholic Tradition," by Thomas A. Shannon and James J. Walter. *Theological Studies* 66 (September 2005).

Introduction

Bioethics as a multidisciplinary field had its origins in the late 1960s and early 1970s. It began in response to two important currents. The first was concerned with the rapid developments that were being made in the scientific and medical arenas, both in medical and biotechnology and in the life sciences. The second was concerned with two cultural realities: the pluralism, with its moral relativism, that was shaping American culture during and beyond the post–World War II era, and the civil rights movement in the 1960s, especially with its emphasis on autonomy and the right to self-determination. Though bioethics in this configuration is relatively recent, the Catholic moral tradition had been discussing issues related to medicine and patient care since at least the sixteenth century. Not only have theologians from this tradition been writing treatises in these areas, but popes in the twentieth century, especially those from Pope Pius XII to John Paul II, have made many pronouncements on issues ranging from assisted reproductive technologies to the forgoing/withdrawing of mechanical ventilators and feeding tubes.

Much of the literature that has been written in recent years in the field of bioethics has come from the disciplines of philosophy and the social sciences. Theological reflection on the complex bioethical issues that confront society has also continued in recent years, but not much attention has been placed on the distinctive contribution that the Roman Catholic moral tradition can make. This book exists to fill this need in that its intent is to demonstrate that the Catholic moral tradition does have resources within itself to address the growing number of issues.

The structure of the book is "issue-oriented." In other words, rather than beginning with some abstract analysis or set of principles and then applying them to concrete issues such as reproductive cloning, we have decided to structure the volume by reference to the issues themselves. By analyzing the issues in their concrete circumstances in culture, we articulate the theoretical underpinnings at work in the analysis.

The book is divided in four parts, and each part seeks to address a series of important issues in contemporary bioethics from the Catholic perspective. The first part addresses the theological issues in bioethics. It studies how religion or theological reflection might contribute to bioethics and clarifies some of the important theological concepts that have been developed in the field (e.g., the concept of "playing God"). The second part focuses on those issues at the beginning of life. It analyzes such important and controversial issues as the moral status of the preimplantation embryo, embryonic stem cell research, human cloning, reproductive technologies, and the issue of abortion. Part 3 seeks to address those complex issues related to molecular genetics and biotechnology and those concerned with the care of critically ill patients. Now that the Human Genome Project has completed its work by mapping and sequencing all the genetic material in the human person, we will be faced with new biotechnologies and genetic medicines that will seek to cure diseases that regularly kill people. But will this search for new cures violate the canons of morality? Will we save these patients' lives only for them now to live in chronic pain and disability? Should one consider "quality of life" as one of the criteria for intervening medically? Finally, part 4 focuses on a range of very complex issues concerned with the end of life. Terminal sedation as a way of dealing with the refractory pain of dying cancer patients, on the one hand, and the forgoing/withdrawal of artificial nutrition and hydration, on the other, are two of the most controversial issues being discussed in contemporary bioethics, especially within the Catholic community.

We would argue that there is really no such thing as "Catholic bioethics" in the sense that only Catholics could do that field or that only Catholics would have access to the knowledge about the issues discussed. However, we will argue in this book that critical reflection on the Catholic moral tradition not only can and does shape and inform our ways of thinking about these important issues but that it also can yield important and valid moral insights as well.

I

THEOLOGICAL ISSUES

Religion and Bioethics: A Value-Added Discussion

Thomas A. Shannon

Two sets of concerns inform this chapter. One is autobiographical and professional and the other is more disciplinary or content oriented. Both dimensions of this topic are critical for me and helped shape my own orientation to various topics in bioethics. Thus, the chapter begins with some reflections on how the field of bioethics was shaped and then moves into how a religious dimension will add to the debate.

THE FIELD OF BIOETHICS

When I received my doctoral degree from Boston University in 1972, the field of bioethics was in its initial phases. I took a course in bioethics offered through the Boston Theological Institute, the consortium of theology schools in the Boston area. Joseph Fletcher was one of the instructors, and Robert Veatch made a guest appearance. Other guest instructors from various divinity schools in the area gave presentations as well. In this course some attention was given to the religious dimension of the various problems we discussed, but philosophical and social analysis also played an important part of the discussion. I wrote a paper on the moral status of the fetus using the Thomistic theory of delayed animation further developed and applied to contemporary embryology by Joseph Donceel. But in all of this, the orientation was mainly philosophical rather than religious.

Yet in the development of bioethics there is a very long tradition of reflecting on these issues in religious categories and within religious communities. Many religions, such as the Catholic tradition, use a philosophical framework for such discussions, but the thrust of the analysis is informed by theological principles or faith-derived values. Topics such as humans created in the image of God, stewardship, human finitude, the value of community, and immortality inform these discussions in critical and profound ways. And this is reflected in the fact that many seminaries or divinity schools treated such topics in their curricula, mainly under the rubric of pastoral care, a course on the administration of the sacraments, or as part of the general curriculum in moral theology. Thus, questions of ordinary and extraordinary means of treatment would be treated under the fifth commandment: Do not kill. Abortion would be treated there also. Issues having to do with reproduction were treated in Catholic moral theology in the course on the sacrament of matrimony. Although divinity schools offered very few explicit courses that we would today identify as bioethics courses, many of the problems we discuss today have a long history of debate in moral theology. For example, the discussion of ordinary and extraordinary means goes back, in the Catholic tradition, to at least the sixteenth century.[1]

In the early days of bioethics, it should come as no surprise that many of the individuals teaching in this area came out of seminaries or divinity schools. The Catholic side had both Gerald Kelly and John Ford. Kelly wrote a medical ethics text as well as frequent articles addressing such topics. Richard McCormick, Warren Reich, and Charles Curran picked up where Kelly and Ford left off. Other Catholic theologians followed their lead: James J. Walter, Lisa S. Cahill, Richard Gula, and James Keenan. On the Protestant side were individuals such as Joseph Fletcher (at least in his time as an Episcopalian priest) Paul Ramsey, William F. May, Robert Veatch, James Childress, Stanley Hauerwas, and Karen Lebacqz. Although these individuals incorporated philosophical analysis into their courses and writings, they also were informed by their religious traditions or religious values. Particularly in the Catholic tradition, new topics and problems were incorporated into an existing framework that was then re-articulated in light of the new problems. Professionally trained philosophers generally were not part of these early discussions, although such individuals (Daniel Callahan in particular) were eventually to play a major role.

My strongest memory about this phase of the development of bioethics—this would be in the mid-1970s—is that many professionally trained philosophers were not interested in this field or such problems because the focus was practical problem solving rather than broad, theoretical philosophical analysis. The few philosophers who became engaged in the bioethics discussion were referred to as "applied philosophers," and that phrase was frequently pronounced with a certain level of condescension, if not outright disdain. At that time, analytic philosophy still was the dominant methodology in many graduate schools of philosophy, so there was little professional incentive to think about such practical and conceptually messy problems as whether to turn off a respirator. Thus, the interest in thinking about such problems came primarily from individuals trained in religious studies or theology and who grew up in a tradition that was open to practical problem solving. Although theology and religious studies had their theoretical and historical debates, they also had space—mainly in the disciplines of moral theology, pastoral studies, and pastoral counseling—for practical problem solving. In addition, Catholicism brought to the discussion its own practical history of case discussions both from the tradition of casuistry and the training of confessors. Many religious orders, for example, had the practice of holding weekly or monthly discussions of "cases of conscience," in which a case was presented and then the members of the community discussed various resolutions of it. Such was the fertile ground in which the field of bioethics developed.

What changed to bring in the philosophers and recast the nature of the field? One major element was the foundation of the Hastings Center by Daniel Callahan, a professionally trained philosopher—but with a strong Catholic heritage sharpened during his years as editor of *Commonweal*—and Willard Gaylin, a psychiatrist who remained agnostic on religious issues. The founding of the Hastings Center coincided with technological developments in medicine such as various forms of life support and organ transplantation, as well as the prolonged debate over the recombinant-DNA technology. The Hastings Center validated the public discussion of these questions and conducted a discussion of the many sides of these issues. Many of the individuals who formed the research teams developed by the Hastings Center were the individuals named above. But others were also brought in because, by definition, the Hastings Center was not an advocacy center. It was not to represent a point of view other than an informed, critical discussion that would be helpful in forming public policy. Thus, although many of the individuals spoke from a religious tradition, they had to recast that tradition when speaking to public policy issues. The focus was on a debate accessible to the larger community rather than one directed to a particular religious tradition. Thus, the focus of the Hastings Center changed how bioethical issues were presented and debated. Although religion and religious issues were not eliminated, the priority was the development of an analysis for use in public policy debate.

A second major change in the field of bioethics was the inclusion of professionally trained philosophers in the discussion. These individuals brought with them the methodology, terminology, and viewpoint of their own professional training. And their contributions added significantly to the analysis of various topics in bioethics. So one major reason for philosophers' inclusion was the contributions they could make from their particular perspectives. But another reason is a bit more cynical. The disdain in which some held the developing field of "applied philosophy" was overcome by the availability of grant money and jobs. As bioethics came more and more to the public's attention and the problems became issues of public policy, academics became more interested. Centers were established; professional journals were founded; grant money became available; and universities, colleges, and medical schools began offering courses. Suddenly, applied philosophy looked pretty good, particularly when the job market at universities in the 1970s and early 1980s was tight and jobs in bioethics were available. Today the term *applied philosophy* has almost vanished, and the consideration of problems in a variety of professions—medicine, law, business, engineering, and journalism, to name a few—is regarded as routine and appropriate in graduate philosophy programs.

The point of these comments is not to express dismay at philosophy's entering the bioethics debate, but rather to note its late entry and its need first to validate in some fashion the consideration of practical problems as a legitimate part of the discipline. At one meeting, Al Jonsen described working in a medical school as "doing philosophy in the trenches." Another philosopher told of defining a philosopher as a "professional bullshit detector" during an interview at a medical school. Such descriptions accurately capture critical elements of the practice of bioethics, but they are a far cry from various metaethical considerations or discussions of the fine points of various methodologies. And while a philosopher who is not carefully trained in the fine points of his or her discipline will not get very far as a professional philosopher, neither will that person succeed at bioethics if he or she cannot translate these concepts and methods into a language and analysis to shed light on problems that desperately need such illumination. Thus, rather than seeing philosophy as wasted on such practical discussion, the revised version correctly sees the value that systematic discussion and analysis can bring to complex and value-laden discussions that are a routine, but often confused, part of daily decision making in the practice of medicine.

A third factor that brought philosophers to the fore was the increased recognition of the pluralistic nature of the bioethics debate. An additional dimension of this was the shift to a more procedural resolution of problems— deciding them on the basis of whose right it was to make the decision rather than evaluating the merits of a decision. Recognition of pluralism and procedural resolution helped decrease the role of religion in public policy debates because, rightly or wrongly, religion was seen as partisan and imposing solutions from a faith-based perspective that was not subscribed to by the citizens at large. Or, to paraphrase the argument of the time, to use the position of a particular religion on a specific topic as public policy was to impose its solution on people who were not members of that religion. In the vacuum that followed this debate, philosophy quite naturally stepped in and offered itself as a more neutral approach to considering the issues; at least philosophy could spell out the arguments and show what was at stake without necessarily committing itself to a particular conclusion. In short, religion was seen as advocacy, philosophy as analysis.

The consequences of the introduction of philosophy into the bioethics discussion were quite significant. One was the development of the "Georgetown mantra" of *autonomy, beneficence, maleficence*, and *justice*. Each of these four concepts is quite important, and their application to various problems in bioethics has been significant in illuminating and resolving many problems. The doctrine of informed consent, for example, would probably not have the significant place in the practice of modern medicine that it does had it not been for the development of a strong concept of autonomy.

Ironically, two of the major contributors to this "mantra"—Veatch and Childress—were trained in divinity schools. One might think that, given the academic backgrounds of these early bioethicists, their analysis of these core ideas might have turned out a little differently. Yet the context in which these core ideas were developed was significantly different than a religious context: the focus was the individual and his or her rights in a public policy context. That is, given the context of pluralism, the strategy of proceduralism for problem solving, the primacy of argument over advocacy, and the focus on rights rather than duties, these four concepts were used to think through the decisions of individuals. In informed consent, the issue was the primacy of patient choice, not medical judgment, family, or social obligations. With beneficence or maleficence, the primary issue was goods or harms to the patient, not necessarily social benefits or social harms. With justice, the main consideration was fairness to the individual, not to society. Now to be sure, there were and are many discussions that also included a social dimension; the distribution of scarce resources continues to be a major theme in many debates. But the critical point of departure, and frequently the sole controlling factor for these discussions, was the individual and his or her rights. Again I cannot emphasize enough the importance of that contribution to the various debates, but the problem is that such viewpoints came to be seen as the only ones or as the only normative ones.

Thus the role of family, community, religion, social needs, and medical judgment fell to the side of the road—if not off it completely. Many of the discussions in bioethics focused on the protection of the individual and the attainment of his or her rights as the main, if not sole, agenda. That such an agenda is skewed is now becoming obvious, socially, philosophically, and religiously. Part of this broader discussion is being driven by the shift in the practice of medicine from more or less private practice to some sort of health-maintenance organization (HMO) or other social institutionalization of the practice of medicine. Here, social and systemic issues quickly come to the fore, and analysis of individual needs is inadequate. To be sure, individual needs continue to be critical, but other needs that are socially driven also must be incorporated into the debate.

We are also beginning to recognize the limits of the philosophy of individualism that has been so strong in U.S. culture. Although we will continue to celebrate the individual and recognize the strengths and contributions of our celebration of individual freedoms, we are also recognizing that *individual* and *community* are not mutually exclusive terms and that communities can contribute to individual well-being. We are also learning that resolving the needs of many individuals does not necessarily contribute to social well-being, in spite of almost two centuries of tutoring by Adam Smith and his invisible hand. That is, the social good is not necessarily served by each seeking his or her individual good; in fact, harm can be caused to society in this way. An individual requesting and receiving a full range of services for a particular problem may not be socially harmful, but when everyone seeks the same level of treatment—whether appropriate or not—then society's resources can be strained.

Philosophy itself is turning to the direction of community as a critical resource in the resolution of problems, but we are only at the beginning of that journey.

Finally we are recognizing that, as it is important to treat individuals justly, there are also implications of justice for society in how we resolve such individual needs. The point is not to cast this discussion as a "win-lose" formula, but rather to note that the resolution of individual problems has social consequences, which are also subject to justice considerations. We all recognize the importance of an organ transplant for an individual dying of kidney or heart failure. But we also recognize that how one gets to a particular place on the waiting list is as much a matter of social justice as of individual justice. So, too, the perception of health care is shifting from a private good owed in justice to the individual to a social good owed in justice to the community. The consequences of this shift will be significant in how health-care services are provided, but this is a clear issue of social justice.

Thus, we are coming to recognize the limits of the philosophical concepts and methodologies we have relied on in the past. As valuable and critical as they have been and still are, they cannot resolve all problems nor can they fully analyze the changing shifts in the delivery of health care in this country.

Additionally, the needs of the community are coming to the fore, and we are recognizing that social justice is as important as individual justice. Finally, we are seeing that the individual cannot stand totally alone but needs grounding in the resources that a community can provide.

Religion is one resource that we can use in this rethinking of fundamental bioethical problems as well as the new challenges facing us. I am not arguing for religion as deus ex machina but as a resource available to help extend our analysis and to ground our arguments.

RELIGION AND BIOETHICS: ADDING VALUE TO THE DEBATE

The point of departure for this section is two experiences I had where religion added a value to the discussion. One occurred several years ago when my wife and I (Catholics) were invited to a discussion group whose members (Jewish) had been meeting off and on for many years. I was invited to give a presentation on withdrawing life support. The discussion that followed was lively and very moving. Finally, one person asked how my religion had influenced my discussion. In my typical academic fashion I began by saying how the discussion of forgoing extraordinary treatment was a centuries-old part of Catholicism. "No, no!" he said. "You must believe in immortality; otherwise you could not speak as you do." And then the discussion got very interesting because many others declared that they too did not believe in immortality, which was why so many of their decisions to end treatment had been so difficult. To withdraw treatment was to say an ultimate farewell. And then we discussed how, even if one believed in immortality, such discussions were also difficult, but that while one dimension of one's relation was over, the belief in the possibility of another remained. As one of the prayers in the Catholic liturgy for the dead says: "Life is changed, not taken away."

If one had directly asked me independently of this discussion group if I believed in immortality or some form of personal post-death survival, I would have said yes, but I probably would have qualified that whole topic in a variety of ways so that even I would be unsure of its meaning when finished. But in the context of this discussion, I learned how deeply such a belief was part of me and how that belief has conditioned my thinking about such decisions.

A second experience is more recent. Ray, a friend who was a priest and campus minister among many other incarnations, was diagnosed with a virulent brain tumor. He died seven weeks later. My wife and I were unable to attend the funeral, but my sister-in-law sent us a tape of the funeral, which more than two thousand people attended. Two things stood out for me. One came from the homily that was preached by a colleague of Ray's who accompanied him in this last journey. Of particular interest was their discussion of how in some ways this illness was like the testing of Job—random, unfair, and unintelligible. Yet what came ringing through so clearly was the grace and graciousness with which Ray responded to this, a response born of a depth of spirituality that was supported and nourished by a loving and attentive community. The other element of religion came from a letter to Ray that was read during the homily. Ray pursued peace and justice with the same zeal that he brought to an even earlier incarnation as a Marine. The letter stated that the author simply could not get Ray out of his mind, that he had emblazoned a message in him about justice that he could not rid himself of. This was a message that was so clearly much more than a discussion of "to each his or her own." The preferential option for the poor based on Hebrew and Christian scriptures does not put forth the image of justice as a scale, but rather a concern for the marginalized. And so a religious perspective transformed Ray and those he met.

The sections that follow in the physician-assisted suicide/euthanasia debate and on the provision of health care present two issues for which, like the examples above, religion can add value to the debate.

THE PHYSICIAN-ASSISTED
SUICIDE/EUTHANASIA DEBATE

Although it is probably impossible to argue a listener into a change of position on the topic of physician-assisted suicide and euthanasia, it is possible to suggest gaps or deficiencies in arguments. The technique is to be respectful of the arguments and beliefs of others, to avoid proselytizing or appearing condescending, and at the same time to show how belief changes an argument or an attitude and can add different elements to the debate.

An important and influential text with which to begin is Daniel Callahan's *The Troubled Dream of Life*.[2] This book is one of the strongest arguments against physician-assisted suicide and euthanasia I have seen. But what is most interesting is that it argues the case on secular or philosophical grounds. While Callahan does not deny religious arguments or seek to remove religion from the debate, he does not see them as meaningful for him and he seeks arguments elsewhere. Essentially the argument is grounded in dying a death both reflective of and worthy of the life one has lived. What emerges from the argument is a kind of Camus-like stoicism in the face of the inevitable. One takes what comes and deals with it as best as one can, hoping for a community that supports one, and for personal resources to make one's dying bearable. Yet even in this, Callahan does not shut the door. "I watch and I wait," he says.[3]

An irony found in the book is that although Callahan rejects a religious element to his argument, primarily on personal grounds, the whole tenor of the book reflects a type of secularized Catholicism. The religious roots of the book are closer to the surface than he admits. To lead a life worthy of one's dying or to have one's death reflect one's life is one of the most traditional of Catholic perspectives on death. One is admonished by the tradition to live in a state of constant preparedness, for "one does not know the hour or place." And when one does know this, there is a whole theology of redemptive suffering derived from the tradition of the suffering servant in the books of Isaiah the prophet and from the life of Jesus. The teaching is not a refined sadomasochism, but a gesture of solidarity and service to the community, in terms of the inspiration of the personal example of the one dying and also of a change in how members of the community see themselves and their lives.

Additionally, Callahan's discussion of the value and significance of the distinction between ordinary and extraordinary means of treatment is surely informed by traditional Catholic teaching. Callahan sharpens this distinction in his usual perceptive style, but the teaching is of a piece with the Catholic tradition. So too his argument coheres with the Catholic tradition's teaching on the value of the community and seeking the common good of the community.

Would Callahan's argument be any different if he had not had an earlier exposure to a religious tradition? Perhaps not, for one can find other philosophical arguments making many of the same points. But Callahan came to this argument with a mind-set that already had a fair amount of spade work done and with much ground prepared. The main line of the argument did not have to be rethought from scratch. Additionally his argument was pointed in certain directions—the relation of one's life and death and the role of community—by exposure to his religious tradition. Clearly Callahan went beyond this tradition, refined it, and added other elements to his argument. But a tradition was already present that added important dimensions to his argument.

The religious tradition can provide a needed critique of elements of the physician-assisted suicide/euthanasia debate. This debate is cast in a variety of ways—relief from unbearable pain, an end to incurable terminal disease, a resolution of the uncertainties of the inevitable progress of a disease. But a core feature of the debate, in the judgment of many, is autonomy—the right to control one's destiny. The life I live is mine and mine only, and I choose the circumstances under which I live or—in this debate—die. The mythology underlying this value is at the core of American life—rugged individualism, self-sufficiency, the need to "do it my way."

This element of the debate is central to all dimensions of the physician-assisted suicide/euthanasia debate. This is because of the central role autonomy has rightly played in bioethics almost since the inception of the field. Many of the philosophical and policy gains have in no small measure been due to the significance of autonomy. And we are now coming to realize how deeply autonomy fits into the core values and mythology of American life. Thus the stage was set for this next application of autonomy in the physician-assisted suicide/euthanasia debate. For surely the right to end one's life at the time and circumstances of one's choosing is but a logical application of the right to choose in general and the right to determine one's life circumstances in particular. And this is a difficult argument to overcome. The major fights in bioethics ranging from abortion to the right to refuse unwanted treatment have all been based on autonomy; appeals to it are almost a philosophical knee-jerk reaction. When all else fails, autonomy is the ultimate trump.

But think of the image of autonomy and the mythology underlying it: the solitary individual, the one unknown to all others, the only one who can speak for one's self, the only one who can be trusted with one's self and one's deepest desires, the self-made person. The price of autonomy is quite high—an ultimate aloneness. For truly no one can know me or what is good for me or what I might want in particular circumstances. Only the autonomous self can know this.

What religion can offer here is a correction of autonomy—a reminder that there is a reality called community in which we are born, nourished, educated, sustained, and ultimately flourish. This is not a rejection of autonomy or a tyranny of the many over the one. Rather, it is a recognition that at our deepest levels we are not self-made individuals. Everything we bring to our existence we have received from others—our existence, our language, our education, our food, our clothing, our shelter. As we mature, we assume many of these responsibilities for ourselves and begin to build on these resources and gifts from the community in which we live. We also find a degree of fulfillment in our relations with others whether in friendship or in other forms of committed relations. Here we find new dimensions of fulfillment and even self-discovery. But these new discoveries come as a gift of the relationship itself. We are much more with and a part of a community than the prevailing ideology of autonomy would suggest.

And it is here that I recall various stories of my friend Ray's last weeks. For while surely Ray had a deep devotion to self-reliance and a strong sense of initiative and individual responsibility, he also recognized that his life was not totally of his own making. He knew that although he had an agenda, there was also a larger scheme in which he was not the only or even the main actor. He knew that receiving was also an act of service and that participating in community also meant receiving from that community. In many ways his self-reliance gave way to trust, his autonomy gave way to companionship in community, and his setting his own agenda gave way to altering his course to fit another.

In all this, religious commitment played a large role. Much of what he did and experienced between the time of his diagnosis and death would be meaningless to someone without such a commitment. Yet Ray's path to his dying reveals dimensions of both living and dying that are important parts of our larger social discussion of these issues, even though one might not be led by the same lights as Ray.

One element common to religion is the role of community and its importance in sustaining and nourishing its individual members. All religions hold some form of a theory of individual accountability, but they also join this to community resources of prayer, service, and ritual to aid members in their individual journeys. Additionally religions affirm the value and frequently the necessity of service both to the members of the religious community and to all members of society. This is expressed in the mandate to assist others, to give alms, or to engage in other forms of volunteer work in the community. While religions affirm the value of the individual and strong theories of personal accountability for one's life, they also recognize that communities offer resources to individuals to make such responsibility more possible—more possible precisely because one engages in this process with and for others. Thus, community is not only a locus in which one acts out major elements of one's religious commitments, it is also reality that sustains and nurtures us in our journey.

Two areas of application follow. First, even in the strongest forms of the physician-assisted suicide/euthanasia debate, autonomy fails at a critical level. That is, after all the rhetoric and ideology settles, the argument is that individuals really cannot do it by themselves. They have neither the resources nor access to them, and they are physically unable to do the act by themselves. The only means available are unaesthetic, particularly for survivors. Thus the debate is over physician-assisted suicide or euthanasia administered *by another*. At a very deep level this debate seems to be an appeal to a community for assistance in carrying out one's desires, and the limits and even failure of autonomy as the keystone of the argument are clearly revealed. At a critical juncture in the debate, autonomy fails and the necessity of the community is implicitly invoked, although this is in no way acknowledged by the proponents of physician-assisted suicide and euthanasia.

Second, the notion of community invoked in the physician-assisted suicide/euthanasia argument is a strange one. The community or representative of the community is to serve the individual by helping that individual end his or her life rather than by assisting that person in living, the usual role of community. The image of the individual seeking assistance in dying is usually a person who is alone or certainly feels alone. In the literature on this debate, seldom does one find discussions of individuals who have resources other than themselves, even when these are available. Even in the Dutch film that shows a man being euthanized, his removal from the community is apparent. Certainly this man has community resources—an excellent health-care system, a personal physician who makes house calls, a comfortable house and physical resources, and a loving wife. But the dominant image in the film is withdrawal. The husband does not touch his wife and vice versa, they do not speak of friends, and medical assistance is absent. At the end, the physician puts his arm around the wife and repeats over and over: "Isn't this beautiful? Isn't this better?" And the isolation of each is never stronger than in that moment.

And this is where other memories of my friend Ray return. Granted, Ray was a priest and a member of a religious community with a lot of built-in care and support, but he also had a number of other friends outside the religious community who drove him to radiation treatment, visited him, and provided various forms of service. And what is interesting is that Ray, a very take-charge kind of person with the Marine Corps overlay, accepted the service with grace and graciousness. And in being served himself in his illness, he also served others.

Many will argue that this death is the exception and that it idealizes pain and suffering. Some made the same arguments about the dying of Cardinal Joseph Bernardin. My friend Ray and Cardinal Bernardin had health-care and personal resources not available to most. But that truth stands as a judgment on the physician-assisted suicide/euthanasia debate and the treatment of many of the dying. Our culture frequently isolates the dying, we tend to overtreat and undermedicate them, and we do not provide a space for their dying other than the most technologically advanced. Our culture is a death-denying culture. One almost has the feeling at times that dying is somehow un-American, an affront to our standard of living. Thus, when dying rears its ugly head—and we must never forget its head is ugly—we seek to get it done as quickly and painlessly as possible, efficiency and comfort being other critical American values.

Thus, at a critical moment the individual is alone. The presence of community will not remove the terror, eliminate pain and suffering, or remove the burden. But a community may ease these, relieve the aloneness, bring comfort, and most importantly assure the dying person that he or she is not abandoned. Community certainly does not solve all problems associated with dying, but a community does hold the patient in its midst and show that the patient is valued and not alone. Certainly this vision of community permits a variety of modes of dying, but the context in which they occur is radically different than in the traditional philosophical debate. Religion offers a critical change in perspective in the dying process, a perspective that will not eliminate the reality of death and its terrors but that offers many more options. To eliminate the role of a community—whether of immediate family, friends, or voluntary organizations to which one belongs—from the debate, regardless of how that debate is ultimately resolved, is to shortchange both the individual and the community.

THE PROVISION OF HEALTH CARE

This section is also inspired by my friend Ray and his passion for justice and his commitment to the poor—a message he communicated to others and one that some could not forget. This is a message we too need to hear in our rethinking of health care in the United States.

That we are undergoing a revolution in the provision of health care is apparent to anyone who has been to a physician lately or to anyone who has been without insurance. The general verdict thus far is that the changes are not good, and many are dissatisfied with the way HMOs provide services. The so-called drive-through deliveries that limited care to an overnight stay after normal childbirth was a focal point that sparked a major debate.

Some background features of this debate are important. First, there are two major ways of receiving health insurance. Most Americans obtain medical insurance as a benefit of employment. Employers bear a large share of the cost of medical insurance, although a greater share of these costs is being transferred to workers. Also if one is poor or elderly, insurance comes through government programs, and here too one's copayment is increasing and fewer benefits are available. Consequently, for most unemployed, the underemployed, and many of the nation's poor, there is no medical insurance. The same is frequently true for those who are determined to have a "medical predisposition" to a disease, which disqualifies them from many insurance programs.

Second, we have some rather strange beliefs about medical care in this country. We seem to think, for example, that quality medical care means as much as possible for as long as possible. We seem to think that medical resources are infinite and need not be paid for. And we seem to think that because we have insurance, we are entitled to as many tests and opinions as possible. Health care thus seems to be for many an infinite supply of increasingly high-tech interventions that are very expensive and require an increasingly sophisticated cadre of individuals to use them. Such a vision, even given some degree of exaggeration, is coming up against some realities that are *very* hard for Americans to accept. Resources are not infinite; a plethora of equipment does not necessarily mean quality care; prolonged use of various therapies or technologies is not necessarily in the patient's best interest; and payment for services is becoming complicated, to say the least.

These two situations are creating a very hostile atmosphere around the issue of the provision of health care. Traditionally health care was provided in a fee-for-service model in which many of the costs were underwritten by employment-derived insurance. Here the physician was essentially a small-business person who contracted directly with the patient, who came to the physician. The predominant ethic was that the physician acted in the best interest of the patient; although fees were derived from such transactions, predominant weight in the equation was given to the physician's judgment. Because of this factor, costs escalated and began to go out of control. Thus, there was a shift to HMOs or other managed-care programs. Managed-care organizations used market forces to help solve the cost problem by developing incentive programs for physicians to be efficient in the care they provided (only tests or treatment actually needed and provided as cost effectively as possible) or by developing capitation programs (specific allocations for various diseases or services with cost overruns taken from the operating budget of the HMO). Thus the *culture* of the provision of health care changed rapidly. The word *culture* is emphasized advisedly because, anecdotal reports to the contrary, Americans do not seem to be less healthy than before.

Nonetheless, some features remain that raise critical problems. First, many are still uninsured or have coverage that is inadequate. Second, coverage is still linked to employment. Third, the focus is still on high-tech interventions or rescue medicine rather than prevention. Fourth, many see the changes coming from the shift to an HMO model as radically unfair. These issues need serious and sustained discussion, and religion can bring at least two contributions to this discussion.

First, many religions, and here the discussion focuses on Roman Catholicism, have a concept of justice. The bishops of the United States presented their understanding of justice in the 1986 pastoral letter "Economic Justice for All."[4] In the approach of the bishops, justice mandates specific responses to the individuals we meet within our daily lives. Here, justice as participation and as the preferential option for the poor would focus on the needs of individuals and ensure their participation within the decision-making structure of society. Justice would ensure that individuals are not marginalized because of their income or social status. Justice would ensure that the poor or disenfranchised are not the one who receive less or inferior treatment because of their inability or reluctance to speak out.

The vision of justice offered by the bishops has five basic dimensions.

1. It is necessary to develop a cultural consensus that places economic rights in the same position of honor enjoyed by other social rights such as civil rights, the right of free speech, and the right to privacy. Here, human dignity is protected by ensuring adequate participation in the resources of the community.
2. Justice is realized when individuals and groups actively participate in the life of the community. Justice seeks to give voice and choice and to diminish social, political, or economic marginalization as much as possible.
3. Justice is to be reciprocal. That is, justice is served not only when individuals' needs are fulfilled, but also when individuals are enabled to be active and productive within the community. Thus, justice demands contributions to the common good as well as contributions from it.
4. Justice does not focus on the production of goods and services only. It also must evaluate the sources of production, the means of production, and patterns of distribution.
5. With regard to distribution of resources, unequal distributions must be evaluated with particular attention to their impact on those whose basic human needs are unmet. Also unequal distributions based on characteristics such as race, sex, or other, arbitrary standards cannot be justified.

What is critical in this orientation toward justice is its focus on both the dignity of the person and the construction of social structures that enable participation in as well as reception from society. Additionally, the vision of justice looks to the poor and mandates that their needs be met. In fact, the letter says that the increased economic participation of the marginalized takes precedence over the preservation of privileged concentrations of power and wealth.

One can ask how this type of preferential option for the poor shapes our attitude toward the provision of health care. One response is to recognize the breadth of the mandate. This was aptly summarized by Cardinal Bernardin when he said, "Our moral, political and economic responsibilities do not stop at the moment of birth! We must defend the *right to life* of the weakest among us; we must also be supportive of the *quality of life* of the powerless among us, . . . the sick, the disabled, the dying."[5]

What this discussion of justice brings to the table is an expanded understanding of justice, one that sees the inclusion of all members of the community so that they can both receive from the community and contribute to it. The provision of health care to all is one way in which quality participation within a community is ensured.

A second concept related to this discussion of justice is the common good. Considerations of the common good have largely fallen by the wayside in the last several decades in mainstream discussions of social and political ethics. In part this has been because, as Bellah phrases it, "American culture has focused relentlessly on the idea that individuals are self-interest maximizers and that private accumulation and private pleasures are the only measurable public goods."[6] Downplaying the common good is also reflected in our reliance on cost-benefit analysis for social decision making. What is given priority here is social efficiency and a neglect of the social consequences that follow from such decisions. Finally, we continue to hear the rhetoric that the government and our institutions are the enemy of the individual. Although the Reagan mantra of "Get government off our backs" is not as frequently invoked as it was in the 1980s, the sentiment remains alive; it can be seen particularly in many of the critiques of the Clinton health proposal as well as in the rhetoric that drives the "reform" of welfare. What we seem to have forgotten is that "even autonomy depends on a particular kind of institutional structure and is not an escape from institutions altogether."[7] And we have further forgotten that autonomy is "only one virtue among others and that without such virtues as responsibility and care . . . autonomy itself becomes . . . an empty form without substance."[8]

In discussing the common good, a double nostalgia must be resisted and ultimately rejected. The American version is derivative from a vision of rural or small-town America as seen through the idealization of the early days of the founding of our republic or the paintings of Norman Rockwell. Another version is papal and longs for the Middle Ages. According to Pius XI,

> At one period there existed a social order which, though by no means perfect in every respect, corresponded nevertheless in a certain measure to right reason according to the needs and conditions of the times. That this order has long since perished is not due to the fact that it was incapable of development and adaptation to changing needs and circumstances, but rather to the wrongdoing of men. Men were hardened in excessive self-love and refused to extend that order, as was their duty, to the increasing numbers of the people; or else, deceived by the attractions of false liberty and other errors, they grew impatient of every restraint and endeavored to throw off all authority.[9]

To be sure, there are virtues to be admired and emulated in both visions, but our world is largely industrialized and urban. Our problems, although similar to those of past generations, cannot rely on the solutions of our fore-bears because our times and social context are quite different.

In Roman Catholic social theory, from which I derive my perspective, the concept of the common good has a rich and varied history. In "Rerum Novarum," the 1891 encyclical by Leo XIII that began the tradition of Catholic social thought, Leo defined the common good as that for the sake of which civil society exists and "is concerned with the interests of all in general, and with the individual interests in their due place and proportion."[10] More specifically, Pius XI, in "Quadragesimo Anno," stated that "Those goods should be sufficient to supply all needs and an honest livelihood, and to uplift men to that higher level of prosperity and culture which, provided it be used with prudence, is not only no hindrance but is of singular help to virtue."[11] Both of these conceptions of the common good are derived from the static and hierarchically structured society in which these popes lived. Additionally, as Dennis McCann notes, these writers assumed that the common good derived from such a society was "self-evidently substantive, objectively knowable, and indivisible."[12] Such a perspective is overly optimistic at best and epistemologically naive at worst, but nonetheless such a concern for the good of society and all of its members stays at the heart of the encyclical tradition.

John XXIII began a shift from such a hierarchical and static vision of society and the common good by identifying the foundation of the common good as the human person who has rights and obligations flowing from his or her nature.[13] This vision moved the focus from the structure of society to the person and used the concept of rights to ensure the protection and enhancement of the individual in society and the concept of obligation to guarantee that the person actively participate in the development of society. Such thinking led John to a vision of the common good that did not stop at national boundaries but included "the entire human family."[14]

The Second Vatican Council, in its pastoral constitution, "The Church in the Modern World," continued this line of thought by recognizing that "the concrete demands of this common good are constantly changing as time goes on."[15] This important document recognizes that the common good is a dynamic concept and one that must be responsive to the changing needs of human society.

The American Catholic bishops then used this perspective to develop a vision of social justice that "implies that persons have an obligation to be active and productive participants in the life of society and that society has a duty to enable them to participate in this way."[16] Here, they follow Pius XI, who said, "It is of the *very* essence of social justice to demand from each individual all that is necessary for the common good."[17] Thus, the bishops envision justice as a means through which the person achieves the perfection of his or her self through contributing to the well-being of society. In the perspective of the bishops, then, the core of justice is the establishment of "minimum levels of participation in the life of the human community for all persons"[18] rather than establishing zones of privacy whereby individuals attempt to seek their private good independently of the community.

The American Catholic bishops make the following affirmation: "The common bond of humanity that links all persons is the source of our belief that the country can attain a renewed public moral vision."[19] And finally, the bishops state, "The dignity of the human person, realized in community with others, is the criterion against which all aspects of economic life must be measured."[20]

This orientation presents a vision of justice and the common good that is not quite in the mainstream of America libertarian theory. The bishops recognize this and argue that the next phase of the American experiment needs to secure for this vision of social justice the same status as the other rights we correctly celebrate. The significant difference is that the bishops' vision orients the person to his or her role in the community whereas our traditional vision focuses on the autonomous individual.

This vision, based in a particular religious tradition, can make a valuable contribution to the public debate over health care and particularly the question of insurance. Although one can argue that this vision supports a variety of particular policies in the general health-care debate, its more important function is to be a kind of searchlight that illumines aspects of the debate frequently ignored. That is, this perspective mandates that a key element of the provision of health care be the inclusion of those who are marginalized or in the greatest need of health-care services. It argues that the well-being of society can be achieved only when those at the margins are brought into the mainstream and enabled to make their contributions to the common good of all. One key element in this strategy is to ensure that such individuals receive appropriate health care. Such policies not only respect and promote the dignity of all citizens but also guarantee a more just society in which the good of society prospers through the participation of the many in its goals.

The contribution of religion to this aspect of the debate is not to propose particular policies or strategies, but to make sure the debate addresses the needs and concerns of all, to ensure that the needs of the voiceless are given voice, and to ensure that the marginalized are protected and thus enabled to make their contribution to society. The role of religion here is to guarantee a broad social debate and the representation of the needs of all.

CONCLUSION

This chapter has reviewed some historical aspects of the development of bioethics that suggest why religion has been put to the side of much of the bioethics debate: the use of philosophical analysis, the focus on analysis of issues rather than advocacy, and the pluralistic nature of the public policy debate. This marginalization of religion was not necessarily intentional or motivated by hostility to religion. Rather, it began happening gradually, and then religious voices began to be perceived more as sectarian critiques rather than as contributions to the mainstream discussion. Such an understanding of religion as sectarian, at least in its politics if not its theology, was certainly helped by the blatantly partisan alignment of several religious organizations with the Republican agenda and their sponsorship of individuals for public office. The rise of the "Moral Majority" set the discussion of religion and public policy back several decades.

In bioethical discussions, religion should not necessarily or primarily focus on making public policy proposals—although religious bodies and individual members of religious organizations are certainly entitled to do this as members of our society. Rather, religion can identify aspects of the bioethics debate not highlighted by customary political or philosophical analysis, it can help ensure a wider agenda of public policy discussion, and it can argue for the inclusion of a broader constituency in the provision of health care.[21]

What religious traditions have to offer is a broader vision of both individuals and society, a more inclusive vision of justice, an inclusive vision of the common good, and a view of human dignity that argues that individuals should receive from the community as well as participate in its well-being. This contribution does not directly translate into a set of policy recommendations, but it does serve as a lens with which we can sharpen our view of various debates and critique them when appropriate.

ENDNOTES

1. D. A. Cronin, "The Moral Law in Regard to the Ordinary and Extraordinary Means of Conserving Life," in *Conserving Human Life* (Braintree, Mass.: Pope John XXIII Medical-Moral Center, 1989).

2. D. Callahan, *The Troubled Dream of Life* (New York: Simon & Schuster, 1993).

3. Callahan, *The Troubled Dream*, 371.

4. This letter as well as other papal encyclicals can be found in D. J. O'Brien and T. A. Shannon, eds., *Catholic Social Thought: The Documentary Heritage* (New York: Orbis Books, 1992).

5. J. Bernardin, "The Consistent Ethic of Life and Health Care Systems," in *Consistent Ethic of Life* (Kansas City, Mo.: Sheed and Ward, 1988), 52. Italics in the original.

6. R. Bellah et al., *The Good Society* (New York: Alfred A. Knopf, 1991), 50.

7. Bellah, *The Good Society*, 12.

8. Bellah, *The Good Society*.

9. Pius XI, "Quadragesimo Anno," see note 4 above, 64.

10. Leo XIII, "Rerum Novarum," see note 4 above, 33.

11. Pius XI, "Quadragesimo Anno," see note 4 above, 59.

12. D. McCann, "The Good to Be Pursued in Common," in *The Common Good and U.S. Capitalism,* ed. O. Williams and J. Houck (Lanham, Md.: University Press, 1987), 164.

13. John XXIII, "Pacem in Terris," see note 4 above, 132.

14. John XXIII, "Pacem in Terris," 147.

15. Vatican II, "Gaudium et Spes," see note 4 above, 220.

16. American Catholic bishops, "Economic Justice for All," see note 4 above, 595.

17. American Catholic bishops, "Economic Justice for All," see note 4 above, 595.

18. American Catholic bishops, "Economic Justice for All," see note 4 above, 596.

19. American Catholic bishops, "Economic Justice for All," see note 4 above, 584.

20. American Catholic bishops, "Economic Justice for All," see note 4 above, 584.

21. Many of my ideas about the common good and the relation of religion to society have been shaped by M. Himes and K. Himes, *Fullness of Faith: The Public Significance of Theology* (New York: Paulist Press, 1993).

2

Playing God or Playing Human?

Thomas A. Shannon

This chapter will examine a few senses in which the term "playing God" is used and the connotations they suggest. After these considerations, I wish to reflect on the usefulness of this term and suggest some other directions.

EXAMPLES OF THE USES OF
THE TERM "PLAYING GOD"

Paul Ramsey

In his book *Fabricated Man*, Ramsey presents a vision of what God does and in this context then discusses the implications for us of playing God. Given that this book focuses on ethical issues in genetics, Ramsey takes God's action in reproduction as the paradigm.

Ramsey says, "We procreate new beings like ourselves in the midst of our love for one another, and in this there is a trace of the original mystery by which God created the world because of His love."[1] He adds, "Men may be able to subdue the mystery of procreation, they may be able to subdue all the wonders of human sexual response, in their sciences. But they cannot subdue the mystery in the fact that eminently human communications of marital love are also the places where we engage as procreators, and establish and step into the covenant of parenthood."[2] Ramsey then states his ethically decisive observation: "To put radically asunder what nature and nature's God joined together in parenthood when he made love procreative is to disregard the

23

foundation of the covenant of marriage and the covenant of parenthood in the reality that makes for a least minimal loving procreation . . . is inevitably to fall far below—into a vast technological alienation of man. Limitless domination over procreation means the boundless servility of man-womanhood."[3]

These quotes show the extremely strong linkage Ramsey asserts between acts of human procreation and divine creation, between human love and divine creation. In procreating—and Ramsey vigorously rejects the term reproduction because of its mechanistic overtones—humans do not act on their own; they act in concert with God.

Thus Ramsey argues in his famous statement, "Men ought not to play God before they learn to be men, and after they have learned to be men they will not play God."[4] At its most basic level, this means we ought to learn and respect our roles as creatures and to keep in mind that science and medicine serve human life. Theologically, the phrase suggests that we need to determine the significance of the ultimate religious context in shaping human acts. And Ramsey further specifies what learning to be human entails when he says, "We ought rather to live with charity amid the limits of a biological and historical existence that God created for the good and simple reason that, for all its corruption, it is now—and for the temporal future will be—the good realm in which man and his welfare are to be found and served."[5]

In spite of these statements, Ramsey is not a biological Luddite. He does argue that there are very important interventions that can be morally justified and morally required given that we now possess certain capabilities. He has two points of critique. First, there are things we can do that we ought not do. Second, we need to resist the impulses and capacities of what he would call a morally blind technology. Both of these orientations coalesce around procreation in which humans join their powers with divine powers in the mystery of the creation of another life. With rhetorical flourish, Ramsey states, "I do not believe men should enslave themselves to an acknowledged minority of scientific saviors, or any man make himself willing to reduce another fellowman to a 'thing in the world' over whom benefits are to be 'wrought,' while unfurling the banner of man's future triumph over natural forces."[6]

The diatribe—and that is the only word to use for this, I think—is directed against a spirit of positivism and reductionism that Ramsey saw as an ideological component of the developing genetics as well as a kind of messianic positivism that guided many of what he considered the dystopic statements of the social speculations of biologists. To play man—to use his phrase—is to respect the limits of biology created by God; thus, in playing man we learn not to play God. We neither destroy what God has united, nor do we overstep our limits.

Joseph Fletcher

To move into the world of Joseph Fletcher in his book *The Ethics of Genetic Control* is to move to the other extreme; indeed, it is to move into the world Ramsey condemns. Fletcher celebrates our new powers and calls for their implementation, yet he does not do this uncritically. While he acknowledges that our new knowledge and ability to control nature have taken us beyond our wildest dreams, we do have the obligation to "try as imaginatively as we can to foresee the consequences of 'stealing such powers from the gods.'"[7]

Yet here is a first cut at defining playing God: to steal the powers of the gods, which he understands as a Promethean gesture. Fletcher further specifies this by describing playing God as "trying to invade God's privileges and prerogatives."[8] This is done primarily by interfering with nature that is understood to be God's creation and plan. To interfere is "an artificial contrivance [and] is a presumptuous form of playing God, especially if it takes the place of natural modes and processes—for example, coital conception."[9]

The critical problem for Fletcher is that our traditional understanding of God is gone. Because of pluralism, mobility, and new information and capacities, we can no longer think the way we used to nor can we continue to have the luxury of a religiously based morality. And while Fletcher still holds to the religiously grounded imperative of neighbor love, "How to do this is no longer prescribed in codes but is open-ended and up to responsible moral agents."[10] Thus, for Fletcher, the issue is not whether we might play God, but as he phrases it in a subheading in a chapter "Let's play God."[11]

And so he does. Fletcher argues that there are no longer any acts of God, for the world is not "run from outside by God's will, in any case."[12] We are now responsible for our world and for what goes on in it. Here, Fletcher acknowledges that the "death of the old God"[13] does not make our life easier for we do not have the omniscience people once attributed to that "old God." But act we must, and Fletcher illustrates what this means when he argues that having children the old-fashioned way through what he calls the sexual roulette or potluck of random combinations through sexual intercourse is irresponsible. He says, "As we learn to direct mutations medically we should do so. Not to control when we can is immoral."[14] Such design ensures that the children born through such genetic planning will be wanted because they are born through rational processes and intentionally.

Thus, to play God for Fletcher is to act as a human, to take the powers and capacities we have discovered through our intellect and apply them to our everyday life. The old God is gone, displaced by our newly discovered capacities—and we must step forward and take responsibility for our lives.

Splicing Life: 1982 President's Commission Report

This report, which focused on religious and ethical issues in genetic engineering, specifically addressed the term "playing God." The commission identified three specific meanings associated with the term.

First, playing God is an expression of wonder or awe at the new powers that we have. It is a reaction "to the realization that human beings are on the threshold of understanding how the fundamental machinery of life works."[15] Thus, in this sense the term "playing God" is not an objection to modern science; rather, it is an expression of appreciation of what possibilities lie before us. It is a descriptive phrase, not an evaluative one.

The second sense of the term is an expression of an abuse of powers through interfering with nature. The strong version of this phrase states that such interventions violate "God's prescriptive nature or go against God's purposes as they are manifested in the natural order."[16] The commission, however, does not argue that all interventions into nature are an abuse of one's powers or a violation of limits. Moreover, scholars studying this issue for the commission argued that none of the religions represented thought that genetic engineering per se violated such a natural law.

A third meaning looks to the capacity to create new species by creating new life-forms by gene splicing. The nuance here is that people may now have Godlike powers, but they do not yet have Godlike wisdom to consider "the uncontrollability and uncertainty of the consequences of human interferences in the natural order."[17] Here, playing God makes the point that we had better consider carefully the consequences of what we are doing, for the human race has a history of "fallibility and ignorance."[18]

The commission argues that the term "playing God" in itself is not a prohibition or a condemnation of the scientific capacities we have through modern genetics. Rather, it is an admonition to examine these capacities carefully and to apply them with the utmost wisdom and skill.

REFLECTIONS

Playing

These three perspectives relate the term "playing God" to a certain mode of acting, to an association of human powers with divine powers. To play God is either, from Ramsey's perspective, to abrogate to one's self the powers of God by transgressing God's design or, in Fletcher's terms, to simply acknowledge reality and realize that the old God no longer exists and to begin acting responsibly in the world. The term is conceived of as a power struggle between two worldviews—one that includes the divine and one that does not.

As such, both Ramsey and Fletcher require us to make many assumptions about God, God's work, and human responsibility, and to make these assumptions in a fairly sharp and dramatic way. And because both operate at such an extreme, both are, I think, flawed. Ramsey's perspective makes us almost powerless before nature, even as he acknowledges that interventions are possible. Fletcher assumes there are no limits to intervention as long as we consider carefully the greatest good for the greatest number. Yet both are somewhat uncritical in their orientation and ultimately lead us into dead ends.

Ramsey uses the term "playing God" as a way of arguing that humans have overstepped their boundaries. This suggests that there is a clear and obvious demarcation between the roles of God and humans. There are areas of life where God rules, where God is in charge, and where humans ought not enter. The term evokes an omnipotent God who is the creator of all and is in charge of all. Fletcher's use of the term "playing God" evokes the image of God as a God of the gaps, that is, the God invoked when all else fails, or because our limits are exceeded, our knowledge at an end, and our powers frustrated. Thus, it is most clearly in the gaps of our knowledge or power that God rules and where God's power is most clearly evoked. Here, God reigns supreme and here we cannot play God.

Of course, the gaps grow smaller, boundaries are exceeded, God's reign shrinks, God's power becomes lessened, and eventually God becomes unnecessary. Some draw two consequences from this: 1) there is no God, and 2) there are no inhibitions on interventions. Humans step into the recently vacated gaps and play God by exercising the powers in the gaps where previously only God was thought to exist. I argue that neither of these visions is particularly Christian—or Jewish or Islamic, for that matter. Ramsey's is too biologically deterministic and Fletcher's is too secular. The vision both present is too much dependent on the Greek philosophical and mythological tradition. It is certainly much more resonant with the myth of Prometheus, who in stealing fire from the gods and giving it to humans, became like the gods and thus played God. However, he suffered the fate of one who usurped the power of the gods. Were the God suggested by this version of playing God actually this fearful of sharing creation, assumedly that God would never have created in the first place. Why spoil the way things are!

Perhaps a better rendering of playing God is to learn as much about God as one can and then play God by acting as God acts. Minimally, this might mean that we are to be creative as well as generous in our creativity and to keep covenant with our God and our creations. To affirm this is to surrender full control because we are not God. But it is also to assert a profound relation between humankind and the rest of created reality. We play God by imitating God—no small task.[19]

Two immediate consequences follow from this. First, this image of playing God does not set up a kind of competition between God and humans. The image is stripped of its traditional mythological overtones and given a chance to return to a version much more faithful to the Judeo-Christian tradition. Second, in principle, such an understanding of playing God does not prohibit interventions into created reality. The moral element here would focus on the kind of intervention. And a more helpful hermeneutic for understanding the term "playing God" might in fact be genuine play—and the nuance here is that play cannot be purely instrumental for then it is no longer play, but work. And though creation is described in Genesis as a labor from which God rested, and in Job as a kind of civil engineering project, the book of Wisdom does describe the creative act of God as a form of play.

I would highlight three applications here. First, we need not fear to intervene in nature—that is part of imitating God. Second, when such interventions become primarily instrumental or essentially take on a purely utilitarian or reductionist cast, we have a warning signal that something may be problematic. Third, to play God is to act as God—and a primary reality of that seems to me to be a spirit of generosity, a generosity that ought to mediate our experience of and interactions with creation.

Stewardship

One of the most traditional ways of thinking of human responsibility in the Christian tradition is stewardship. This theological metaphor comes from the book of Genesis in which God places humans in charge of the Garden of Eden and tells them they are to tend it and care for it. The implications are 1) that God is the owner, so to speak, of the garden and humans are to manage it for God; and 2) that human responsibility is limited.

Now this is an excellent metaphor and it has served us well. But it has functioned within a specific framework and that framework had two dimensions. First, the framework is that of a static universe, one that is fixed and stable. There are inbuilt laws within both nature and objects that guide the development of everything according to fixed purposes. This is clearly resonant with the perspective of Ramsey. Second, the stability of the universe was reinforced by the historic fact that humans could not do too much anyway. Interventions into nature were limited by a lack of both knowledge and capacities. And Fletcher shows us the limits of this perspective when knowledge develops almost exponentially as it has in, for example, the biological sciences.

The presuppositions of this framework have changed dramatically. We know that our world is a dynamic, changing, evolving cosmos. What is now has not always been and what has been gave way to what is now. And we can intervene now in many ways: either by screening an individual's genetic profile and accepting or rejecting it or creating a new genotype by recombining genes from different species and creating a transgenic animal. In short, stewardship isn't what it used to be. I would like to suggest a new model of stewardship using the theology of the Franciscan theologian Bonaventure. And though his world is the static and hierarchical world of the thirteenth century, he has an insight about stewardship that I think is worth considering.

Bonaventure grounds human dignity in terms of the location of humans within the created order and our function within that order. For Bonaventure, this means that humans, who were created last according to the biblical narrative, are highest in the order of creation. In this perspective, the function of humans is to be mediators by representing the world before God and ensuring the participation of all reality in redemption, particularly through our bodily dimension. This vision of human dignity allows Bonaventure to affirm humans, but not at the expense of nature; rather, he articulates a vocation for humans inclusive of nature, which can ground an ecological ethic. For Bonaventure, such status is not a claim to power. Rather, it mandates service—to God, to one's neighbor, and to nature. Position, for Bonaventure, does not confer power—it calls to service.

Thus, as we actualize our redemption initiated at baptism, we enter more and more into the order intended by God. As we do this, we begin to actualize this reality in our own lives. This will evoke a response of respect and reverence to nature and one another, not dominion and domination. Stewardship is actualized not by lording it over creation, but by appreciating the goodness of nature and by being its voice before God.

This leads us to see, as the poet Gerard Manley Hopkins phrases it, "the dearest freshness deep down things." Such a perspective does not prohibit interventions in nature. Rather, it cautions us that such interventions must go beyond what is seen or what can be modeled even through the most sophisticated imaging technologies. Such intentions touch but a part of what reality is; to miss that is to miss the potential of reality. Such a recognition of the potentials of nature and our embeddedness within it can lead to a continuous conversion of heart. Then, once again, we can as Bonaventure phrases it, "read the book of Creation, [to] receive the full service of things below him [or her], and to be in this way their decisive mediator on the way to God."

CONCLUSIONS

The framework I have sketched out in these last two sections suggests that we can intervene in nature but that such interventions have limits. Let me use as an example the situation of cloning as a form of assisted reproduction to ensure that a couple has a child with a genetic relation to one of the partners.

I think it is important, first, to distinguish between the means of reproduction and the context in which those means are used. I would argue that cloning as a means of reproduction for humans in not inherently immoral. As a means, I do not think that cloning undermines human dignity or violates the dignity of the embryo so generated. I do think there are serious safety issues that need to be examined before any attempts at cloning as a means of human reproduction would go forward. Thus, I think a first layer of moral analysis of cloning as a means of reproduction ought to be the very traditional one of safety, as is the case with the development of any new intervention on human subjects.

Second, the critical moral analysis ought to focus on an assessment of the context in which cloning might be used as a form of assisted reproduction. First, we know that assisted reproduction is a very lucrative and competitive multimillion dollar per year business. This means there is keen competition between clinics for clients and their money. This in turn gives rise to a strong incentive to implement immediately any new technology that might give one clinic an edge. Lori Andrews quotes one fertility clinician as saying, "We go from mindside to bedside in two weeks. We make things up and try things on patients. We never get their informed consent, because they just want us to make them pregnant."[20] One would hardly expect responsible research on cloning in such a success-driven context, particularly when such clinics have no obligation to have an ethics review board of any type.

Second, this drive for success will be reinforced by the joint presumptions that autonomy reigns supreme here, as in all other areas of American life, and that since such reproductive choices are private, these choices are immune from any social evaluation. Relying on autonomy in this fashion begs the question of whether individual choice is the only morally relevant value at stake in the discussion. The private-choice assumption ignores the social costs of pregnancy: higher insurance premiums for plans that would subsidize highly experimental forms of reproduction such as cloning, the increased use of monitoring technologies to track such an experimental pregnancy, increased use of NICUs (neonatal intensive care units) resulting from multiple pregnancies should many clones be generated and implanted, and the cost of such a procedure that would continue to exacerbate the class divisions between those who can and cannot afford the technologies.

Third, cloning in particular would reinforce the increasing instrumentalization of reproduction. While affirming that I do not think there is anything inherently wrong with such means of reproduction, there is a danger that we may lose the sense of a child as gift and look upon children as a means to an end, an end that is as carefully designed and programmed as possible. A correlative danger here, a danger particularly associated with cloning and its tie-in with genetic determinism, is that of a closed future for a child.

The concept of stewardship that emphasized service and respect for nature rather than dominion and domination that I developed from Bonaventure would also suggest a backing off from cloning as a reproductive technology. Many of our ideas about various relationships, including marriage and family, are often narrowly drawn, held morally hostage by a view of a biologically based morality, and a focus on individual desires and wants. The vocation of service that our place in creation confers upon us leads us to see beyond these narrow boundaries to the needs of others. Thus, one could argue for adoption rather than cloning as an appropriate way to actualize one's service to others. One could also foster a respect for nature by choosing not to focus so many resources on a technology such as cloning that may benefit only a few. Such an attitude of service leads us to think more of the needs of the many rather than generating an attitude of dominion that thinks of the wants of the few.

Although I am not persuaded that cloning as a means of reproduction is inherently immoral, I am persuaded that we would not necessarily use such a means wisely and that the social costs of such a procedure would be extremely high. I conclude by arguing that cloning as a form of assisted reproduction not go forward and that any research related to human cloning be supported with federal money to ensure that there will be some monitoring of the research and that its applications will be subject to some public scrutiny before cloning becomes another unmonitored means of reproduction offered through private clinics. Such a recommendation comes neither from an assumption of biological boundaries, as Ramsey would have, nor from fear of the uses of human powers, as Fletcher would have. Rather, it comes from the sense that we have limits based on responsibility to our children, society, and nature as well as the sense that playing God in the best understanding of the term suggests genuine play and less control.

ENDNOTES

1. P. Ramsey, *Fabricated Man* (New Haven, Conn.: Yale University Press, 1970), 88.
2. Ramsey, *Fabricated Man*, 88.
3. Ramsey, *Fabricated Man*, 89.
4. Ramsey, *Fabricated Man*, 138.
5. Ramsey, *Fabricated Man*, 149.
6. Ramsey, *Fabricated Man*, 151.
7. J. Fletcher, *The Ethics of Genetic Control: Ending Reproductive Roulette* (Garden City, N.Y.: Anchor Books, 1974), 6.

8. Fletcher, *The Ethics of Genetic Control*, 127.

9. Fletcher, *The Ethics of Genetic Control*, 127.

10. Fletcher, *The Ethics of Genetic Control*, 127.

11. Fletcher, *The Ethics of Genetic Control*, 126.

12. Fletcher, *The Ethics of Genetic Control*, 200.

13. Fletcher, *The Ethics of Genetic Control*, 200.

14. Fletcher, *The Ethics of Genetic Control*, 158.

15. President's Commission for the Study of Ethical Problems in Medicine and Bio-medical and Behavioral Research, *Splicing Life: The Social and Ethical Issues of Genetic Engineering with Human Beings* (Washington, D.C.: U.S. Government Printing Office, 1982), 54.

16. President's Commission, *Splicing Life*, 55.

17. President's Commission, *Splicing Life*, 58.

18. President's Commission, *Splicing Life*, 59.

19. A. D. Verhey, "'Playing God' and Invoking a Perspective." *Journal of Medicine and Philosophy* 20 (1995): 347–64.

20. L. Andrews, "Human Cloning: Assessing the Ethical and Legal Questions," *Chronicle of Higher Education* (February 13, 1998): B5.

3

Horizon Analysis and Moral Stance: An Interpretation of Cardinal Bernardin's "Consistent Ethic of Life"

James J. Walter

Cardinal Joseph Bernardin's speeches on the consistent ethic of life that occupied much of his attention before his death have definitely challenged much of the Catholic moral theology that has developed before and since Vatican II. My interest in his speeches is to apply a specific type of analysis to his notion of a consistent ethic in order to interpret what his intentions were in developing this provocative challenge. The particular type of analysis I will rely on is "horizon analysis" or "intentionality analysis," which has been used by such scholars as Edmund Husserl, Martin Heidegger, Maurice Merleau-Ponty, Paul Ricoeur, Karl Rahner, and Bernard Lonergan.[1] My own interpretation of this type of analysis will draw principally from the thought of Lonergan.

A FRAMEWORK

Let me begin with the central thesis of this chapter. My focus is descriptive and analytic, not evaluative. To use a metaphor, I seek to use a hermeneutic key to unlock the inner intentionality of what I think Bernardin meant by the "consistent ethic of life." I do not seek to appraise and evaluate its validity or adequacy; that is a task for another time or for others to undertake. The argument of this chapter is that what Bernardin intended by his consistent ethic was essentially to develop a "moral stance." In other words, the cardinal most often described what he meant by a "consistent ethic of life" by reference to a "vision"[2] or a "framework"[3] that could be used across a wide range of concrete issues affecting the dignity or sacredness of human life, especially innocent human life. He believed that all the moral issues from "womb to tomb" (i.e., issues from abortion to capital punishment to policies on health care and warfare) should be placed within a comprehensive "framework" or "vision" to formulate a normative judgment on the issues. "Vision" and "framework" render in another way what I call moral stance or horizon. This vision or framework (stance) that he sought to articulate was comprehensive in scope,[4] consistent in application,[5] analogical in character,[6] and dialogical in its culture and social policy.[7] Each of these descriptions of his vision is important in itself to understand and appreciate, and I will return to each of them shortly. However, before moving directly to an analysis of the descriptions, I need to develop more thoroughly what horizon analysis is and how one might use it in both general theological and ethical discourse. In other words, by articulating what horizon analysis can contribute to theological and ethical analyses I will be able to articulate better what this analysis can contribute to Bernardin's consistent ethic of life.

Bernard Lonergan has made use of horizon analysis to clarify the nature and importance of both a theological and a moral stance. He used a heuristic metaphor, namely "horizon," to describe the context of all human cognition. For him, horizons can be understood literally as the line where earth meets the sky and where they limit our field of vision. In this ocular model, horizons change when we move from one position to another.[8] So, if I am standing in a valley the furthest point that I can see is bounded by the hills that block my vision of what might lie beyond them. Though I might be able to ask questions about what may lie beyond the hills, I am not able to answer such a question. The answer simply lies beyond my horizon. If I then move to the top of one of the hills, my vision is expanded and more of the terrain that lies before me comes into view. What was once hidden from me is now within my horizon or grasp, and consequently I now have an answer to my former question about what might lie beyond the hills.

If one makes a transition from an ocular to a disclosure model of conceiving horizon, however, we can grasp that, for Lonergan, there are also horizons to our knowledge and desires, and they too can change on the basis of what we care to know and love. In other words, what I am interested in knowing or caring about (values) are likewise bounded. Simply stated, my ability to know certain things or my ability to commit to values has limits. These limits can be exceeded when I am willing to ask different kinds of questions or willing to dedicate myself to new sets of values that have hitherto been beyond my horizon. Similar to the ocular model where I made a change from one location to another, what now comes within my grasp with these new questions and commitments is a different range of data or sets of experiences to reflect on. When one uses a disclosure model of horizon as a way of understanding stance, then, one understands that all stances imply two necessary and interrelated poles: a subject pole and an object pole. Both a theological stance and a moral stance are formed through the interaction between a subject pole, which involves the existential questions of the agent about his or her commitments, attitudes, lived values, actions, and social policies, on the one hand, and an object pole, which involves the range of data (a text, an experience, a collection of statistics, etc.) or "world" that comes into view for the agent to interpret, judge, and act on, on the other. In essence, the interaction between these two referents fashions how one looks on reality, and it structures one's understandings of and moral judgments about the world, God, and self. To understand how stance can help to interpret theological interpretations, let's turn our attention to the nature of disclosure models and the five models of theological inquiry.

THE NATURE OF DISCLOSURE MODELS

There are several kinds of models. Scale or picture models copy an object exactly, according to a measure that miniaturizes or enlarges the image, such as the architectural model of a building or the representation of the DNA molecule. On the other hand, disclosure or analogue models do not provide exact details, but like the drawing for a sculpture, they evoke the final product. They are a basic sketch, a guiding tool for inquiry, simplifying for the sake of identification. Their imaginative configuration approximates the result and invites understanding. In the investigation of models of both general theological interpretations and ethical interpretations below, I use the second notion. In disclosure models, one distinguishes two poles: the subject investigating and the object or world disclosed by the study. In the analysis below I will first begin with general theological models developed through horizon analysis and then I will turn my attention to ethical models that serve as a moral stance.

Five Models of Theological Inquiry

There have been five basic models of theological inquiry in the history of Christian theology.[9] As we will see, each model places a subject pole (the theologian and his or her questions, interests, values, etc.) in relation to an object pole (the field of data that is consulted or appealed to in the formation of a normative claim to truth or value). It is important to understand that no one theologian or author stands completely in one or another of these models. Rather, the models serve as heuristic devices to help the reader understand the subject and object poles of the author and the meaning of his or her writings. We will see this more concretely when I turn my attention to Cardinal Bernardin and his speeches on the consistent ethic of life.

Classical Model

In the mode of theology that reigned supreme for some eighteen hundred years, the theologian was a believer who used various philosophic tools (Platonic, Neoplatonic, Augustinian, Aristotelian, etc.) within a particular confessional tradition to investigate the belief within the church. His (during this time, the theologian was almost always male) task was to express a carefully formulated tradition to the world. The world's understanding of itself had no explicit "internal" relevance in theological reflection. As examples, we might think of Thomas Aquinas, Bonaventure, Martin Luther, and John Calvin. Though it can be said quite justly that a theologian such as Aquinas included the intellectual concerns of Muslims and Jews, classical thinkers had as a goal the conversion of others. Their heirs during the later scholastic period—such as the Jesuit Francesco de Suarez (1548–1617) and the Lutheran Johann Gerhard (1582–1637)—exemplified an often logically brilliant organization, together with strict confessional polemics.

Liberal Model

In reaction to the academic form of Christian theologies, the period from 1750 to 1840 experienced an explosion of religious devotion as well as radical cultural departures in painting, poetry, music, and other arts. Romanticism in theology hoped to overcome a dry intellectual assent to doctrines through a resurrection of affective attachment to worship, the scriptures, and beliefs. Whether in France (with René Chateaubriand, 1768–1848), in England (with Samuel Taylor Coleridge, 1772–1834; or, later, F. D. Maurice, 1805–1872), in Germany (with Friedrich Schleiermacher), or somewhat later in America (with Horce Bushnell, 1802–1876; and Walter Raushenbusch, 1861–1918), the emphasis in theology shifted from the objective contents of faith to the subjective conditions of beliefs. The emerging sciences, developing political idealism, and artistic subjectivity had inner relevance to faith. Thus, the subject in this theological model is committed to modernity as a personal enterprise and sees the object of theology to be the Christian tradition—but as reformulated for the sake of the claims of the modern world.

Neo-Orthodox model

There were strong responses to the nineteenth century's mode of theological investigation. In the early twentieth century, the Catholic community responded with a broad negative action against what were called modernists (especially Alfred Loisy [1857–1940] and George Tyrell [1861–1909]), condemning any "subjectivization" of Christian doctrines. After the devastating trench warfare of World War I, Karl Barth (1886–1968), especially in his *Commentary on the Epistle to the Romans* (1919) and his *Church Dogmatics* (1932–1967), said a resounding no to the optimistic beliefs of liberal theology. Convinced, as the Catholic antimodernists were, that theological study had collapsed the dialectically critical character of the Christian proclamation into the scientific, cultural, and artistic biases of the age, he proposed a return to the prophetic immediacy of the scriptures with the reformers as the most authentic interpreters of the message. Because of the fall of man, human beings are caught in a realm of sin such that only God's infinite qualitative difference, his radical otherness, can transform our existence.

Reinhold Niebuhr (1891–1971), in *The Nature and Destiny of Man* (1939–1943), mediated the language of dialectical divine presence to the American scene. In a sense, neo-orthodoxy allowed modernity to define the questions of experience, its quest for the infinite, and its sense of sinful personal and social alienation, but maintained that only the unique claims of Christianity could transform the problems into grace. The object pole of theology, therefore, is the wholly other God, a paradoxical mystery whose reality calls into question all our paltry reasoning and religious pretensions. The subject engaging in theology, called into existence by this God, is a human being dedicated to the quest forged by an authentic faith, truth, and love.

Radical model

This theological endeavor looks at the development of postclassical thought and reminds us that modernity will not disappear. Is not the God who is wholly other busy overturning human expectations? Is not this God constantly competing with human projects? And hence, must not believers in this God conclude that our commitment to moral actions is inconsequential at best, sinful at worst? Can language about such a divinity be in any sense truthful, let alone verified? In this model, the concerns of the modern world are paramount; they define both theologians and the world disclosed by their study. The subject is committed to contemporary science, transforming political endeavors and affective honesty; the object remains the Christian message, but this message concerns a person (Jesus), who is the paradigmatic moral person, and doctrines (salvation) without any clearly defined or sharply argued transcendent reference. The theological questions asked use the tools of early linguistic analysis (especially those of Ludwig Wittgenstein [1889–1951] and A. J. Ayer [1910–1989]) and cultural commentary to argue that (at least the old classical or neo-orthodox) God is dead. This primarily American phenomenon is associated with figures like Paul van Buren, Gabriel Vehanian, Thomas J. J. Altizer, and Joseph Fletcher.

Dialogical Model

A proposal that hopes to integrate the concerns of all these models has been suggested by David Tracy and others. It involves commitments at both poles of the model with a correlative process of interaction. The subject/theologian is committed to *both* an authentic public secularity (note: not secularism) *and* an authentic Christian quest for truth, justice, and love. The object disclosed by theology is a critical reformulation of both secular concerns *and* the motifs of Christian doctrine and value. Because faith *and* the world are taken seriously, they involve a mutually corrective interpretation. Faith must listen to both the questions *and* the answers proposed by the world. The truthful character of the investigation is clarified by an examination of the moral claims made for religious as well as worldly "objects." Subject *and* object are correlatively "revised."

These models for theological reflection place the normative dimension, whether of truth or of value, in differing places, but the standards at stake are primarily intellectual values. The models then establish a relationship between the conceptualized norms.

In the classical formula, the norm for truth or for value is to be found in the confessional tradition and its doctrines; in the liberal model, the standard is modernity's teachings as they reformulate Christian experience; in the neo-orthodox model, God's otherness is the normative judgment upon humanity's reasoning powers; and in the radical model, modernity shapes both believer and beliefs. In the final model, there is a dialogical norm: beliefs and reason are mutually related, so that if we say that faith is primary, we must recognize that its expressions are always culturally shaped. Since both faith and the mystery of the wholly other exceed our ability to explicate them, we recognize that the subjective and objective poles of theological investigation—psychologically, socially, and culturally determined as they are—must be willing to "let go" of themselves when more adequate formulations appear.

These five theoretic correlations can also be judged according to their engagement in praxis or informed and committed doing.[10] The classical model focuses on the primacy of theory. "Theory regards objective knowledge as the formulation and verification of intelligibilities; it primarily regards possible, probable, or certain constructs of reality."[11] It mediates doctrines and value judgments in a particular cultural context, so that Christian activity implements good theory. One's religious and moral knowing is not intrinsically changed by doing.

In models in which only praxis is important, Christianity gains an internal relation to human activity, both religious and secular, but at the cost of losing theoretic criticism of itself. Christian service would always be paramount but without a doctrinal spine or theoretic warrants. Praxis should be understood as what we actually do, as involved and committed, the intersubjective home, in which we establish ourselves as authentic or inauthentic subjects. A theology that stresses this dimension tends to think of doctrine as secondary, teaching as second-rate, and noncommitment to sociopolitical transformation as sinful. Many of the forms of liberal or radical theology fall within this category.

There is also a type of praxis theology that stresses the primacy of faith and love. Christianity stands in judgment on both the theoretic formulation and the commitments of human praxis. The primary focus is upon the wholly other God. The prototype remains Karl Barth, for whom theology was always dialectically related to human activity. His Catholic friend Hans Urs von Balthasar can also be understood within this framework.

In the final two models for theology, there is an attempt to include both theory and praxis within religious discourse while maintaining the specific values Christianity has to offer to both. Where theory remains primary, the correlations between life, thought, and Christian conversion are mediated primarily through the extraordinarily tough demands of various contemporary sciences and theoretic disciplines. Matthew Lamb believes that Rudolf Bultmann, Paul Tillich (1886–1965), the Niebuhrs, and Karl Rahner (1904–1984) belong in this category. Here, theoretic issues are mutually and critically correlated, but nonintellectualized praxis becomes largely the application of already constituted theories. Human praxis fails to be the true origin of Christian knowing and loving. However, those who participate in the dialogical model that I have sketched above (e.g., Bernard Lonergan and John Baptist Metz) opt for the primacy of critical Christian praxis in which theoretic and practical reflection are mutually informing. Christian praxis, by its loyalty to the suffering and poor, by its commitment to the radically unloved, by its recognition of atonement within creation groaning to be completed, better informs both thought and action.

Ethical Stance

The search for the "imperative" or normative judgment in both human and Christian moral experience is one of the human desires for meaning. In the moral life, the "ought" is part of the very process of self-transcendence through which we seek to conform our decisions and lives to informed judgments of value. Since judgments are not guesses but probable truths, normative judgments of value are concerned with the way the world and human relations probably ought to be. Yet the discernment of particular imperatives is not enough; there is also the need for coherence among all the normative judgments we make as individuals and as a society. Stated more concretely, it is not sufficient for us to arrive at distinct normative decisions on the issues of the value of human life and the economic policies affecting Third World countries. There must be some congruence, coherence, and consistency between these two sorts of normative value judgments—that is, judgments of virtue, of rightness/wrongness of actions, and of obligation. The desires for coherence and congruence result in what is called a stance. Simply defined, an ethical stance is a coherent combination of value judgments about the world, God, and self. Not only is stance the locus for the determination and justification of value judgments about what is right or wrong, good or bad, virtuous or vicious, stance is also the search for consistency between and among a whole range of judgments of value and oughtness. This search and desire for consistency in the moral life is what ties together one's judgments about abortion and one's judgments about the health-care policies that affect the poor.

An ethical stance, like general theological models, is formed through the interaction between a subject pole (existential questions about our commitments, lived values, actions, etc.) and an object pole (the range of data or "world" that comes into view for us to interpret, judge, and act on). The interaction between these two referents fashions the ways in which we look on reality and structures our understandings and judgments about the world. For example, we have seen the classical theologian's subject pole comprises a commitment to a particular religious-moral tradition, and the furthest range of the object pole—that is, the range of data consulted and acted upon—includes the beliefs of that tradition. The ethical stance of such a theologian, then, represented an almost monolithic way of viewing and structuring the moral life. Specific imperatives, virtues, values, and actions were understood and judged according to the established moral data (doctrines) of the tradition, and alternative ways of understanding and judging were thought erroneous or were beyond the boundaries of the theologian's consciousness.

When we seek to thematize or make explicit in consciousness the contents of a stance, that is, to make explicit both the subject and object poles of the decision maker's stance, we attempt to make explicit the very foundations of the normative judgment itself and its justification. In other words, the normative judgment—that is, judgments about what kinds of virtues we need to live the moral life well, or judgments about the rightness of actions, or judgments about our moral obligations—arises from within the context of a normative stance, and so the stance is actually the ground and justification of the normative judgment itself. For example, for most classical theologians, the ethical imperative or normative judgment arose only from within the confines of their particular religious-moral traditions. This is so because these theologians were committed at the subject pole to the religious tradition and its values, and the object pole was the tradition itself with its doctrinal tradition.

If a theologian was committed to Roman Catholicism, then all ethical imperatives found their ground and justification from within that tradition. Thus, until the middle of the twentieth century, almost all Roman Catholic theologians argued the primary purpose of marital sexual relations was procreation. They were committed to preserving their long-standing understanding of sexuality that can be traced back to Augustine and Thomas Aquinas. This tradition had understood sexual relations between spouses as acts of nature (and not primarily as acts of love) having a moral intentionality or finality (procreation) built into them by God. To act against this moral finality by some form of artificial contraception was tantamount to acting directly against God. We can see, then, that how we discern, argue, and justify the ethical imperative is a function of how we intend and understand the human world.

There have been several normative stances proposed within the Christian traditions.[12] In classical Protestantism, for example, in Martin Luther's writings, faith was considered the stance for the moral life. *Sola fide* (by faith alone) was the fundamental viewpoint from which the ethical imperative was discerned, argued, and justified. Second, in some forms of Protestant liberalism of the twentieth century, love (*agape*) became an alternative stance to faith. For example, Adolf von Harnack (1851–1930) thought that the entire gospel of Jesus could be embraced under the rubric of love without depreciating the gospel message itself.[13] Thus, von Harnack considered the entire moral life to be founded on the single commandment to love in the New Testament.

Some neo-orthodox Protestant theologians proposed a third stance based on Jesus Christ. For example, in reaction to Protestant liberalism, Karl Barth argued that it is only through Jesus Christ that the Christian is enabled to know and do the good. Thus, his ethics is a form of christological monism in that the ethical imperative and all normative judgments must always be founded on Jesus Christ alone and can be authentically discovered and justified only through belief in him.[14]

Against these stances, James Sellers proposed the stance of promise and fulfillment as the normative horizon of the Judeo-Christian moral life. For him, salvation is best understood as "wholeness," but humanity has not yet possessed this wholeness fully and therefore must search for it. Humanity is moving toward the plenitude of salvation (wholeness) that has been promised, and so the best stance from which to discover and justify the ethical imperative is within the horizon of promise and fulfillment.[15]

Finally, Charles E. Curran has proposed a stance based on the fivefold Christian mysteries of creation, fall, incarnation, redemption, and resurrection destiny.[16] For him, each one of these doctrinal themes normatively interprets Christian experience within a comprehensive schema. All these mysteries taken together, then, serve as a way not only to shape and inform the Christian's moral reasoning on concrete issues but also as a way to critique other religious and secular stances in society that underlie and justify normative judgments on moral issues like abortion, capital punishment, and so forth.

As helpful as all these stances might be, all of them seem to be far too content-oriented and doctrinaire in their intent and far too narrow in their scope. In other words, these stances are interpreted through content categories alone, for example, Jesus Christ or love (agape) or the fivefold Christian mysteries, and the content is too indigenous to a specific confessional traditional (doctrinaire). Surely, the content categories of the believer's stance can and should be specifically Christian, particularly when explicit reference is made to Jesus and his teachings of the kingdom, but I argue that the proper category by which one should understand a stance should be formal or structural in nature. In other words, one should understand a stance by reference to the interaction between the subject and the object poles of human knowing. Furthermore, an ethical stance must be as comprehensive as possible to take into view as many elements of moral experience as possible. Nearly all the stances discussed above lack this comprehensive scope. For example, Barth's stance (Jesus Christ) fails to appreciate that in fact nonreligious people do experience an authentic ethical imperative, although they have no reflective experience of God or of Jesus Christ.

CARDINAL BERNARDIN'S "CONSISTENT ETHIC OF LIFE" UNDERSTOOD AS A MORAL STANCE

I have already defined a moral stance as a coherent and consistent combination of normative value judgments about the world, God, and self. It is precisely in the interaction between the subject and object poles that the claim to a normative moral judgment about virtues, moral actions, and obligations in the moral life is discovered, articulated, and justified. Thus, like all stances, Cardinal Bernardin's consistent ethic of life structures one's fundamental understanding of moral experience, serves as a critique of others' interpretations of moral reality, and becomes a source of ethical criteria to evaluate particular actions and social policies across a wide range of moral issues. Though a stance is always logically prior to systematic reflection on specific issues (e.g., abortion), nonetheless it seeks such reflection by its very nature. Because a stance is the foundation of or matrix within which moral imperatives are discovered and ultimately justified, the validity of the imperatives rests on the validity of the stance. Thus, if a stance lacks comprehensiveness, coherence, or authenticity, then so do the moral imperatives or moral judgments of virtue, value, or obligation that have been discerned and formulated from within the stance.

The vision that Bernardin proposes is comprehensive in that it refuses to leave out any life issue that affects the sacredness of persons. At the subject pole where one's attitudes and commitments come into view, he is committed to a full range of issues where human life and dignity are at stake, and these commitments and attitudes are nourished and informed by various theological themes. Though he argues that these themes are specifically grounded in the New Testament, he believes that neither the themes nor the content generated from the themes are specific or unique only to the Christian stance.[17] By arguing in principle that the themes and content are not necessarily specific to Christians, Bernardin is able, at the level of his vision (stance), to dialogue with others in society who are not Christian. At the object pole where the range of data or "world" comes into view, Bernardin's consistent ethic of life is comprehensive in that the vision encompasses all the particular issues from "womb to tomb." Put negatively, his moral stance refuses to exclude any issue that threatens the dignity or sacredness of the human person, and he employs this vision to criticize other groups whose stance is narrowed by commitment to one specific issue, for example, abortion.

On almost every page of his speeches, Cardinal Bernardin calls for a consistency in attitude and in the use and application of certain moral principles. Though I will assess neither the adequacy nor the validity of these moral principles here, what is important for my purposes is to indicate how the consistency he calls for is part of his moral vision or stance. Of course, any particular moral stance can be inconsistent, and to that extent it is incoherent, and possibly even inauthentic. People can hold to one thing, yet incoherently do something else that is inconsistent with their basic attitudes and commitments. Likewise, individuals and whole communities can commit themselves to certain moral principles to inform and direct their behavior, but then they can be highly selective and serendipitous in the application of these principles. One of the hallmarks of an *adequate* vision of moral experience is its ability to tie together attitude and doing, commitment and application. It seems to me that it is this adequacy that Bernardin seeks to achieve in his emphasis on consistency. He will use consistency not only to assess the adequacy of others' stances but also the adequacy of various social attitudes and policies.

The moral stance of Cardinal Bernardin is also analogical in character because it seeks to view issues that are not identical but that have some common characteristics.[18] Though he insists that each issue along the spectrum of life must be considered on its own merits, he believes this should not dull our vision to the possible connections among these distinct concerns. A stance that is analogical, then, approaches the interpretation of moral experience with an eye to possible similarities; it refuses to look on our moral lives as disparate and unconnected. The radical existentialist's or situationist's vision is inspired by the novelty of the individual and the particular. As such, their vision is committed to seeing only the disconnections within moral experience and the uniqueness of each moral issue. Bernardin's stance is quite different from this situationist's view, and it is quite different from other stances. His stance is not as radical as their claim to particularity, and his is not narrowed by a desire to concentrate on the importance of a single issue at the expense of seeing connections to other issues. By paying attention to and focusing on the links that exist among a variety of issues, Cardinal Bernardin's stance can allow him to dialogue and form coalitions with others along a whole spectrum of concerns in order to transform both people's hearts and actions and society's policies.

I indicated above that a moral stance is logically prior to systematic reflection but that it ultimately seeks that kind of reflection. When the contents of a stance are thematized and made explicit, the attitudes and commitments embodied in that vision make their way into and influence systematic reflection on moral experience. Bernardin is certainly correct in describing his consistent ethic as a way (I would say "heuristic device") of defining the problems that confront human dignity.[19] This is precisely what a stance is and does. But he also claims that the consistent ethic is systematic.[20] He links this term to the nature of Catholic theology, which is the systematic reflection on religious-moral experience. As a reflective discipline, theology has the task of drawing out the meaning of each moral principle and the relationships among them,[21] and it refuses to look at and treat moral issues in an ad hoc fashion.[22] I would argue, though, that not all theologies can accomplish what Bernardin seeks. Some types of theology that have a narrow stance that lies behind them will not in fact look at and treat moral issues in any other way than ad hoc. Because a moral stance is not only the foundation of systematic reflection but also of the moral imperative and normative judgment discoverable by that reflection, the adequacy of a theology will depend upon the comprehensiveness and authenticity of the stance that gives rise to that discipline.

When we turn our attention to placing Bernardin and his writings into one or more of the general models of theological discourse, what we find with him, like with most other authors, is that he does not neatly fit into any one of the models. Rather, he seems to move between two of the general models: the neo-orthodox and dialogical models. Though we find Bernardin in each of these models, I would argue that his consistent ethic of life was in fact an attempt on his part to change his stance from the neo-orthodox to the dialogical model.

In some of his earlier speeches, especially those dealing specifically with the moral issue of abortion, Cardinal Bernardin appears to fit more squarely into the neo-orthodox model that I had described above. It seems that what he is committed to and the kinds of questions that he asks are determined principally, if not entirely, by the moral tradition of the Roman Catholic Church and its doctrinal tradition. Thus, the range of data that comes into view for him tends to be the doctrinal content of this tradition, though some opening is made to other considerations. On the other hand, Bernardin also adopts the dialogical model in which he regularly reformulates his commitments and questions to include those concerns, values, and normative claims of both secular society and of other religious traditions. Consequently, we find that the range of data that he consults and is interested in investigating begins to change in that his data now comprise the experiences of people, including the experience of women, and the values and data of secular society. For example, when Bernardin held open sessions for his "Common Ground" initiative or interviews prior to the writing of the pastoral letter *The Challenge of Peace*, he sought input from various secular sources, some of whom for the latter sessions were either military strategists or others who had an expertise in matters of warfare.[23] He did not limit his data at the object pole solely to the contents of the doctrinal tradition of the Roman Catholic Church on issues of peace and warfare. In these instances, Bernardin is committed to dialogue. As he states in the Gannon lecture,

> As we seek to shape and share the vision of a consistent ethic of life, I suggest a style governed by the following rule: We should maintain and clearly articulate our religious convictions but also maintain our civil courtesy. We should be vigorous in stating a case and attentive in hearing another's case; we should test everyone's logic but not question his or her motives.[24]

What we find here is Bernardin's commitment not only to the values and normative claims of the Catholic tradition but also a commitment to a dialogue with others and their values and normative judgments. When one is invested in true dialogue, one must suspend for the moment one's own taken-for-granted assumptions and normative judgments and allow the conversation with the other and his or her values and judgments to be included as new data for further reflection. Bernardin's questions about and commitments to including the experiences and judgments of others in society beyond his own ecclesial community and religious tradition were the conditions of the possibility for him to formulate the consistent ethic of life. Had he remained, as head of the Office for Pro-Life Activities of the United States Conference of Catholic Bishops, only within the neo-orthodox model of theological discourse—with its commitments to the established tradition and its content only—it is quite possible that he would never have articulated the need for the consistent ethic of life—with its commitments to dialogue with others outside the tradition. As he changed his commitments and questions about a wide range of issues that confront the sacredness of life, the data (people's experiences, scholarly documents, etc.) that came into view for him to consult and reflect upon also changed. As we recall, when the subject pole changes, there is a corresponding change at the object pole. Such an important change both signaled and marked his movement from the neo-orthodox model of normative judgment making to the dialogical model. In moving from one model to another, Bernardin was able to challenge two different groups. The first group was the pro-life movement within his own Catholic tradition that had a tendency to focus on only a single issue—namely, abortion—and thus not see how a normative judgment on this issue must be consistent with other normative judgments on a wide range of other moral issues that affect the sacredness of human life—for example, capital punishment, delivery of health care to the poor, warfare, and so forth. On the other hand, his consistent ethic was also a challenge to secular society to change its attitudes, practices, and social policies on these same issues related to the sacredness of life.

CONCLUSION

In the end, Cardinal Bernardin has left us with a great challenge. Understanding the nature or inner intentionality of that challenge as the systematic development of an authentic, comprehensive, analogical, and dialogical stance is the first task in taking up the charge that Bernardin has placed before us. His commitment to placing into dialogue both the legitimate secularity of society with its values *and* the authenticity of the Christian tradition and its values is the nexus and challenge of his consistent ethic of life.[25]

ENDNOTES

1. See David Tracy, *The Achievement of Bernard Lonergan* (New York: Herder and Herder, 1970), 8.

2. For examples where Bernardin describes the consistent ethic as a "vision," see "A Consistent Ethic of Life: An American-Catholic Dialogue" (Gannon Lecture, Fordham University, 1983); "A Consistent Ethic of Life: Continuing the Dialogue" (Wade Lecture, St. Louis University, 1984); "National Consultation on Pornography, Obscenity and Indecency" (Cincinnati, 1984); "Address at Seattle University" (1986); and "Address at Consistent Ethic of Life Conference" (Portland, Oregon, 1986). Martin Kenny, in his licentiate dissertation at Weston Jesuit School of Theology, also claims that Bernardin's consistent ethic attempted to develop a "moral vision." See Martin Kenny, "A Critique of Joseph Cardinal Bernardin's Proposal of the Consistent Ethic of Life" (licentiate dissertation in sacred theology at Weston Jesuit School of Theology, 1997), 20.

3. For examples of the consistent ethic as a framework, see "The Consistent Ethic of Life and Health Care Systems" (Loyola University of Chicago, 1985); "Address at Seattle University"; and "Address at Consistent Ethic of Life Conference."

4. For examples, see "The Challenge and the Witness of Catholic Health Care" (Catholic Medical Center, Jamaica, New York, 1986) and "Address at Consistent Ethic of Life Conference."

5. Almost every page of Cardinal Bernardin's speeches makes reference to the necessity for "consistency" in the ethic that he proposes.

6. For example, see "Address at Seattle University" and "Address at Consistent Ethic of Life Conference."

7. Though Bernardin does not use the word "dialogical" to describe his stance, this word certainly renders his intent to "cast our case in broadly defined terms, in a way which elicits support from others." For examples, see "Linkage and the Logic of the Abortion Debate" (Kansas City, 1985) and "Address at Consistent Ethics of Life Conference." In addition, Bernardin's constant reference to culture and what is going on in culture not only indicates that cultural facts are relevant to his analysis at the level of the object pole, but these references also clearly manifest his desire to dialogue with various groups within society.

8. See Bernard Lonergan, *Method in Theology* (New York: Herder and Herder, 1972), 235–44.

9. These models are based on David Tracy, *Blessed Rage for Order: The New Pluralism in Theology* (New York: Seabury Press, 1975), 24–63.

10. See Matthew Lamb, *Solidarity with Victims: Toward a Theology of Social Transformation* (New York: Crossroad, 1982), 61–99; and Francis Schüssler Fiorenza, *Foundational Theology: Jesus and the Church* (New York: Crossroad, 1984), 5–55.

11. Lamb, *Solidarity*, 62.

12. For a more complete discussion of the stances that have been proposed within the

Christian traditions, see James Sellers, *Theological Ethics* (New York: Macmillan, 1966), 31–68.

13. Adolf von Harnack, *What Is Christianity?* trans. T. B. Saunders (New York: Harper & Brothers, 1957), 70–74.

14. Karl Barth, *Church Dogmatics II/2*, trans. G. W. Bromiley et al. (Edinburgh: T. & T. Clark, 1957), 509–49.

15. Sellers, *Theological Ethics*, 55–65.

16. Charles E. Curran, "The Stance of Moral Theology," in *New Perspectives in Moral Theology* (Notre Dame, Ind.: Fides, 1974), 47–86.

17. See "The Death Penalty in Our Time" (Criminal Court of Cook County, Ill., 1985); "Address at Seattle University"; and "Address at Consistent Ethic of Life Conference."

18. See "Address at Seattle University." Though the analogical character of Bernardin's vision is present, albeit implicitly, throughout all his speeches, he begins to make explicit reference to it only in his later speeches.

19. For example, see "A Consistent Ethic of Life: Continuing the Dialogue." Bernardin also uses his vision as a way (heuristic device) for testing public policies, party platforms, and candidates. See "A Consistent Ethic of Life: Continuing the Dialogue"; "Address at Seattle University"; and "Address at Consistent Ethic of Life Conference."

20. See "Address at Seattle University" and "Address at Consistent Ethic of Life Conference."

21. See "Address at Consistent Ethic of Life Conference."

22. See "Address at Consistent Ethic of Life Conference."

23. See National Conference of Catholic Bishops, *The Challenge of Peace: God's Promise and Our Response* (Washington, D.C.: United States Catholic Conference, 1983), especially the footnotes to part 2: War and Peace in the Modern World: Problems and Principles, 39–62.

24. "A Consistent Ethic of Life: An American-Catholic Dialogue," 10.

25. I have used some of the material in this chapter that I originally wrote for a "Consistent Ethic of Life" symposium at Loyola University Chicago. That original material was published as "Response to John Finnis: A Theological Critique," in Thomas G. Fuechtmann, ed., *Consistent Ethic of Life* (Kansas City, Mo.: Sheed & Ward, 1988), 182–95. This current chapter was written originally as part of a three-year seminar on Cardinal Bernardin's speeches under the direction of Thomas Nairn.

4

The Communitarian Perspective: Autonomy and the Common Good

Thomas A. Shannon

AUTONOMY AND ITS CONTEXTS

Autonomy

Together with respect for persons, justice, and beneficence, autonomy has been a major workhorse in bioethical analysis over the past several decades. From issues like abortion to euthanasia, advance directives to artificial reproduction, we have relied almost exclusively on autonomy as the cornerstone of ethical analysis. Let any challenge to personal freedom or private decision making be made and almost immediately, in the wonderful phrase of Art Caplan, the "autonomy drum begins banging." Think, for example how autonomy functions as the main line of defense against any attempts to qualify or regulate access to or use of reproductive technologies, including, but not limited to, artificial insemination, in vitro fertilization (IVF), surrogate motherhood, and abortion. Autonomy has had a profound impact on the practice of medicine and on how medical ethics as a discipline has developed.

The issue of autonomy was highlighted in a dramatic way in the play and later the movie *Whose Life Is It?*, the tragic story of a young and competent man who wishes to end his life because he will remain a quadriplegic. The story of Dax Cowart, the victim of severe burns over almost his entire body, is another widely documented case of a competent patient refusing lifesaving treatment. Both cases were resolved by the continuation of treatment and by cries of outrage because of such blatant overrides of autonomous judgments.

This should be no surprise, for autonomy is the "All American" value. Almost from conception we have had drummed into us the message that we must be the master of our fate, the captain of our ship, the one to forge our own destiny with our own hands, and that we are the one solely responsible for our own fate. The myth of the self-made person has taken strong root in our culture.

And to be sure, there is a very positive dimension to that myth. It is clearly the source of creativity, energy, and initiative. Americans do have a strong sense of responsibility and that has spurred us to action, to seize our destiny, to realize that the future is of our making. The new world is a world of opportunity, a world of improvement, a world of possibility.

Two Case Studies

Let me present two cases in which autonomy structures major elements of decision making in medical ethics. First, I will consider some ethical issues in guardianship of the elderly. Then I will consider some issues in artificial reproduction. Analysis of the issues will follow later.

Adult Protective Services

I begin with some comments in an essay entitled "Ethical Issues in Adult Protective Services" by Jane Boyajian. Privacy is defined here as the right to make one's own decisions and decide what is in one's best interests. We would all agree to this. But what is interesting and relevant are the conclusions drawn from this principle. Privacy involves respecting the decision of another, leaving them alone and free from interference. Finally, it means letting people "live according to a lifestyle others find repulsive, even harmful, without interference from others. Potentially vulnerable adults can refuse social services which caseworkers believe will improve their quality of life."[1]

Another issue raised in the article is what the author calls an obligation in a democratic society to promote autonomy over protection and intervention. The issue here is a critical one, because there has been a history of paternalistic abuse of the elderly, the mentally ill, and others with diminished competence. One needs to remember that to assert a priority is not to establish that such a priority actually exists.

A third issue raised in this article is professional conduct. The author states that "the first step in promoting an ethically responsible professional practice is separating personal values from professional assessments. . . . Personal considerations have no place in professional decision-making."[2] The comment raises, but does not resolve, issues related to personal values and professional ethics.

Artificial Reproduction

Let me now turn to some issues raised with respect to artificial reproduction. The area of human reproduction presents a very focused area of tension between the wishes of the individual and social norms, restraints, and resources.

Legally the issue came into clear focus with the 1968 Supreme Court decision in *Griswald* v. *Connecticut*. The court determined that the state had no business involving itself in a couple's decision of whether or not to have a child. Another dimension was added in the 1973 *Roe* v. *Wade* case that decriminalized all state abortion laws. The basis of this decision was that the right of privacy was broad enough to encompass a woman's decision to abort.

Such control over one's body as the basis for the validation of surrogacy is highlighted by Lori Andrews in her book *Between Strangers*. She notes her and others' surprise at some women's opposition to surrogacy, particularly since it was women who argued for and supported the control of women's bodies by women. Such a qualification of autonomy, by prohibiting surrogacy, could open the door to other forms of reproductive regulation. Thus, she argues, autonomy forms a strong defense against bodily intrusions.

BEYOND AUTONOMY: A RETURN TO THE COMMON GOOD

A Critique of Autonomy

Shortcomings in the Myth of Autonomy

As powerful and positive as the myth of autonomy is, there is a downside to it. I argue that the foundations of it are false. There are no self-made people. No one of us starts from square one in anything. At birth we are given a language, a culture, education, socialization, and all manner of skills. We are born into a community that to some extent nourishes us and gives us the foundation on which we build. How far we take that is, indeed, to a large extent, up to us, but we must not forget that we began in a community that formed us and gifted us.

It is also the case that we, as a culture, have taken the concept of individualism about as far as it can go. We understand autonomy to be a situation in which I am so individual, so idiosyncratic that I, and only I, can know what I think, what I feel, and what is good for me. We seem to have taken the philosophy of individualism to its logical conclusion and affirmed that indeed we are all islands, apart from each other. Very little, if anything, unites us. What we share is our separateness, not our common good or common destiny. Many in our culture no longer assume that parents know what is good for their children, that teachers know what is good for students, that spouses know what is good for each other, that physicians know what is good for patients.

Perhaps this degree of the emphasis on autonomy and individualism is symbolized by the most common expression of contemporary relations: the contract. A relation frequently consists only of what is expressly specified by the terms of the contract. If it is not expressly stated, then we do not have to do it, nor should there be any expectation of our doing it. Perhaps the most interesting form of this is the prenuptial contract. No longer is it for better or worse or richer or poorer but rather for "*x* percent" of actual and anticipated income, together with wages lost because of time invested in the relationship instead of one's career. The marriage contract has replaced the marriage covenant because of the priority of autonomy over the community. This cultural situation has left us quite alone, with few, if any, to know our interests, what is good for us, or what might help us to mature as a healthy member of our society.

The consequence of the recent dominance of autonomy, located in a rapidly increasing technological arena, has been a profound isolation of the individual from the family and the community. The rights of the individual or the autonomous choices of the individual are essentially trumps that the individual can use either to demand or to reject relations. But such relations are a function of autonomous choice, not a consequence of living in community. The autonomous individual stands in final and total judgment of all that impacts him or her.

The immediate shortcoming of this position is manifestly clear and most problematic when the patient is unable to speak on his or her own behalf, that is, when he or she is comatose, unconscious, or in some other way incompetent. Resolutions of this situation range from advance directives of one sort or another, trying to specify the patient's best interests, or substituting judgment of what the patient would do if he or she knew of this situation for the judgment that the patient needs to make but cannot. All of these are ways to preserve autonomy by replicating the patient's autonomy in situations in which the exercise of autonomy is impossible. They are based on the perception that incompetence is not a disqualification for the exercise of autonomy. One retains one's rights and the right to exercise these rights in such a condition of incompetence.

However, a soft underbelly of autonomy is beginning to be revealed. We

are beginning to recognize that some requests or demands made by autonomous individuals can be problematic. The fact that someone chooses a therapy does not automatically qualify one for that therapy. The fact that one
chooses a therapy does not mean that the therapy will be successful. The fact
that one rejects a therapy does not mean that such a decision was an appropriate one. And even the fact that one has the right to make an autonomous
decision does not mean that the impact on others or the community should
not be taken into account.

We are beginning to recognize that the social impact of individual, autonomous choices has profound significance. One such area of impact is the cost
of health care. The sum of autonomous choices in medical care is staggering.
Not all do—or even can—receive the same medical therapy, even though
needs may be similar. The shortage of organs for transplantation continually
brings this problem to public awareness. Yet another area is the increasingly
strident debate over euthanasia—whether done in an individual act, or with
the assistance of a physician. Finally, given that health insurance in America
is largely private and to a large degree contingent on one's employment, we
find autonomy confronting a rather insurmountable corporate barrier.

The upshot of all this is that autonomy, though an important and critical
value in our society and the practice of medicine, is proving itself inadequate
to help us resolve critical social issues. In particular, our overreliance on
autonomy has seduced us into thinking problems such as the ones described
above are individual problems and can be resolved on the individual level.
Our captivation by autonomy has also led us to think of the individual as an
isolated being, complete in his or her own self. In this view, the community
is frequently seen as an obstacle—if not an outright barrier—preventing the
individual from achieving his or her desires or goals. However, some, myself
included, say that America at the present time is living proof of the falseness
of the claim that individual choices to promote one's own good lead to the
good of all.

The Paternalistic Response

Questioning autonomy typically leads to cries of paternalism and violations of liberty. Paternalism—either doing something for someone without
his requesting it or not cooperating with someone when she requests our
help—has gotten quite bad press, particularly in our country, and particularly
in the helping professions. The professionals in these areas actually thought
they had some good ideas about how to help people and tried to put them
into practice. The doctrine of informed consent was a strong and appropriate

protest to inappropriate and unwarranted interventions into people's lives, bodies, and value systems.

There certainly were and are abuses of paternalism. Much reform and creativity in various fields—education, medical training, and the arts—were stifled because a certain group knew how to do it and knew what all the students needed. Much personal growth was thwarted because parents and educators had certain goals in mind to which individuals had to conform for their own good. People have been prevented from following their interests because what they wanted to do was too dangerous, too risky, too new, perhaps too exciting. And so initiative was stopped.

But now, as I have indicated, autonomy holds sway and almost any intervention to help someone—even when he or she needs it—falls under the suspicion or condemnation of paternalism. We have almost worked ourselves into a position in which we think that we as humans share nothing in common, that we have no common values, needs, aspirations, or goods. In the interest of promoting autonomy, we have talked ourselves into a denial of any commonality of interests with the consequence that practically any intervention is an invasion of individual privacy.

James Q. Wilson, in his recent book *The Moral Sense*, asks the interesting question, "Are we prepared for the possibility that by behaving as if no moral judgments were possible, we may create a world that more and more resembles our diminished moral expectations. We must be careful of what we think we are, because we may become that."[3]

Response to Autonomy in Adult Protective Services

In my earlier comments about adult protective services, I presented several issues derived from autonomy, including the right to lead a repulsive lifestyle, the right to refuse medications, and professional ethics. Let me make some comments about those issues.

I would think that in adult protective services, many of the individuals, while moderately autonomous, also need a lot of protection. Perhaps that's why this area is referred to as protective services. I think one can promote and respect autonomy while still providing appropriate and adequate levels of service. The issue is not to do for others what they can and ought to do for themselves; it is to recognize that providing help and assistance are not *automatically* violations of autonomy. Instead of thinking in terms of rights of autonomy and prohibitions against paternalism, instead of thinking in a conflict model, why not think in terms of a cooperative or collaborative model in which both the patient and guardian work toward mutually desired goals? Shifting the model will not resolve conflicts—and conflicts there will surely be—but a shift in frame of reference will help rethink the strategies we use to achieve our goals.

I should think we would want professionals with strong values and beliefs. And I should think we would want the value-laden professionals to bring the best of their values to bear on the resolution of a case. Of course we don't want someone coming in and taking over and telling us to put sweaters on because they know we're cold. But if someone is not formed and developed in a value context, that person isn't going to be very good at recognizing anyone else's values. Also, someone who has a strong value perspective in his or her own professional life is going to recognize a conflict of values and is going to be sensitive to the problems in particular situations. We might disagree about the solutions and resolutions, but at least we will know what the debate is about: it's about the ethical response to a human being in need, and not some technical debate about procedures.

I find the statement that someone has the right to lead a repulsive lifestyle rather appalling. This is the conclusion to which we have been led by an exaggerated sense of autonomy and privacy: individuals have the right to lead repulsive lifestyles while we stand by and applaud such exercises of autonomy. This is particularly ironic when medications that could help that person by resolving elements of a depression that might be causing the lifestyle are available. This is not an argument for simply going in and taking over someone's life. It is an argument that when we can figure out why someone is leading a basically destructive lifestyle and can intervene in a moderate way through medication, autonomy may fall to beneficence. Why continue to let someone harm himself to the point of either causing irreversible physical damage so he is permanently bedridden, or cause himself to become incompetent and then, and only then, provide the appropriate medication? I genuinely think that the good of intervention in cases like these accomplishes more good than harm.

One of the first cases described to me when I began to work in bioethics was of a woman who was severely depressed. While depressed, she always refused medicine, and because she would forget to take her medicine, she always refused the medicine. But when she had been taking the medicine, she always consented to it. The way the case was resolved was that the team decided the person who chose the medication and lived without depression was her better self, and so they assumed she would always want her medicine. That solution makes sense to me. The good to be achieved and the harm to be avoided, particularly in the areas of physical and mental illness, seem to me to outweigh the harm, if any, done through a modest violation of autonomy.

Autonomy and Artificial Reproduction

Even though we live in a culture that generally supports almost unlimited reproductive rights, there are proposals that argue that access to the new reproductive technologies be qualified. For example, some propose that only married heterosexual couples should have access to IVF. Others argue that commercial surrogacy, in particular, should be prohibited altogether. Such suggestions are, at least prima facie, violations of autonomy and a restraint of an individual's reproductive freedom. Are there justifications for apparent restrictions such as these?

A critical dimension of autonomy is freedom. If one does not have the capacity to choose or to remain constant in one's choices, then one can hardly be thought of as free. Yet freedom is somewhat of a confusing reality, particularly in our culture.

Freedom has certainly played a major part in the establishment of our nation. The Bill of Rights, in particular, is an ongoing, living testimony to some of our most cherished freedoms. Yet there are debates about those freedoms: Does free speech include the right to destroy the flag? Can song lyrics be censored? Can a woman's reproductive decisions be qualified? All of these raise profound issues about one of our most treasured gifts.

One of the critical ethical dimensions of freedom in our culture is our seeming equation of freedom with the capacity to choose. That is, freedom consists in either the fact of a choice or the capacity to choose and the protection of freedom consists in protecting choice. Such a position suggests that what is chosen is not central to the ethical analysis. If one couples this with our primarily procedural legal system, guaranteeing the capacity for choice discharges our ethical and legal duty.

Such a position on freedom is important because it ensures that a critical capacity will be safeguarded from unwarranted intrusions or interferences. Autonomy is at its core the capacity to be ourselves. The protection of freedom of choice ensures the protection of a core element of that autonomy. Yet I am uncomfortable with that position. It is reminiscent of Bentham's position that there is no moral difference between playing push-pin and doing philosophy. What is morally relevant is reduced to what one has chosen instead of whatever value, or lack thereof, might be associated with either choice.

To some extent we need to at least consider the value of what is being chosen. Not to do so would be to accept a position of total value neutrality or to assume that all realities are of the same value. Either position fails to discriminate where discrimination is indicated. A richer concept of freedom would incorporate the value of what is chosen. Such a position is derivative from the medieval philosopher Scotus who argued that the essence of freedom was not merely the capacity to choose but rather adherence to the good that one chooses.

Such a position automatically raises profound concerns in our culture—what is the good and who defines it, for example. Nonetheless, there is an element in this perspective that we need to reincorporate into our ethical analysis—the recognition that the fact that something is chosen neither ends the ethical discussion nor makes that choice worthwhile. While we need to protect the procedural dimension of freedom, we also need to evaluate what we choose, lest we fall into an ethical or cultural indifference.

Minimally, then, I argue that the fact of being chosen does not ethically ensure that reality's worthwhileness or that all objects of choice are thereby ethically valuable. Assumedly, one would choose something because of a value in that reality and this would be done after some comparison. Thus choices are value laden though such values can be argued about. Additionally, one could be asked to justify and/or defend one's choice.

Such a position does not require that there be a test of values either by an institution or individuals. Rather it seeks to acknowledge that choices convey values and that their worthwhileness can and ought to be debated. Additionally, while it is also clear that an object increases or decreases in value in relation to its desirability to me, such objects have a meaning and value in themselves, a premoral goodness or badness that is then factored into the moral decision. Thus, choice occurs within a context that is already value laden, though the reality of choice further articulates those values.

This perspective does not seek an end to reproductive rights. Rather, it seeks to examine those rights in relation to the good they hope to actualize and the overall significance of that good. While not all will agree on the same goods or the same priority of goods, at least the debate will be moved to the values at stake. At some point, a discussion such as this is necessary to move us beyond the procedural conundrums in which we find ourselves.

A Reconsideration of the Common Good

Considerations of the common good have fallen by the wayside in the past several decades in mainstream discussions of social and political ethics. In part this has been because, as Bellah phrases it, "American culture has focused relentlessly on the idea that individuals are self-interest maximizers and that private accumulation and private pleasures are the only measurable public goods."[4] Another dimension of this is a shift from the family's being child centered to its being adult centered.[5] This shift reflects a priority of personal fulfillment over the good of family members and an understanding of the family as a locus for individual fulfillment over development of an identity through social interactions. Downplay of the common good is also reflected in our reliance on cost-benefit analysis for social decision making. What is given priority here is social efficiency and a neglect of the externalities that follow from such decisions. Finally, we continue to hear the rhetoric that the government and our institutions are the enemy of the individual. While the Reagan mantra of "Get government off our backs" is not as frequently invoked, the sentiment remains alive, particularly in many of the critiques of the Clinton health proposal.

What we seem to have forgotten is that "even autonomy depends on a particular kind of institutional structure and is not an escape from institutions altogether."[6] We have further forgotten that autonomy is "only one virtue among others and that without such virtues as responsibility, and care . . . autonomy itself becomes . . . an empty form without substance."[7]

As a way of responding to the issues raised thus far, I want to propose a reconsideration of the common good as a critical component of personal and social decision making. In doing this, I want to recognize two caveats. First, I want to affirm, following the wisdom of Joseph Pieper, that it is "definitely not possible to define the *bonum commune,* in this sense, with any comprehensiveness and finality."[8] Thus I do not conceive of the common good as a type of institutional or repressive Procrustean bed with which to trim excesses of autonomy. Second, again following Pieper, "the 'good of a commonwealth' includes the inborn human talents, qualities and potentials, and part of the *justitia distributiva* is the obligation to protect, preserve, and foster these capacities."[9] The positive contribution of the concept of the common good is, as I see it and as I understand how it is located in the Catholic social ethic, to encourage and enhance participation in the community so that individual action will benefit both.

The Common Good: The Lure of Nostalgia

In discussing the common good, a double nostalgia must be resisted and ultimately rejected. One version is American and is derived from a vision of rural or small-town America as seen through the idealization of the founding of our republic or in the paintings of Norman Rockwell. Another version is papal and longs for the idealized Middle Ages.

At one period there existed a social order which, though by no means perfect in every respect, corresponded nevertheless in a certain measure to right reason according to the needs and conditions of the times. That this order has long since perished is not due to the fact that it was incapable of development and adaptation to changing needs and circumstances, but rather to the wrongdoing of men. Men were hardened in excessive self-love and refused to extend that order, as was their duty, to the increasing numbers of the people; or else, deceived by the attractions of false liberty and other errors, they grew impatient of every restraint and endeavored to throw off all authority.[10]

To be sure, there are virtues to be admired and emulated in such visions but our world is, to a large degree, industrialized and urban. Our problems, though they may be similar to those of past generations, cannot rely on the solutions of our forebears for our times and social context are quite different.

A Constructive Reconsideration of the Common Good

Following the lines of thought developed by Michael and Kenneth Rimes in their book *Fullness of Faith: The Public Significance of Theology*, I would like to present some constructive proposals for reconsidering application of the common good in our situation.

In Roman Catholic social theory, from which I derive my perspective, the concept of the common good has a rich, varied history. In "Rerum Novarum," the 1891 encyclical by Leo XIII that began the modern tradition of Catholic social thought, Leo defines the common good as that for the sake of which civil society exists and "is concerned with the interests of all in general, and with the individual interests in their due place and proportion."[11] More specifically Pius XI, in "Quadragesimo Anno," stated, "Those goods should be sufficient to supply all needs and an honest livelihood, and to uplift men to that higher level of prosperity and culture which, provided it be used with prudence, is not only no hindrance but is of singular help to virtue."[12] Both of these conceptions of the common good derived from such a society were "self-evidently substantive, objectively knowable, and indivisible."[13] While such a perspective is overly optimistic at best and epistemologically naive at worst, nonetheless such a concern for the good of society and all of its members stays at the heart of the encyclical tradition.

John XXIII began a shift from such an hierarchical and static vision of society and the common good by identifying the foundation of the common good as the human person who has rights and obligations flowing from his or her nature.[14] This moved the focus from the structure of society to the person and used the concept of rights to ensure the protection and enhancement of the individual in society and the concept of obligation to guarantee that the person actively participate in the development of society. Such thinking led John to a vision of the common good which did not stop at national boundaries but also included "the entire human family."

The Second Vatican Council, in its pastoral constitution *The Church in the Modern World,* continued this line of thought by recognizing that "the concrete demands of this common good are constantly changing as time goes on."[15] This important document recognizes that the common good is a dynamic concept and one that must be responsive to the changing needs of human society.

The American Catholic bishops continued this line of thinking in their pastoral letter "Economic Justice for All." The bishops say, for example, that "human dignity, realized in community with others and with the whole of God's creation, is the norm against which every social institution must be measured."[16] Again they affirm that "[t]he common bond of humanity that links all persons is the source of our belief that the country can attain a renewed public moral vision."[17] And finally, the bishops state, "The dignity of the human person, realized in community with others, is the criterion against which all aspects of economic life must be measured."[18]

The bishops then use this perspective to develop a vision of social justice that "implies that persons have an obligation to be active and productive participants in the life of society and that society has a duty to enable them to participate in this way."[19] Here they follow Pius XI, who said, "It is of the very essence of social justice to demand from each individual all that is necessary for the common good."[20] Thus the bishops envision justice as a means through which the person achieves the perfection of his or her self through participating in the well-being of society. In the perspective of the bishops, then, the core of justice is the establishment of "minimum levels of participation in the life of the human community for all persons,"[21] rather than establishing zones of privacy whereby individuals attempt to seek their private good independent of the community.

This orientation presents a vision of justice and the common good that is not quite in the mainstream of American libertarian theory. The bishops recognize this and argue that the next phase of the American experiment needs to be securing for this vision of social-justice-as-participation the same status as the other rights we currently celebrate. The significant difference is that the bishops' vision orients the person to his or her role in the community, whereas our traditional vision focuses on the autonomous individual.

Refashioning the Common Good

This emphasis on community, social justice, and human dignity realized in community leads to a certain shaping of an understanding of the common good that has a different emphasis than in the past. This shift looks to freedom, equality, and participation as core elements. I will touch on each of these in relation to the encyclical tradition as well as independent of it.

As I noted earlier, the American experience of freedom in general is "freedom from." And, typically, what we most desire to be free from is coercion, particularly any institutional coercion. While that perspective has contributed significantly to advances in our society, the question of the object of our freedom remains undeveloped in our society. Thus we need to focus on what I call "freedom for." This is the issue of the significance and value of our choices. Minimally we need to recognize that choices are not value neutral. Though sometimes what we do is whimsical, most of the time our choices reflect preferences and priorities with respect to some good we wish to achieve. We also need to reconsider the reigning assumption that the fact of my choosing an option makes that option worthwhile or free from critique. As I say this, I hear the autonomy drum beginning to beat in the background. But I think we need to seriously consider the values behind the choices we make. For while the choices are undeniably ours and ours alone to make, some are harmful to ourselves and society. To say this is not to give free reign to censorship or invite a new wave of Puritanism. Rather, it is to recognize that what we choose has a significant effect on who we become, and who we become has a powerful effect on what society becomes. Perhaps rather than prohibit actions, we need to begin to model appropriate behavior to show the positive consequences that can accrue for ourselves and society.

Equality resonates strongly within our culture and vast social and personal energy has been spent in achieving greater degrees of equality for all citizens. Yet we face a dual danger now with respect to equality. First, some may think that equal means *same* or *identical* and attempt to locate criteria for equality on quantitative measures. Second, others may identify equality with freedom from all norms in the name of idiosyncrasy or autonomy.

The social norm of equality of persons is derived from our common dignity and value as persons. Such dignity "need[s] to be incarnated in social policies and practices."[22] Most critically this means that we must strike the proper balance between a false uniformity and a destructive utilitarian individualism. We must recognize the value and uniqueness of each person and the wealth of riches they bring but must also remember that our origin and development as persons is communal. To seek equality for oneself is also to affirm the same for one's neighbor.

The emphasis on participation in society as a means of achieving the common good is a traditional theme in the encyclical tradition being reiterated in a different context. Formerly, participation meant living out the duties of one's state in life. These duties were derived and defined from the hierarchical society in which one lived and found one's purpose. Thus, participation was mainly passive and culturally proscribed.

Participation now reflects self-determination both through individual choices concerning, for example, one's lifestyle or career, and through participation in the development of the community. Participation is individual and social, political and economic. Michael and Kenneth Himes state well the implications of this reimaged pluralism.

> This call for active participation implies subsidiarity and pluralism. What is needed for healthy social life is that an abundance of human associations and groups be allowed to flourish so that persons will be able to find a wide array of institutions that give form and structure to participatory community in the various realms of human existence. Furthermore, the bias is toward the grassroots in deciding at what level decision-making should occur in an organized group. This is to insure that even a well-meaning paternalism does not eviscerate the participation of people in the life of the community.[23]

CONCLUSIONS

Michael and Kenneth Himes argue that, according to the communitarian perspective, liberalism has failed in five significant ways:

1. It has led to the decline of civic virtue, the practices encouraged by what has been called the tradition of republicanism or civic republicanism;
2. Liberalism fosters a political community that speaks of an individual citizen's right but downplays civic duties;
3. There has been a disappearance of public space where common life can occur;
4. There is a marked lack of participation in the political activities necessary for democracy to flourish;
5. Endemic to liberalism is a failure to acknowledge that social life is constitutive of the human person resulting in the neglect of important social institutions.[24]

Embedded in such a critique, of course, are other assumptions about society and the human person. The assumptions and values derivative from them have formed the basis of my critique of autonomy and my suggestions for a different social agenda. Yet I want my comments to reflect an appreciation for and commitment to a rightful freedom, equal regard, and broad participation in the way we organize society.[25] I want to reintroduce the concept of the common good, not to serve as a repression of individual or communal aspirations but rather to invite us to reconceptualize our society and the good we need to share in common so that such a society can be viable.

Here I follow Dennis McCann's suggestion that the concept of the common good must be procedural, not substantive; partial, not universal; consensus based, not hierarchically imposed. Broad social participation in such a quest can check efforts of power blocs who attempt to impose their vision of the good on others. Conflict is not eliminated here but is seen as part of a larger process of the definition of self and community rather than individuals and groups carving out zones of privacy or lifestyle enclaves.

Finally, in the words of Michael and Kenneth Himes,

> The common good must not be seen as so specific in detail that diversity within society is repressed. What must be sought instead is an open, informed, civil discussion by citizens so that consensus on what Murray called the orders of justice, peace and morality in public life might be attained through persuasion, not coercion.[26]

This chapter is an invitation to begin such a discussion.

ENDNOTES

1. J. Boyajian, *Minnesota Adult Protective Services Guide*, 2–6.
2. Boyajian, *Minnesota Adult Protective Services Guide*, 2–6.
3. J. Q. Wilson, *The Moral Sense* (New York: Free Press, 1993), 220.
4. R. Bellah, *The Good Society* (New York: Alfred A. Knopf, 1991), 50.
5. Bellah, *The Good Society*, 46.
6. Bellah, *The Good Society*, 12.
7. Bellah, *The Good Society*, 12.
8. J. Pieper, *Joseph Pieper: An Anthology* (San Francisco: Ignatius Press, 1989), 65; emphasis in original.
9. Pieper, *Joseph Pieper*, 66; emphasis in original.
10. Pope Pius XI, "Quadragesimo Anno," p. 64.
11. Leo XIII, "Rerum Novarum," in *Catholic Social Thought: A Documentary History*, edited by D. O'Brien and T. A. Shannon (Maryknoll, N.Y.: Orbis Books, 1992).
12. Leo XIII, "Quadragesimo Anno," in *Catholic Social Thought: A Documentary History*, edited by D. O'Brien and T. A. Shannon (Maryknoll, N.Y.: Orbis Books, 1992).
13. D. McCann, "The Good to Be Pursued in Common," in *The Common Good and U.S. Capitalism*, edited by O. Williams and J. Houck (Lanham, Md.: University Press, 1987), 164.
14. John XXIII, "Pacem in Terris," in D. O'Brien and T. A. Shannon, *Catholic Social Thought: A Documentary History*, edited by D. O'Brien and T. A. Shannon (Maryknoll, N.Y.: Orbis Books, 1992), 132.
15. Vatican Council II, "The Church in the Modern World," in *Catholic Social Thought: A Documentary History*, edited by D. O'Brien and T. A. Shannon (Maryknoll, N.Y.: Orbis Books, 1992).
16. United States Catholic Conference (USCC), "Economic Justice for All," in *Catholic Social Teaching: A Documentary History*, edited by D. O'Brien and T. A. Shannon (Maryknoll, N.Y.: Orbis Books, 1992), 584.

17. USCC, "Economic Justice for All," 584.
18. USCC, "Economic Justice for All," 584.
19. USCC, "Economic Justice for All," 595.
20. USCC, "Economic Justice for All," 595.
21. USCC, "Economic Justice for All," 595.
22. M. J. Himes and K. R. Himes, *Fullness of Faith: The Public Significance of Theology* (New York: Paulist Press, 1993), 41.
23. Himes and Himes, *Fullness of Faith*, 36.
24. Himes and Himes, *Fullness of Faith*, 36.
25. Himes and Himes, *Fullness of Faith*, 42.
26. Himes and Himes, *Fullness of Faith*, 44.

II

ISSUES AT THE BEGINNING OF LIFE

5

Reflections on the Moral Status of the Pre-embryo

Thomas A. Shannon and Allan B. Wolter, OFM

In this chapter, we wish to review contemporary biological data about the early human embryo in relation to philosophical and theological claims made of it. We are seeking to discover more precisely what degree of moral weight it can reasonably bear. While other ethical conclusions might well be drawn from the results of such a reflective investigation, we limit ourselves to a few moral considerations based on our current knowledge of how human life originates. As Catholics, we too believe that "from the moment of conception, the life of every human being is to be respected in an absolute way because man is the only creature on earth that God 'wished for himself' and the spiritual soul of each man is 'immediately created' by God."[1] But we are also vitally concerned as to when one might reasonably believe such absolute value could be present in a developing organism. We would also like to defuse some of the polar opposition fanned by the rhetoric of both pro-life and pro-choice advocates that creates a legislative dilemma for morally and religiously responsible politicians. We even hope that a rational analysis of available scientific data might lead to some broad consensus among concerned citizens that the term "human life" is not necessarily a univocal conception.

All life is a many-splendored creation on the part of God; this is especially true of human life at any stage of its development. But we suggest that appropriate protection of the human organism changes with its developmental stages. We wish to present a theory that recognizes the right of every potential mother to a meaningful life and a healthy personality development[2] but condemns irresponsible destruction of fetal life.

One of the hallmarks of the Catholic tradition, with certain conspicuous exceptions, has been to be in dialogue with the philosophy and science of its day and to use such insights in articulating the vision of Catholicism. Such efforts have been done better and worse. Many have taken time to evaluate the correctness or usefulness of a particular articulation. But in almost all cases, because of new discoveries in science, changes in scientific theory, and the use of new philosophical frameworks, the insights and articulation of the faith of one generation have differed from those of another. Sometimes such differences have led to severe conflict. One remembers the Copernican revolution, the case of Galileo in the seventeenth century, and the tensions introduced by the rediscovery of Aristotelian science in the thirteenth century. Nor can historians of medieval theology forget that certain philosophical views of Aquinas himself were regarded as theologically dangerous by two successive archbishops of Canterbury and condemned by the bishop of Paris in 1277 on the advice of the prestigious university theological faculty, a condemnation that was lifted insofar as it applied to St. Thomas only two years after the saint's canonization in the fourteenth century.

Anyone who has studied the history of ideas—scientific, philosophical, or theological—knows that there is a usefulness in reviewing the theoretical conceptions of the past, since they have a habit of recurring cyclically in new and useful scientific garb.[3] The same is true of the theoretic conceptions used by theologians in articulating their faith. We argue that the most recent scientific discoveries fit in more admirably with the epigenetic conception of how a human being originates that was held for centuries by the great theologians and doctors of the Church than does the more recent and now more commonly accepted—though happily not defined—moment of fertilization as coincident with the time of animation. The widespread acceptance of the theory of immediate animation is of post-Tridentine origin,[4] having entered into the tradition only in the early seventeenth century, and in 1869 the distinction between the formed and unformed fetus was no longer canonically recognized. This assumption about immediate animation still plays a large part in contemporary ecclesiastical documents, as do references to the scientific literature purporting to buttress arguments supporting the theory, as we will discuss later.

We would also like to remind our readers, however, that some forty years ago two learned priests from the University of Louvain,[5] where this theory of immediate animation was originally introduced, repudiated its scientific standing and went to some lengths to explain historically how this mistaken interpretation of empirical data was initially accepted. We claim that the most recent scientific evidence concerning fertilization and the development of the very early human embryo does even more to reinforce their view that any theory of immediate animation seems to have become as untenable today as it was commonly held to be for centuries by Catholic thinkers. We think that since scientific observations, now recognized as erroneous, played such a historical role in the development of the position favoring such a theory, new and respected scientific evidence should be used by Catholic theologians when they discuss the process of fertilization and conception to determine its moral implications.

We hope our analysis will be welcomed because of our acceptance and use of the methodology of the tradition and because we take seriously the role of science in helping articulate the context of moral problems, as do current ecclesiastical documents. While our conclusions may differ from those of these documents, we think such differences are to be cherished because they help the community understand its beliefs and values at a much deeper level and allow some of the forgotten riches of our Catholic tradition to be expressed to a new audience.

This rearticulation needs careful examination, however, because the fact that something is new does not ipso facto make it good or correct. Thus a careful and prayerful process of discernment should also be an important part of the way we rearticulate our tradition, for the community must genuinely receive the reconceptualization of the tradition before it is authentic. This chapter is an attempt at such a process of discernment by setting out an account of the process of individuation in the early human embryo in light of modern biology and reflecting on it in the light of some important theological and philosophical insights that seem to have perennial vitality.

The medieval and post-Renaissance theologians articulated their theory of the person, the body, and ensoulment in light of the biology and philosophy of their day. On the basis of this they appropriately drew moral conclusions. We know now that biology used at any one time, if not out of date, may well need updating. But the philosophy and history of science also make it clear that there is a significant difference as to how our scientific knowledge of the wonder of God's creation grows. We believe that such a moment of review is necessary today if we are to give a reasonable defense of the respect Catholics have traditionally had for human life. We know that in the male seed there is no homunculus, but it was not until the 1700s that mammalian sperm was discovered, and not until the 1800s that the mammalian egg was found and its role revealed. Modern diagnostic technologies such as ultrasound and fetoscopy have given us a whole new perspective on the development of the human embryo. Thus, while we can correctly say that the biological data of a past era are inadequate in light of the discoveries of modern science, we cannot dispose as easily of the basic philosophical or theological way our scholastic predecessors interpreted those data. And we certainly cannot fault their use of the most advanced scientific knowledge available to them as a necessary condition for articulating any rational philosophico-theological conception of the person, the body, and ensoulment. It is in that spirit that we present this brief review of what embryology has to tell us today.

CONTEMPORARY PERSPECTIVES
ON THE HUMAN EMBRYO

The Pre-embryo

In mammalian reproduction an egg and sperm unite to produce a new and almost always genetically unique individual.[6] The process, how this occurs, is undergoing tremendous reconceptualization and remodeling in the light of new studies and new diagnostic technologies that allow access to this entity.

A critical discovery of the past two decades in that of capacitation, "the process by which sperm become capable of fertilizing eggs"[7] and that human sperm need to be in the female reproductive tract for about seven hours before they are ready to fertilize the egg. This process removes or deactivates "a so-called decapacitating factor that binds to sperm as they pass through the male reproductive tract."[8] This permits the acrosome reaction to occur, which is the means by which lytic enzymes in the sperm "are released so that they can facilitate the passage of the sperm through the egg coverings."[9] Then the sperm are able to penetrate the egg so fertilization can begin.

Fertilization usually occurs in the end of the Fallopian tube nearest the ovary. Sperm usually take about ten hours to reach the egg, and if not "fertilized within 24 hours after ovulation, it dies."[10] Fertilization, however, is not just a simple penetration of the surface of the egg. Rather, it is a complex biochemical process in which a sperm gradually penetrates various layers of the egg. Only after this single sperm has fully penetrated the egg and the diploid female nucleus, one having only one chromosome pair, has developed, do the cytoplasm of the egg and the nuclear contents of the sperm finally merge to give the new entity its diploid set of chromosomes. This process is called syngamy. It takes about twenty-four hours to complete and the resulting entity is called the zygote. Thus the process of fertilization (and it is important to note that it is a process) generally takes between twelve and twenty-four hours to complete,[11] with another twenty-four-hour period required for the two diploid nuclei to fuse.

Fertilization accomplishes four major events: giving the entity the complete set of forty-six chromosomes; determination of chromosome sex; the establishment of genetic variability; and the initiation of cleavage, the cell division of the entity.

Now begins a very complex set of cell divisions as the fertilized egg begins its journey down the Fallopian tube to the uterus. About thirty hours after fertilization, there is a two-cell division; around forty to fifty hours there is a division into four cells; and after about sixty hours the eight-stage cell division is reached. "When the embryo approaches the entrance to the uterus, it is in the 12–16 cell stage, the morula. This occurs on the fourth day."[12] Although the cells become compacted here, there is yet no predetermination of any one cell to become a specific entity or part of an entity. On around the sixth or seventh day the organism, now called the blastocyst, reaches the uterine wall and begins the process of its implantation there so that it can continue to develop. Here we have a differentiation into two types of cells: the trophectoderm, which becomes the outer wall of the blastocyst, and the inner cell mass, which becomes the precursor of the embryo proper. This process of implantation is completed by the end of the second week, at which time there is "primitive utero-placental circulation."[13]

Critical to note is that from the "blastocyst state to the completion of implantation the pre-embryo is capable of dividing into multiple entities."[14] In a few documented cases these entities have, after division, recombined into one entity again. Nor must this particular zygote become a human; it can become a hydatidiform mole, a product of an abnormal fertilization that is formed of placental tissue.

Note also that the zygote does not possess sufficient genetic information within its chromosomes to develop into an embryo that will be the precursor of an individual member of the human species. At this stage the zygote is neither self-contained nor self-sufficient for such further development, as was earlier believed. To become a human embryo, further essential and supplementary genetic information to what can be found in the zygote itself is required, namely

> the genetic material from maternal mitochondria, and the maternal or paternal genetic messages in the form of messenger RNA or proteins. In terms of molecular biology, it is incorrect to say that the zygote has all the informing molecules for embryo development; rather, at most, the zygote possesses the molecules that have the potential to acquire informing capacity.[15]

That potential informing capacity is given in time through interaction with other molecules. This new molecule with its informing capacity was not coded in the genome. Thus, the determination to be or to have particular characteristics is given in time through the information resulting from the interaction between the molecules.[16]

The development of the zygote depends at each moment on several factors: the progressive actualization of its own genetically coded information, the actualization of pieces of information that originate *de novo* during the embryonic process, and erogenous information independent of the control of the zygote.

The Embryo

The next major stage of development is that of the embryo. This is the beginning of the third week of pregnancy and "coincides with the week that follows the first missed menstrual period."[17] This phase begins with the full implantation of the pre-embryo into the uterine wall and the development of a variety of connective tissues between it and the uterine wall. Eventually the placenta develops and is the medium through which maternal-embryonic exchanges occur.

Two major events now occur. The first is the completion of gastrulation, "profound but well-ordered rearrangements of the cells in the embryo."[18] This process results in the development of various layers that ultimately give rise to the tissues and organs of the entity and is completed by the third week. At this time all expressions of the genes are switched off, except those that determine what a particular cell will be. There are now three layers present that are responsible for the development of much of the organism.

> The embryonic ectoderm gives rise to the epidermis; the nervous system; the sensory epithelitim of the eye, ear, and nose; and the enamel of the teeth. The embryonic endoderm forms the linings of the digestive and respiratory tracts. The embryonic mesoderm becomes muscle, connective tissue, bone and blood vessels.[19]

The second major event, the process of embryogenesis or organogenesis, now begins and is completed by the end of the eighth week. This process results in the development of all major internal and external structures and organs.

By the end of the third week the primitive cardiovascular system has begun to form with the development of blood vessels, blood cells, and a primitive heart. Since the "circulation of blood starts by the end of the third week as the tubular heart begins to beat,"[20] the cardiovascular system reaches a functional state first.

The nervous system progresses from a neural tube to the essential subdivisions of the brain into forebrain, midbrain, and hindbrain.[21] During this time also the upper and lower limb buds begin to appear. The digestive tract begins to form, as do all the external structures such as the head and the eyes and ears. Hands and feet make their appearance, as do, by the end of the eighth week, distinct fingers and toes.

The development of the nervous system is critical because this is the basis for the "generation and coordination of most of the functional activities of the body."[22] The rudimentary brain and spinal cord are present around the third week but are as yet "unspecialized or undifferentiated for neural function."[23] Neuron development begins around the fifth week, and around the sixth week the "first synapses . . . can be recognized."[24] Bruce Carlson observes that at about the seventh week "the embryo is capable of making weak twitches in the neck in response to striking the lips or nose with a fine bristle."[25] Clifford Grobstein notes that "the earliest continuous neuronal circuitry for reflex conduction and behavior could be initiated as early as six weeks."[26] Such a pattern, Carlson says, "signifies that the first functional reflex arcs have been laid down."[27]

In a rather thorough review of the literature, Michael Flower describes various embryonic movements and the neural basis necessary for their possibility.[28] Flower notes that the earliest reported elicited reflex response from an embryo occurred at 7.5 weeks. This was a movement away from a stroking stimulus to the mouth. Such movements were typical during this period of the eighth week of development.[29] In the middle of the ninth week the patterns make a transition to whole body responses, and during the twelfth week local reflexes dominate. These data indicate a critical level of integration of the nervous system.

This review of embryonic development up to the eighth week shows a dramatic process of development from the initiation of fertilization to the formation of an integrated organism around midgestation. The rest of the paper will concentrate on examining what moral implications these data might have. The intent is not to draw a moral ought from a biological is, but to reconsider the compatibility of moral and philosophical claims with what we know of developmental embryology.

MORAL CONSIDERATIONS

Conception

A critical finding of modern biology is that conception, biologically speaking, is a process beginning with the penetration of the outer layer of the egg by a sperm and concluding with the formation of the diploid set of chromosomes. This is a process that takes at least a day. This raises a question as to how one ought to understand the term "moment of conception" frequently used in church documents.

One could understand "moment" metaphorically as referring to the process as a whole, or if it is meant to convey an instant of time, then it would seem to refer to either the end of the process of biological conception when the zygote has become an embryo, or to some prior stage of development that has been reached in which this human life form (fertilized egg, zygote, or pre-embryo) has acquired a distinct set of properties. However, it seems that the theologians who framed these carefully crafted documents wished to convey the idea that at the moment of conception (whatever stage of development of human life this is determined to be) everything is present that is required essentially for this human organism to be a person in the philosophical/theological, if not psychological, sense of the term: a rational or immortal soul has been created and infused into the organic body. At the same time, while they wished to set forth guidelines, they declared it was still a theoretically open question and hence they did not want to specify, or define, the moment when such passive conception (as it was called by Catholic theologians for many centuries) took place. Prayerful reflection on what embryology and our Catholic tradition tell us may not yield any direct positive knowledge of when passive conception takes place, but it does seem to throw considerable light on when it has not occurred.

Biologically understood, conception occurs only after a lengthy process has been completed and is more closely identified with implantation than fertilization.[30] The pastoral letter "Human Life in Our Day" speaks of conception "initiating . . . a process whose purpose is the realization of human personality."[31] Such a phrase is biologically correct if applied to implantation and seems to be a reasonable moral description of the typical outcome of conception.

Singleness

Clearly and without any doubt, once biological conception is completed we have a living entity and one that has the genotype of the human species. As Grobstein nicely phrases it, "conception (fertilization) is the beginning of a new generation in the genetic sense."[32] This zygote is capable of further divisions and is clearly the precursor of all that follows. But can we say with "Donum Vitae," quoting the "Declaration on Procured Abortion," "From the time that the ovum is fertilized, a new life is begun which is neither that of the father nor of the mother; it is rather the life of a new human being with his own growth."[33]

How are we to understand this phraseology in the light of the biology of development? For, while it is correct to say that the life that is present in the newly fertilized egg is distinct from the father and mother and is in fact usually genetically unique, it is not the case that this particular zygote is fully formed and it is not a single human individual, an "ontological individual," as Ford suggests.[34] Because of the possibility of twinning, recombination, and the potency of any cell up to gastrulation to become a complete entity, this particular zygote cannot necessarily be said to be the beginning of a specific, genetically unique individual human being. While the zygote is the beginning of genetically distinct life, it is neither an ontological individual nor necessarily the immediate precursor of one.

Second, the zygote gives rise to further divisions "resulting in an aggregate of cells, each of which remains equivalent to a zygote in the sense that it can become all or any part of an embryo and its extra-embryonic structure."[35] Such cells at this stage are totipotent:

> Within the fertilized ovum lies the capability to form an entire organism. In many vertebrates the individual cells resulting from the first few divisions after fertilization retain this capability. In the jargon of embryology, such cells are described as totipotent. As development continues, the cells gradually lose the ability to form all the types of cells that are found in the adult body. It is as if they were funneled into progressively narrower channels. The reduction of the developmental options permitted to a cell is called restriction. Very little is known about the mechanisms that bring about restriction, and the sequence and time course of restriction vary considerably from one species to another.[36]

Such a process of restriction is completed when the cells have become "committed to a single developmental fate. . . . Thus determination represents the final step in the process of restriction."[37] Such determination begins during gastrulation, three weeks into embryonic development.

Genetic uniqueness and singleness coincide on one level only after the process of implantation has been completed and on another after the restriction process is completed. Thus, if we take implantation as the marker of both conception and human singleness, this does not occur until about a week after the initiation of fertilization. If we use determination and restriction, because of their signaling of the loss of totipotency of the cells, as the markers of human singleness, then individuality does not occur until about three weeks after fertilization. Of critical importance is Ford's observation, "The teleological system of the blastocyst should not be identified with the ontological unity of the human individual that will develop from it."[38]

There is, then, a partial answer to the very interesting question[39] "Donum Vitae" asks, "How could a human individual not be a human person?"[40] A Catholic philosopher might well object or reply that this is certainly a very muddied question, for "traditionally speaking" individuality has been considered a necessary, though not sufficient, condition for human personhood. The rational soul has never been considered the formal reason why something human is individual. Obviously, "human individual" can have several meanings. If it refers to a fertilized ovum, this is indeed something both human (qua product) and numerically single. Yet until the process of individuation is completed, the ovum is not an individual, since a determinate and irreversible individuality is a necessary, if not sufficient, condition for it to be a human person.

Something human and individual is not a human person until he or she is a human individual, that is, not until after the process of individuation is completed. Neither the zygote nor the blastocyst is an ontological individual, even though it is genetically unique and distinct from the parents. The potential for twinning remains until the beginning of gastrulation, although it is rare for it to occur this late. Additionally, a zygote that divides can reunite and one individual will emerge. Furthermore, each cell can form a total individual. A human individual, to use the language of the document, cannot be a human person until after individuality is established.

Also, as Grobstein noted, genetic uniqueness does not necessarily imply singleness.[41] That is, when fertilization is complete and the haploid state is reached, the organism has its full complement of genetic information. At this point it is genetically unique. But because of the potentiality for twinning, this uniqueness may be shared by more than one organism. Thus, even though unique, the organism is not necessarily single. Singleness or individuality occurs after the genetically unique organism has implanted and its development is restricted to forming one unified organism.

An individual is not an individual, and therefore not a person, until the process of restriction is complete and determination of particular cells has occurred. Then, and only then, is it clear that another individual cannot come from the cells of this embryo. Then, and only then, is it clear that this particular individual embryo will be only this single embryo.

One can reasonably conclude, then, that if there is no single human entity, there is no person, for the one is the presupposition of the other. Thus, when "Donum Vitae" approvingly refers to the findings of modern science and argues "that in the zygote . . . resulting from fertilization the biological identity of a new human individual is already constituted,"[42] does not this statement of the congregation fail to make a critical distinction between genetic uniqueness and singleness? In using "individual" rather than "person" in this meticulously worded statement, the congregation may have sought to sidestep the controversial question of when personhood begins. But if "individual" be taken in its philosophical or technical meaning, scientific data available today hardly justify the claim that a particular zygote is necessarily both genetically unique and an individual.

This is particularly important in assessing the theological intent of the congregation, particularly since it argues that the "conclusions of science regarding the human embryo provide a valuable indication for discerning by the use of reason a personal presence at the moment of this first appearance of a human life."[43] As the statement stands, three concepts appear to be conflated here: genetic uniqueness, singleness, and personal presence. The argument for the first presence of human and personal life in the zygote relies heavily on scientific claims about the fertilized egg. However, such claims of singleness and personhood cannot be made, the former scientifically and the latter philosophically. We assume that the congregation would want to adjust its findings in the light of these distinctions.

Ensoulment

In this section and elsewhere, we will be discussing the principle of immaterial individuality or immaterial selfhood.[44] In the Catholic tradition, and clearly in many of the sources we cite, the usual term for this is "soul." Our practice will be to use the term "soul" when speaking within a clear traditional context. But when we develop our own presentation, we will use the term "immaterial individuality" or "immaterial selfhood," because the term "soul" has many connotations and images connected with it and in so far as possible we wish to avoid problematic usages and confusing images.

Issues

Although far from being a defined doctrine, there is support in Roman Catholic moral theology for the position that ensoulment is coincident with fertilization or, at least, as early as possible after conception. This position apparently dates from the early seventeenth-century writings of Thomas Fienus, professor on the faculty of medicine at Louvain.[45] This opinion gradually caught on and became the dominant opinion. This position was complemented by teachings that held that the embryo "possesses the essential parts of a human body, though very minute in size."[46] This teaching on immediate animation eventually worked its way into the mainstream of Catholic moral theology. If doctors of medicine were Catholics, explains Dorlodot,

> they were told that the theologians of their time held that the soul is created by God immediately after fecundation. The theologians in turn based themselves on the opinion of the doctors, as these did on that of the theologian. In other words, *caecus caeco ducatum praestat.* Finally, the moral theologians, who completely forgot the

principles, which, according to the great doctors of Catholic morality, render abortion always illicit, invoked the danger of favouring abortive or sterilizing practices.[47]

Additionally, the removal from canon law in 1896 of the distinction between the formed and unformed fetus suggests that there is not a time when the body is unformed.[48] The *Ethical and Religious Directives for Catholic Health Facilities* provide another reason when they include in the definition of an abortion the "interval between conception and implantation."[49] Also, we have the 1981 testimony of Cardinal Cooke and Archbishop Roach in support of the Hatch amendment: "We do claim that each human individual comes into existence at conception, and that all subsequent stages of growth and development in which such abilities are acquired are just that—stages of growth and development in the life cycle of an individual already in existence."[50] Finally, in "Donum Vitae" we read, "Nevertheless, the conclusions of science regarding the human embryo provide a valuable indication for discerning by the use of reason a personal presence at the moment of this first appearance of a human life."[51]

If this statement is to be accepted as it stands, we suggest that the conclusions of science should be interpreted differently, particularly if we reflect on what we know from science in the light of a centuries-long tradition among Catholic philosophers and theologians. For like them we are struck by both the wonder and sacredness of human life even from its obscure beginnings, as well as to when we could begin to suspect a personal presence might be there. Nor can we forget that for some seventeen centuries the Church indeed condemned abortion, but not on the ground that it might by even the most remote possibility be in all cases a question of murder. Certainly some of the greatest minds and doctors of the Church refused to believe, as many today seem to do, that ensoulment is coincident with fertilization or that we must trace the genesis of each human person back to that moment. Obviously, the Sacred Congregation for the Doctrine of Faith had no intention of definitively settling this question, for it stated pointedly, "This declaration expressly leaves aside the question of the moment when the spiritual soul is infused. There is not a unanimous tradition on this point and authors are as yet in disagreement."[52] It did not believe, however, that such theoretical openness should lead to any rash or precipitous practical action, for it goes on to say, "From a moral point of view this is certain: even if a doubt existed concerning whether the fruit of conception is already a human person, it is objectively a grave sin to dare to risk murder."[53]

Several very critical questions arise here, particularly since abortion was traditionally considered a sin against marriage but not homicide. One of them, concerning the moral possibility of acting on probable knowledge, has already been masterfully treated by Carol Tauer.[54] Others concern practical and philosophical issues relating to the development of the pre-embryo and embryo. It is to these issues that we now turn.

The dominant position of the moral tradition on ensoulment was the acceptance of a time during the pregnancy when the fetus was not informed by the rational soul. Two distinctions were used in discussing this. The first distinction is between active and passive conception and is exemplified in "De Testis" of Benedict XIV, in which the pope comments on the doctrine of the Immaculate Conception.

> Conception can have a twofold meaning, for it is either active, in which the holy parents of the Blessed Virgin, joining each other in a marital role, have accomplished those things which have to do most of all with the formation, organization, and disposition of the body itself for receiving a rational soul to be infused by God; or it is passive, when the rational soul is coupled with the body. This infusion and union of the soul with a duly organized body is commonly called passive conception, namely, that which occurs at that very instant when the rational soul is united with a body consisting of all its members and its organs.[55]

Thus the pope would seem to understand active conception, in our terminology, as the physical union of egg and sperm that will become the embryo, while passive conception would be the moment the rational soul is infused into a suitably organized body, one that results from (begins with) organogenesis.

The second distinction is between mediate and immediate animation by such a soul. The theory of mediate animation is succinctly stated as follows:

> Animation by the intellectual soul is impossible so long as the parts of the brain which are the seat of the imagination and the *vis cogitativa* (and we might add the memory) are not suitably organized. But it still is more evident that there cannot be animation by the intellectual soul when the brain is not even outlined, or again, when even the embryo really does not as yet exist. Now that is precisely the case with the ovum, and the morula, and of that which results from its development, so long as there has not appeared, on a particular part of the germ, that which by its ulterior development will become a fetus.[56]

Immediate animation occurs coincidentally with the fusion of egg and sperm, known as the moment of conception. This is the position used in the teachings referred to at the beginning of this section. This distinction is also thoroughly discussed by Donceel, as previously noted.[57]

Medieval theologians were particularly interested in clarifying the technical meaning of "conception" in their justification of the celebration of the popular feast of the Blessed Virgin Mary's conception. Henry of Ghent, following common scholastic reasoning, distinguished between the "conception of the seed when fetal life begins" and the conception of the human soul some "35 or 42 days later [when], depending on the sex, a rational soul is created."[58] Such a position echoes St. Anselm's perceptive judgment, "No human intellect accepts the view that an infant has a rational soul from the moment of conception."[59]

Had this saint known of the empirical data on wastage, he would have considered such a claim not only irrational but blasphemous.[60] Only about 45 percent of eggs that are fertilized actually come to term. The other 55 percent miscarry for a variety of reasons. Some are related to the biochemistry of the uterus, others are a function of low levels of necessary hormones, while yet other reasons have to do with structural anomalies within the pre-embryo or embryo itself.[61] Such vast embryonic loss intuitively argues against the creation of a principle of immaterial individuality at conception. What meaning is there in the creation of such a principle when there is such a high probability that this entity will not develop to the embryo stage, much less come to term?

Also, given the fact that twinning and recombination is a possibility, what is one to say about the presence of immaterial individuality during that process? If this principle is initiated at fertilization and then a twin is formed, how does one explain the relation of the original principle to the zygote that splits off? And should recombination occur, how does one explain coherently the fate of such a principle of immaterial individuality? Should one freeze the pre-embryo, all organic processes stop for the duration. What is the status of immaterial individuation then? It is genuinely unclear what to think of that in terms of the standard theory of immediate ensoulment. Then there is the issue of whether a soul, in the classic sense of the form of the body, is needed for the fertilized egg to develop into its possible subsequent forms.

Commentary

The question of the moral significance of the morula and of embryonic wastage has been noted previously in the moral literature. In 1976, for example, Bernard Häring brought together much of the scientific literature and examined its moral significance. His conclusion concurs with one suggestion in our analysis and opens the door to other issues: "the argument that the morula cannot yet be a person or an individual with all the rights of the members of the human species seems to me to be convincing as long as we follow our traditional concept of personhood."[62] This conclusion opens up several areas for consideration.

First, we concur with Häring and particularly with the analysis of Ford that, given the biological evidence, there is no reasonable way in which the fertilized egg can be considered a physical individual minimally until after implantation. Maximally, one could argue that full individuality is not achieved until the restriction process is completed and cells have lost their totipotency. Thus the range of time for the achievement of physical individuality is between one and three weeks. One simply cannot speak, therefore, of an individual's being present from the moment of fertilization.

Second, given the standard definition of personhood used in Catholic moral theory—an individual substance of a rational nature—questions are raised about the rational nature. When might one consider such a rational nature to be present? Ford suggests the formation of the primitive streak, which coincides with the time of the formation of the neural tube, as an appropriate criterion.[63] Another criterion would be around eight weeks, when the first elicited responses have been recorded. These are the result of a simple three-neuron circuit. Thus, toward the end of the embryonic period, some neural activity is present. A third answer would be the formation of a relatively integrated nervous system, which occurs around the twentieth week of fetal development. Of critical importance here is the connection of neural pathways through the thalamus to the neocortex. This allows stimuli to be received, as well as activities to be initiated.

One can speak of a rational nature in a philosophically significant sense only when the biological structures necessary to perform rational actions are present, as opposed to only reflex activities. The biological data suggest that the minimal time of the presence of a rational nature would be around the twentieth week, when neural integration of the entire organism has been established. The presence of such a structure does not argue that the fetus is positing rational actions, only that the biological presupposition for such actions is present.

Third, the pre-embryonic form as a system is not totally passive, the recipient only of actions from the outside, as it were. It has its own activities arising from the released potencies of the novel combination of its constituent materials. Such potencies are released when these elements form a system, that is, the embryo. This development of new systems gives rise to new activities and possibilities and serves as the foundation or presupposition for other stages of development. Philosophically speaking, we have every reason to believe that the dynamic properties of the organic matter—the elements of the fully formed zygote—owe their existence to their organizational form or the system. Important to note is that "where there are only material powers—that is, the ability to form material systems—there is only a material nature or substance."[64] Thus the material system or form of the developing body can explain its own activity. We conclude that there is no cogent reason, either from a philosophical or still less from a theological viewpoint, why we should assert, for instance, that the human soul is either necessary or directly responsible for the architectonic chemical behavior of nucleo-proteins in the human body.

Among the scholastic theologians and doctors of the Church, perhaps St. Bonaventure has given the most helpful model for what we have in mind. In his interesting Aristotelian interpretation of how St. Augustine's theory of seminal reasons might be explained according to the science of his own day, he argued that if the potencies be understood as active rather than passive, then the Aristotelian formula that the new substantial form "is educed from the potency of matter" made sense. For "the philosopher of nature says that matter first receives the elementary form and by its means it comes to the form of the mineral compound only by means of the latter to the organic form, for he looks to that potency of matter according to which it is progressively actualized by the operation of nature."[65]   ·

If we interpret this in more contemporary terms, it means simply that the new substantial form is nothing more than that of the organic system itself, and that its new and unique dynamic properties stem from the complementary interaction of elements that make up the system. All that is needed is some external agent to bring the elements of that system together, for, as Bonaventure puts it, "in matter itself there is something cocreated with it from which the agent acting in matter educes the form. Not that this something from which the form is educed is such that it becomes some part of the form to be produced, but it is rather that which can be and will become the form, even as a rosebud becomes a rose."[66]

These remarks suggest that the principle of immaterial individuality is indeed the ultimate actualization of all the potencies contained within the forms or systems that constitute the organic life of the human being. Thus, finally, we can say that while it is necessary to recognize the distinctions between higher and lower vital functions in the human being, nonetheless there may be "an area where the biochemical theory is the more plausible explanation, and another area where the animistic position seems to be the only tenable view."[67]

The question of when such a principle comes into being is dependent on which level of the system of the human being one is examining and what activities are performed here. The strong implication of these suggestions is that immaterial individuality comes into existence late in the development of the physical individual.

CONCLUSIONS

Biological Data

Physical Individuality

Two biological data mandate a revision of our understanding of the beginning of individuality: 1) the possibility of twinning, which lasts until implantation, which occurs about a week after fertilization begins; and 2) the completion of the restriction process, which prevents individual cells from forming another individual, about three weeks into the pregnancy. While one can speak of genetic uniqueness, in that the fertilized egg has its own genetic code distinct from any other entity (except an identical twin, triplet, etc.), we simply cannot speak of an individual until in fact that individual is present, and the earliest that can be is about two or three weeks after fertilization begins.

Neural Development

Three markers are significant in neural development: 1) gastrulation, the development of the various layers in the pre-embryo that give rise to the whole organism; 2) organogenesis, the presence of all major systems of the body, occurring around the eighth week; and 3) the development of the thalamus, which permits the full integration of the nervous system, around the twentieth week.

Critical here is the necessity of a functioning and probably integrated nervous system for the possibility of rational activity. For if there is no nervous system functioning, it is not clear that the rational part of the definition of a person can be fulfilled, even though the individual part might be. The functioning nervous system is a necessary condition for the possibility of a new stage of development to emerge and is also a sign that the organism is prepared for this. Thus any of the three markers noted immediately above could serve as an indicator of the capacity for rationality though not necessarily its actuality.

Developmental Autonomy

Given the philosophical discussion on nature and substance, it is reasonable to argue that the developing body as an organized system is a new substance or nature and has the capacity to elicit the potencies within its own reality. That is, a fully formed zygote is a new nature because it has its own actuality and potentiality. It is in itself a sufficient explanation of its own development and activities. The same is true on each new level of development as the zygote becomes an embryo and, finally, a fetus. On a genetic level, the clearest marker of the presence of self-directing activity that would manifest such a new nature would appear in the zygote after it has developed the capacity to manufacture its own messenger DNA and thus be developmentally, though not physically, independent of the mother.

Moral Implications

Physical Individuality

We find it impossible to speak of a true individual, an ontological individual, as present from fertilization. There is a time period of about three weeks during which it is biologically unrealistic to speak of a physical individual. This means that the reality of a person, however one might define that term, is not present at least until individualization has occurred. Individuality is an absolute or necessary condition for personhood.

We conclude that there is no individual and therefore no person present until either retraction or gastrulation is completed, about three weeks after fertilization. To abort at this time would end life and terminate genetic uniqueness, to be sure. But in a moral sense one is certainly not murdering, because there is no individual to be the personal referent of such an action.

Since the zygote is living, has the human genetic code, and indeed possesses genetic uniqueness, this entity is valuable, and its value does not depend on the presence or absence of any or a particular quality or characteristic such as intelligence or capacity for relationships.[68] Thus the zygote and the blastomers derived from it, because they are living, possess ontic value and are in themselves valuable. Thus the general argument made here is not a so-called "quality of life" argument.

Nonetheless, until the completion of restriction or gastrulation, the zygote and its sequelae are in a rather fluid process and are not physical individuals and therefore cannot be persons. The pre-embryo at this state, we conclude, cannot claim absolute protection based on claims to personhood grounded in ontological individuality. Yet, since the pre-embryo is living and possesses genetic uniqueness, some claims to protection are possible. But these may not be absolute and, if not, could yield to other moral claims.

Immaterial Individuality

If one assumes, as we think correct to do, that the potencies actualized in the formation of the new nature of the fertilized egg have the inherent capacity to ground its growth and development, then there is no need to posit a principle of individual immateriality, understood as the Aristotelian *nous* or as the entelechy of the body, in pre-embryonic development.

Since the evidence for such a principle comes from the internal evidence of those who experience it, it is difficult at best to ground any speculation as to when it comes into existence. We would make this argument: On the one hand, the developing pre-embryo as a new nature has within it the potential for future development. On the other hand, if the will as a rational potency is what genuinely distinguishes the person from a nature, then one needs to look to biological presuppositions that enable such a potency to exist. We would argue that the earliest time is around the eighth week of gestation, because then the nervous system is fully integrated.

Summary

We have reviewed some of the salient biological data about the initial stages of the development of human life, with a view to evaluating the philosophical and theological claims made of them. Reflecting on these from a historico-theological perspective, we have tried to discover whether there exists some rational justification for the absolute value that is attributed to the zygote or pre-embryonic state based an claims to personhood, or whether our earlier long-standing Catholic tradition of mediate animation by a rational soul does not provide a more satisfactory philosophical and theological account. For if we consider judiciously what the great scholastic doctors had to say about the "moment of conception," we seem to have good reason to reintroduce, in interpreting the data of present-day science, the theological distinction between active and passive conception made by Pope Benedict XIV in discussing Mary's immaculate conception.

We thus affirm that any abortion is a premoral evil. That is, it is the ending of life. Consequently, we do not want to be understood as proposing or supporting an "abortion on demand" position or assuming that early abortions are amoral. Abortion is a serious issue, because life is involved and one needs always to respect life. We have made one major argument, however, in this chapter. Given the findings of modern biology, there is no evidence for the presence of a separate ontological individual until the completion of either restriction or gastrulation, which occurs around three weeks after fertilization. Therefore, there is no reasonable basis for arguing that the pre-embryo is morally equivalent to a person or is a person as a basis for prohibiting abortion. That is, there is no biological support for the position that the fertilized egg is from the beginning of the process of fertilization a distinct individual needing no outside agency to develop into a person. Neither is there good philosophical evidence that the principle of immaterial individuality need be present from the beginning to explain the physical development of the pre-embryo.

This position obviously does not support the argument that abortion is to be prohibited because a person is present from the beginning of fertilization. The earliest such an argument could reasonably be made is after the completion of gastrulation. We recognize that this argument will dismay many and comfort others. Our intention in proposing the argument of this chapter is to gain a greater coherence between moral theology and modern embryology.

In this sense we are complementing the work of the Roman congregations and bringing it up to date. We also wish to test the strength of our argument, already subjected to review by several colleagues, in review by a wider and more diverse audience. Additionally, our intention is to develop a position that is reasonable and can be reasonably defended in the public sector.[69] Finally, we think our position on the pre-embryo and embryo can stand rigorous scrutiny and we propose it as a factor in developing a feasible state and/ or national policy on abortion.

One is reminded here of Henry de Dorlodot's evaluation of immediate animation made more than fifty years ago in his seminal work *Darwinism and Catholic Thought*: "We are not exaggerating in the least when we regard the fact that this theory [of immediate animation] should still find defenders long after the experimental bases on which it was thought to be founded have been shown definitely to be false, as one of the most shameful things in the history of thought."[70]

ENDNOTES

1. See "Donum Vitae," quoting "Gaudium et Spes," in Thomas A. Shannon and Lisa Sowle Cahill, *Religion and Artificial Reproduction* (New York: Crossroad, 1987), 147.

2. We are concerned here especially with victims of rape, incest, or sexual abuse.

3. Philosophers of science have stressed the important difference between the linear growth of scientific data and theoretic conceptions used to interpret them, for important theories have a life of their own that ensures their perenniality. Or, as Santayana put it, those who forget history are condemned to repeat its mistakes.

4. Theologians at the Council of Trent, in contrasting the virginal conception of Christ with the ordinary course of human nature, asserted that normally no human embryo could be informed by a human soul except after a certain period of time "cum servato naturae ordine nullum corpus, nisi intra prasecriptum temporis spatium, hominis anima informari queat" (*Catechism of the Council of Trent*, part 1, art. 3, n. 7) cited in E. C. Messenger, *Theology and Evolution* (Westminster, Md.: Newman, 1949), 236.

5. We refer to Dr. Messenger and Canon Henry de Dorlodot.

6. The term *pre-embryo* is being used to describe this entity from the zygote state to the beginning of the formation of the primitive streak during the third week; see Keith L.

Moore, *Essentials of Human Embryology* (Philadelphia: Decker, 1988), 16. The primitive streak gives rise to other structures that continue the physical development of the embryo. The purpose of using this term, as well as other terms such as zygote, embryo, and fetus, is to integrate scientific descriptions into the moral discussion. These terms, as used in this chapter, beg no moral questions but help us clearly identify the entity we are discussing. See Clifford Grobstein, *Science and the Unborn: Choosing Human Futures* (New York: Basic Books, 1988), 62. But see "Donum Vitae," which also uses these terms but attributes "to them an identical relevance in order to designate the result (whether visible or not) of human generation from the first moment of its existence until birth" (introduction 1, n). The text of *Donum vitae* can be found in Shannon and Cahill, *Religion and Artificial Reproduction*, 140ff. All references will be to this text.

7. Steven B. Oppenheimer and George Lefever Jr., *Introduction to Embryonic Development*, 2nd ed. (Boston: Allyn and Bacon, 1984), 87.

8. Oppenheimer and Lefever, *Introduction*, 87.

9. Bruce M. Carlson, *Patten's Foundations of Embryology*, 5th ed. (New York: McGraw-Hill, 1988), 134.

10. Oppenheimer and Lefever, *Introduction*, 175.

11. Oppenheimer and Lefever, *Introduction*, 176.

12. Oppenheimer and Lefever, *Introduction*, 175.

13. Moore, *Essentials*, 14.

14. Carlson, *Patten's Foundations*, 35.

15. Carlos A. Bedate and Robert C. Cegalo, "The Zygote: To Be or Not to Be a Person," *Journal of Medicine and Philosophy* 14 (1989): 642–43.

16. Bedate and Cegalo, "The Zygote," 644.

17. Moore, *Essentials*, 16.

18. Carlson, *Patten's Foundations*, 186.

19. Moore, *Essentials*, 18.

20. Moore, *Essentials*, 24.

21. Carlson, *Patten's Foundations*, 296.

22. Carlson, *Patten's Foundations*, 456.

23. Grobstein, *Science*, 47.

24. Grobstein, *Science*, 48.

25. Carlson, *Patten's Foundations*, 457.

26. Grobstein, *Science*, 48.

27. Carlson, *Patten's Foundations*, 458.

28. Michael J. Flower, "Neuromaturation of the Human Fetus," *Journal of Medicine and Philosophy* 10 (1985): 237–51.

29. Flower, "Neuromaturation of the Human Fetus," 238–39.

30. Norman M. Ford, *When Did I Begin? Conception of the Human Individual in History, Philosophy and Science* (Cambridge: Cambridge University, 1988), 176–77. This outstanding and comprehensive analysis of the biological data came to our attention after we had completed much of our own research for this article. We wish to acknowledge how much we have learned from it and to commend it for its exceptionally thorough review of the biological data and philosophical analysis. We also wish to acknowledge the earlier contribution of James J. Diamond, M.D., to this topic; "Abortion, Animation, and Biological Hominization," *Theological Studies* 36 (1975): 305–24.

31. "Human Life in Our Day," United States Conference of Catholic Bishops, 1969, par. 84.

32. Grobstein, *Science*, 25.

33. "Donum Vitae," I, 2, in Shannon and Cahill, *Religion and Artificial Reproduction*, 148.

34. An ontological individual is defined as a "single concrete entity that exists as a distinct being and is not an aggregation of smaller things nore merely a part of a greater whole; hence its unity is said to be intrinsic" (Ford, *When Did I Begin?* 212).

35. Grobstein, *Science*, 235.

36. Carlson, *Patten's Foundations*, 23.

37. Carlson, *Patten's Foundations*, 26.

38. Ford, *When Did I Begin?* 158 (italics added).

39. Although any conclusions should not be laid at his door, Richard McCormick started Shannon thinking about this problem and was suggestive in phrasing the question.

40. "Donum Vitae," I, 2, in Shannon and Cahill, *Religion and Artificial Reproduction*, 149.

41. Grobstein, *Science*, 25.

42. "Donum Vitae," I, 2, in Shannon and Cahill, *Religion and Artificial Reproduction*, 149.

43. "Donum Vitae," I, 2, in Shannon and Cahill, *Religion and Artificial Reproduction*, 149.

44. There is much literature on this, but two interesting articles that are extremely useful for their summaries are Joseph Donceel, "A Liberal Catholic's View," in *Abortion in a Changing World*, edited by Robert E. Hall (New York: Columbia University Press, 1970), and Carol Tauer, "The Tradition of Probabilism and the Moral Status of the Early Embryo," *Theological Studies* 45 (1984): 3–33. Both articles can be found in *Abortion and U.S. Catholicism: The American Debate*, edited by Patricia B. Jung and Thomas A. Shannon (New York: Crossroad, 1988).

45. Henry de Dorlodot, "A Vindication of the Mediate Animation Theory," in *Theology and Evolution*, edited by E. C. Messenger (Westminster, Md.: Newman, 1959), 271.

46. Dorlodot, "A Vindication," 273.

47. Dorlodot, "A Vindication," 273.

48. See also John Connery, *Abortion: The Development of the Roman Catholic Perspective* (Chicago: Loyola University Press, 1977), 212.

49. *Ethical and Religious Directives for Catholic Health Facilities* (Washington, D.C.: United States Catholic Conference, 4.

50. Archbishop John Roach and Cardinal Terence Cooke, "Testimony in Support of the Hatch Amendment," *Origins* 11 (1981): 357–72; also in Jung and Shannon, *Abortion*, 15.

51. "Donum Vitae," I, 1, in Shannon and Cahill, *Religion and Artificial Reproduction*, 149.

52. *Declaration on Abortion* (Washington, D.C.: U.S. Catholic Conference, 1975), 13.

53. *Declaration on Abortion*, 6.

54. See n. 44 above. While many have been unhappy with Carol Tauer's article and have dismissed it, Shannon has not yet seen a substantive refutation of her argument that the "application of the probabilist methods would permit some early abortion." Jung and Shannon, *Abortion*, 79.

55. "Conceptio dupliciter accipi potest: vel enim est activa, in qua Sancti B. Virginis parentes opere maritali invicem convenientes, praestiterunt ea quae maxime spectabant ad ipsius corporis formationem, organizationem et dispositionem ad recipiendam animam rationalema Deo infundendam; vel est passiva, cum rationalis anima cum corpore copulatur. Ipsa animae infusio et unio cum corpore debite organizato vulgo nominatur Conceptio passiva, quae scilicet fit illo ipso instanti quo rationalis anima coprori omnibus membris ac suis organis constanti unitur." Benedict XIV, "De Testis," lib. II, c. 15, n. 1 in *Opera Omnia* 9, edited by J. Silvester (Prato: Aldina, 1843), 303a.

56. Dorlodot, "A Vindication," 266. It was here that Messenger and Dorlodot recalled that the only theological attempt to define the role of the rational soul as the substantial form of the body was made by the council of Vienne (DS 481) and that the fathers and theologians of that council did not subscribe to the immediate animation theory. Dorlodot uses the definition of the council as the major premise of his argument vindicating the mediate animation theory. See Messenger, *Theology and Evolution*, 259.

57. Donceel, " A Liberal Catholic," 48ff.

58. *Quodlibet* 1, 5, g. 13; cited in *John Duns Scotus: Four Questions on Mary*, trans. and intro. by Allan B. Wolter (Santa Barbara, Calif.: Old Mission, 1988), 6. It is interesting to note that Henry breaks with the tradition and ascribes a longer period of gestation before animation to the male rather than the female, as had been customary since Aristotle.

59. Anselm of Canterbury, *De conceptu virginali et de originali peccato, c. 7 in Anselmi Co antuariensis archiepiscopi opera omnia* 2, edited by F. S. Schmitt (Stuttgart-Bad: Cannstatt, 1968), 148 (Anselm of Canterbury, 3rd ed., trans. Grasper Hopkins and Herbert Richardson (Toronto: Edwin Mellen, 1976), 152. It is important to keep in mind that the Archbishop of Canterbury in arguing as to when it is possible to contract original sin, something that all theologians in his day agreed required only the existence of a human soul, not any consciousness or voluntary activity on the part of an infant. As he puts it, "Either from the very moment of his conception an infant has a rational soul (without which lie cannot have a rational will) or else at the moment of his conception he has no original sin. But no human intellect accepts the view that an infant has a human soul from the moment of his conception. For from this view it would follow that whenever— even at the very moment of conception—the human seed perished before attaining a human form, the [alleged] human soul in this seed would be condemned, since it would not be reconciled through Christ—a consequence which is utterly absurd." Today we may have different conceptions as to the nature of original sin and how it is contracted, but we have even less reason than Anselm to believe that there is the remotest possibility of a human will present in what he calls "human seed" at the moment the zygote is formed, or that there is any less rather than a substantially greater amount of "human seed that perishes before attaining a human form."

60. Those who see no insuperable difficulty for the theory of immediate animation in the fact that twins can come from a single fertilized egg should find considerable difficulty in the problem of wastage. To ascribe such bungling of the conception process to an all-wise Creator would seem almost sacrilegious; one would have to assume that God in his foreknowledge would create souls only for those he foreknew would eventually be born, an argument a pro-choice advocate might well apply to aborted fetuses. On the other hand, Catholics, on the basis of rational argument, can hardly hope to argue for anything more

than a suitable level of protection warranted by the development stage of the pre-embryo and its sequelae.

61. Clifford Grobstein, Michael Flower, and John Mendeloff, "External Human Fertilization: An Evaluation of Policy," *Science* 222 (October 14, 1983): 127–33.

62. Bernard Häring, "New Dimensions of Responsible Parenthood," *Theological Studies* 37 (1976): 127. This article is also a good review of the scientific literature of that time period and contains references to other articles that discuss our theme.

63. Ford, *When Did I Begin?*, 171ff.

64. Allan B. Wolter, "Chemical Substance," in *Philosophy of Science* (Jamaica, N.Y.: St. John's University, 1960), 108. This citation is an excerpt from a seminal article originally titled "The Problem of Substance." Its primary aim was to present a cosmological account of how mechanical and natural systems differ, why various forms of living substances arise from nonliving matter, and how traditional scholastic philosophical insights and theories such as both the pluriform and uniform hylomorphic conceptions might be helpful as partial insights to a more complex philosophical theory. The psychological role of the rational soul was discussed peripherally to show how medieval scholastics fitted it into their theories of mediate animation.

65. See John F. Wipple and Allan B. Wolter, *Medieval Philosophy: From St. Augustine to Nicholas of Cusa* (New York: Free Press and Collier Macmillan, 1969), 325.

66. Wipple and Wolter, *Medieval Philosophy*, 320.

67. Wolter, "Chemical Substance," 126–28.

68. For a further discussion of the concept, see James J. Walter, "The Meaning and Validity of Quality of Life Judgments in Contemporary Roman Catholic Medical Ethics," *Louvain Studies* 13 (1988): 195–208 (see also chapter 12 of this volume). Another discussion can be found in Thomas A. Shannon and James J. Walter, "The PVS Patient and the Forgoing/Withdrawing of Medical Nutrition and Hydration," *Theological Studies* 49 (1988): 623–47 (see also chapter 14 of this volume).

69. We suggest that something of the violence between extreme pro-life or pro-abortionists might be defused, and the political dilemma of Catholic politicians seeking more rational options might be solved, if one were to recognize that the moral status of, and hence the protection appropriate for, a fetus changes with its developmental stage.

70. Quoted by Messenger, *Theology and Evolution*, 219.

6

A Catholic Reflection on Embryonic Stem Cell Research

James J. Walter

The focus of my analysis is to frame what I believe to be the key theological and ethical issues related to the production and use of embryonic stem cells in both research and therapy from the perspective of the Roman Catholic tradition. The theological issues that I raise shape and inform the tradition's process of moral reasoning about this topic but do not by themselves determine the morality of stem cell research. From these key theological issues I move to two sets of ethical issues: the first is concerned with what might be called micro issues and the second is concerned with the macro or key social issues. In the conclusion I offer two of my own recommendations on the topic.

THEOLOGICAL ISSUES

There are two theological themes that inform and shape the Catholic community's moral reasoning about stem cell research. The first is the traditional interpretation of the doctrine of creation and the moral implications of such a doctrine. All that is created is considered to be good, and illness and death are viewed as lacking the intrinsic goodness of creation. In addition, the divine has created us to pursue a range of goods or values, the acquisition of which defines human well-being and flourishing. Health is certainly one of these goods that we naturally seek, but so also are the goods of security, culture, art, education, and so forth. The reason this theme is informative is because it helps us think about our moral duties that correspond to each one of these goods or values. We have the duty to heal the sick, but we also have the duty to educate, to protect members of society, and so on. The question here is whether the duty to heal deserves some type of special moral priority over other duties to pursue goods. Is the good of health an absolute good or is it a relative good? Asked in another way: Is the duty to heal an absolute duty or is it a relative duty subject to other duties that are competing with it? Should we grant the duty to heal Parkinson's patients or to alleviate the suffering of injured patients a special duty that overrides or trumps all other moral duties? For example, Glenn McGee and Arthur Caplan have argued that the moral imperative of compassion is what compels us to sacrifice human embryos and to move forward with stem cell research.[1] As the Lutheran theologian Gilbert Meilaender has remarked about their moral justification for stem cell research, "McGee and Caplan never consider analogous possibilities. Only unconditional surrender of Parkinson's disease will do. Progress at relieving human suffering does not seem to be an optional goal. Nor apparently is slower progress, achieved by research techniques not involving the destruction of embryos, acceptable."[2] If there are multiple goods that humans should be seeking on behalf of themselves and society, then it might be dangerous to single out one of these goods (health) and pursue it, as the late Paul Ramsey used to call it, with "messianic ambition."[3]

The second, and related, key theological theme that is derived from the doctrine of creation is concerned with the view that humans are created in the image and likeness of God (Gen. 1:26–27). Though Catholics have interpreted this belief somewhat differently, nonetheless each of the interpretations frames the extent or range of our moral responsibilities as humans for making sure that the human future turns out well. Asked in the form of a question, how much moral responsibility should be accorded to our medical scientists to make sure that all human suffering and illness that result from disease, injury, infertility,[4] and cancer are ameliorated? If stem cell research can or might cure these misfortunes, then has God given us the absolute moral responsibility to make sure that they are treated and/or cured? Or, are our moral responsibilities somewhat different—that is, do we have the moral duty to make sure disease and injuries are cured to the extent that we honor our other moral duties to humanity and the nonhuman world?

The third theme related to the doctrine of creation is concerned with the notion of a common good for society. Many times we focus our attention only on the individual's good in society and do not also consider our moral responsibilities to a common good of society. It is obvious that the Catholic tradition grounds its understanding of the human person in a communitarian anthropology in which we all have moral responsibilities to the good of the whole. Again, this theme focuses the key issue of our duties to heal and cure the sick and injured. If we consider only the individual's good of healing, then we might not respond to the competing duties that we have to all of society and the just relations among individuals and structures in society.

In addition to the doctrine of creation there is also the theological theme of the solidarity with the poor and with those who are most vulnerable in society. The Catholic tradition has regularly argued in its recent social teachings for a commitment to or option for the poor and disadvantaged.[5] This theological commitment, as we will see, will have an important impact on the way that Catholics go about reasoning morally about such issues as stem cell research and the equitable distribution of medical resources in society. To the extent that the poor and disadvantaged are left out of the picture entirely or their interests not protected, it is to that extent that the Catholic tradition would morally question the research under consideration.

MICRO-ETHICAL ISSUES

Although there are many ethical issues at stake in this topic, I will briefly note only four. First, there is the key issue of the moral status of the embryo, whether embryos are used from in vitro fertilization (IVF) labs or whether they are created for research purposes. There are three prevailing views in society about the embryo's status: 1) the view that holds that the embryo possesses no inherent worth; 2) the view that holds that the embryo possesses some pre-personal status but not the worth of a person; and finally 3) the view that the embryo ought to be treated as a person, a position that official Catholic teaching has adopted.[6] For official Catholic teaching, and for some others in society, this crucial ethical issue settles whether or not one may destroy the embryo to derive the pluripotent stem cells for therapeutic goals. Though the tradition does not philosophically define exactly when the embryo becomes a person, nonetheless it has consistently argued in the past several decades that the embryo must be treated as a person from the moment of conception.[7]

Some contemporary Catholic theologians disagree with this position, and their disagreement is based on embryological data.[8] They argue that the pre-implantation embryo deserves respect because it possesses a pre-personal status, but since developmental individuation has not yet occurred, the embryo does not warrant the respect due to persons. It is important to note this theological disagreement with the teaching office of the Catholic Church, but it is also important to note that it would be shortsighted to accord this ethical issue the final say in the debate. Although the moral status of the embryo is certainly an extremely important ethical issue, it is by no means the only one that is relevant to this topic.

The second key ethical issue is concerned with whether there are other, less morally controversial, options that could be pursued for procuring stem cells for therapeutic ends. Margaret Goodell and scientists at the Karolinska Institute in Stockhom were able to differentiate adult mice stem cells in May 2000, which captured the interest of many scientists to begin research on human adult stem cells, for example, hematopoietic stem cells.[9] Another alternative course of research might be with multipotent adult progenitor cells (MAPCs), which were discovered by Catherine Verfaillie and her colleagues at the University of Minnesota in 2002. She found that these cells co-purifying with mesenchymal stem cells in bone marrow could differentiate at the single-cell level not only into mesenchymal cells but also cells with visceral mesoderm, neuroectoderm, and endoderm characteristics in vitro.[10] Umbilical cord blood also seems to contain stem cells that be can differentiated into other types of cells,[11] and lastly there is the possibility of using parthenotes. In mice, parthenogenesis has successfully produced embryos that matured long enough to grow embryonic stem cells in the labs at Advanced Cell Technology in Massachusetts.[12] Because parthenotes seem to lack the intrinsic capacity to successfully survive the process of embryogenesis, I would not consider them to be embryos. Consequently, I do not see any special moral problem with using these cells, as long as a woman has given the appropriate permission to use her eggs for such research. My point here is to suggest from the Catholic perspective that we should not move vigorously forward with embryonic research before becoming clearer about the feasibility of using alternative sources of human stem cells.

The third micro-ethical issue deals with the success of this research. We have seen in the past that a lot of hype had been given to other research projects that did not in the end offer any therapeutic benefit to patients. For example, fetal tissue implants were promised to offer Parkinson's patients, spinal cord-injured patients, and others hope of rehabilitation or cure back in the 1980s and 1990s. However, as we have recently discovered, none of the patients with Parkinson's disease who had fetal tissue cells implanted in their brains reported any benefit in the control of their symptoms. In fact, 15 percent of these patients actually showed rapidly worsening symptoms of Parkinsonism.[13] In addition, notwithstanding the recent protocol for human gene transfer in the case of X-SCID syndrome in London, it does not appear that there has been one unambiguous success with all the attempts to insert genes to correct genetic diseases. In fact, we are discovering that many patients have been harmed by these experiments or even killed (e.g., Jesse Gelsinger at the University of Pennsylvania). This extremely low rate of success should give us some humility and pause in rushing forward into another avenue of research that many find morally problematic.

Finally, at the micro level there is the type of moral reasoning that seems to undergird the efforts to push forward with this research. There is a certain strong utilitarian calculus that is used to justify these scientific efforts—that is, we need to push forward in order to benefit so many sick patients.[14] Other moral concerns and issues also need to be considered in properly assessing any new medical research (e.g., human rights, moral obligations, virtues). I find that this utilitarian calculus is essentially the only reason given to sacrifice the human embryo. As I had discussed earlier in this analysis, I question whether our moral obligations to the sick and injured are as absolute as some lead us to believe. Of course, we have strong moral obligations to these patients, but do these obligations trump all other obligations that we have to them and to society?

MACRO (SOCIAL) ETHICAL ISSUES

There are several socio-ethical issues that need to be raised, but I will focus on only four. The first is concerned not with the moral status of the preimplantation embryo but with the public funding of research that would destroy the embryo. As many recent national polls have shown, there are a substantial number of U.S. citizens who oppose the use of public money to fund research that destroys the human embryo.[15] In other words, if we use public funds to support such research, we are asking people to contribute money for what they believe to be immoral research. We are asking them to cooperate in something that they frankly judge to be wrong to do. Some Catholic ethicists have tried to justify cooperation in the use (not derivation) of already existing cell lines according to President Bush's plan,[16] but this is quite different from either deriving the cell lines or creating research embryos in order to derive pluripotent stem cells.

Second, we should be concerned about claims to intellectual property rights for medical discoveries and the profit motive that is driving much of contemporary medical research, especially by the large pharmaceutical companies. We will need to navigate these important issues so that we are able to balance the rights of the researcher with the needs of those who will not be able to pay for these advances.

Third, we as a society should be concerned about the next logical and sociological steps that might occur as a result of going forward with this research. The National Bioethics Advisory Commission (NBAC) under the Clinton administration made several important recommendations at the end of its report on stem cell research in September 1999. Two recommendations are particularly important:

Recommendation 3: Federal agencies should not fund research involving the derivation or use of human ES cells from embryos made solely for research purposes using IVF.
Recommendation 4: Federal agencies should not fund research involving the derivation or use of human ES cells from embryos made using somatic cell nuclear transfer into oocytes.[17]

In just a few years since this report was written, scientists are claiming that they now need to create research embryos and to use somatic cell nuclear transplant cloning techniques to carry out their research.[18] We are beginning to commodify human eggs; will we soon be willing to buy and sell human embryos to carry on research? This issue, of course, is concerned with the "slippery slope," so we will need to have clear plateaus where we know we will not go any further. I am not encouraged about the future, especially given the fact that we have been so quick to overturn NBAC's clear recommendations.

The last socio-ethical issue may be one of the most important key issues. It is concerned with social justice and the equitable distribution of health care in this country. It is also concerned with social justice and our moral responsibilities to prevent fatal illnesses that take the lives of millions around the world every year.[19] Pluripotent stem cell research, like the human genome project, with all its importance, tends to continue the standard paradigm of contemporary medicine: high-tech, interventionist, and rescue medicine. Preventative medicine is understressed in this paradigm, and the rich are chiefly the only ones who get access to these cutting-edge technologies. The Roman Catholic tradition is committed to the moral principles of the common good, on the one hand, and solidarity with the poor and oppressed, on the other. Thus, this tradition raises important questions about the justice of our current health system and its future embodiments. How will future healing possibilities, which might become available through stem cell research, benefit those who are marginalized in society and the uninsured?[20] When the U.S. bishops fashioned their document on the economy back in 1986, they made several recommendations about economic policy in our country. One of these key recommendations was that "the impact of national economic policies on the poor and the vulnerable is the primary criterion for judging their moral value."[21] We as a society need to use a similar criterion whenever we are about to embark on a new frontier of medical science.

TWO CONCLUSIONS

Though several conclusions might be drawn from my analysis, I briefly discuss only two. The first is that we need to think much more clearly about how to balance the good of health with the other goods that we pursue—for example, the creation of a more just society. Our obligations to the sick are indeed enormous, but they should not be viewed as near absolute such that they almost always trump all other moral obligations to other goods in society. Second, we are at a point in our history in medical research in this country where we have the opportunity to engage in a "teaching moment." We should pause and reflect much more than what we have done about our priorities in both society and in medical research and then raise the question about whether or not our taken-for-granted medical paradigm is in fact the one we should be promoting in the future. Thus, rather than continuing the standard paradigm, should we not question its validity and then possibly fashion a new way of conceiving our moral responsibilities for a more just society. This is certainly one of the challenges that I see the Roman Catholic tradition puts before us on the issue of pluripotent stem cell research.

ENDNOTES

1. Glenn McGee and Arthur Caplan, "The Ethics and Politics of Small Sacrifices in Stem Cell Research," *Kennedy Institute of Ethics Journal* 9 (1999): 153.

2. Gilbert Meilaender, "The Point of a Ban: Or, How to Think about Stem Cell Research," *Hastings Center Report* 31 (January–February 2001): 12.

3. Paul Ramsey, *Fabricated Man: The Ethics of Genetic Control* (New Haven, Conn.: Yale University Press, 1970), 92–96.

4. I list infertility in this context because in May 2003, U.S. scientists had managed to grow egg cells from early mouse embryonic stem cells, and in the same month Japanese scientists found that they could use ES cells to produce immature sperm cells. Thus, some believe that human embryonic stem cells could become a cure for some types of infertility, especially in cases where the woman does not produce her own eggs or the man does not produce any or enough sperm.

5. This "option" or "preference" for the poor and oppressed has become a regular theme in nearly all Catholic social teaching (encyclicals) since the Second Vatican Council in 1965.

6. For a further discussion of each one of these views, see Michael R. Panicola, "Three Views on the Preimplantation Embryo," *The National Catholic Bioethics Quarterly* 2 (Spring 2002): 69–97.

7. In the *Declaration on Abortion* from the Sacred Congregation for the Doctrine of the Faith in November 1974, it is stated in footnote #19, "This declaration expressly leaves aside the question of the moment when the spiritual soul is infused." The same congregation in its *Instruction on Respect for Human Life in its Origin and on the Dignity*

of Procreation in March 1987 reiterated this view on the beginnings of personal life, but then claims, "The human being is to be respected and treated as a person from the moment of conception and therefore from that same moment his rights as a person must be recognized" (sec. I, 1). See also Pope John Paul II's encyclical *Evangelium Vitae*, sec. 60.

8. For some recent examples, see Margaret Farley, "Roman Catholic Views on Research Involving Human Embryonic Stem Cells," in the National Bioethics Advisory Commission's report *Ethical Issues in Human Stem Cell Research, Volume III: Religious Perspectives* (Rockville, Md.: National Bioethics Advisory Commission, June 2000): D-3–5; Norman Ford, "The Human Embryo as Person in Catholic Teaching," *National Catholic Bioethics Quarterly* 1 (Summer 2001): 155–60; and Thomas A. Shannon and Allan B. Wolter, "Reflections on the Moral Status of the Preembryo," in Thomas A. Shannon and James J. Walter, *The New Genetic Medicine: Theological and Ethical Reflections* (New York: Sheed and Ward, 2003), 41–63.

9. For example, see Richard M. Doerflinger, "The Ethics of Funding Embryonic Stem Cell Research: A Catholic Viewpoint," *Kennedy Institute of Ethics Journal* 9 (June 1999): 137–50.

10. Catherine M. Verfaillie et al., "Pluripotency of Mesenchymal Stem Cells Derived from Adult Marrow," *Nature* (June 20, 2002): 1–9.

11. See Nicanor Pier Giogio Austriaco, "Notes on Bioethics," *National Catholic Bioethics Quarterly* 3 (Summer 2003): 367–70.

12. Aaron Zitner, "Scientists Try Unfertilized Eggs as Source of Stem Cells," *Los Angeles Times* (August 12, 2001): 1, A20. Also, in September 2003, Wake Forest University Baptist Medical Center in North Carolina used parthenogenesis to extract stem cells from monkey eggs and then grew them into a variety of different cells, including heart, nerve, and muscle cells.

13. See *New England Journal of Medicine* 344 (2001): 710–14; and Arthur Caplan and Glenn McGee, "Fetal Cell Implants: What We Learned," *Hastings Center Report* 31 (May–June 2001): 6.

14. See Meilaender, "The Point of a Ban," 10–11.

15. For example, the International Communications Research survey in June 2001 showed that 69.9 percent of those polled opposed the use of public money for purposes of destroying the human embryo for such research. See www.usccb.org/comm/archives/2001/01.htm.

16. See Mark S. Latkovic, "The Morality of Human Embryonic Stem Cell Research and President Bush's Decision: How Should Catholics Think about Such Things? *Linacre Quarterly* 69 (November 2002): 289–314, especially 295–97.

17. National Bioethics Advisory Commission, *Ethical Issues in Human Stem Cell Research: Executive Summary* (Rockville, Md.: National Bioethics Advisory Commission, September 1999), 5.

18. On the issue of using somatic cell nuclear transplant cloning (SCNT) in stem cell research, see two important scientific reports: Committee on Stem Cells and the Future of Regenerative Medicine, Board on Life Sciences and Board on Neuroscience and Behavioral Health, *Stem Cells and the Future of Regenerative Medicine: Report of the National Academy of Sciences and the Institute of Medicine*, September 2001; and the National Academy of Sciences, *Scientific and Medical Aspects of Human Reproductive Cloning*, 2002. Both committees recommended the creation of embryos by using SCNT cloning

techniques for research purposes on stem cells. The recent President's Council on Bioethics report *Human Cloning and Human Dignity: An Ethical Inquiry* (2002) discussed the possibility of using SCNT cloning for stem cell research, but the majority recommendation was to establish a four-year moratorium on this type of research.

19. Around the world, 1.1 billion people are without clean water and 2.4 billion people are without sanitation. The result is that more than 2.2 million die each year from both of these preventable factors. Furthermore, approximately two-thirds of the world population (4 billion people) is without adequate nutrition at some point during the year, which can be the cause of many preventable illnesses.

20. For a further discussion of this issue, see Andrea Vicini, "Ethical Issues and Approaches in Stem Cell Research: From International Insights to a Proposal," *Journal of the Society of Christian Ethics* 23 (Spring–Summer 2003): 71–98.

21. U.S. bishops, "Economic Justice for All: Catholic Social Teaching and the U.S. Economy," in *Origins* 16 (November 27, 1986): 443.

7

Cloning, Uniqueness, and Individuality

Thomas A. Shannon

Cloning has once again appeared on the American scene, only this time not as a specter haunting the laboratory, but as a reality. The report of the experiments done at George Washington University gave rise to renewed fears of photocopied people, the storage of clones as replacement parts, and other yet-to-be-imagined assaults on human dignity and the value of the individual.

Such fears are augmented when related to other suggestions about possible consequences of the genome project, the development of a map of the complete human genome. Specifically some fear that the genome, when fully mapped, might serve as a type of template for future humans. That is, the genome will be used as a type or pattern against which a particular individual's genes will be measured. Thus, uniqueness and individuality will give way to the generic, the average, the lowest common denominator. This augurs poorly for individual variation and diversity, as well as for the value given at least verbally to the individual in our culture.

For a culture such as ours where the individual is celebrated as the primary social actor and indeed has priority over institutions, such possibilities threaten core values. The value of the individual, celebrated in our myths of rugged individualism, the self-made person, and the master of one's destiny, is challenged by the possibility of replicating the same genetic structure over and over again—as is done with prized cows.

Two sets of biological data are important for setting the context for this chapter. Each also has philosophical and social implications that will be the subject for consideration in this chapter.

THE HUMAN GENOME

A general definition of the genome is

> The totality of the DNA contained within the single chromosome of a bacterial species (or an individual bacterium) or within the diploid chromosome set of a eukaryotic species (or an individual eukaryote). The human genome, for example, consists of approximately 6 billion base pairs of DNA distributed among forty-six chromosomes. Sometimes the term "the human genome" is used to refer instead to the approximately 3 billion base pairs of DNA within the twenty-two different human autosomes and the human and Y chromosomes.[1]

The genome is, in effect, the totality of the genetic information of the organism. Since the genome project is the attempt to map the three billion base pairs of DNA within the human chromosome structure, one can see that this is a fairly extensive project. The question is, what will be gained? On the one hand, learning the location of the base pairs—which is, after all, the primary purpose of the mapping project—will simply answer the location question, not the function question. Other issues are the organization of the genes, how the messages are coded and transmitted, and the function of "junk DNA," which appears to have no function.

These are technical questions and will take time to examine and answer. But there is one issue that occasionally emerges in discussions of the genome project that has to do with the status of the human genome. This question is: Will the human genome take on a normative status? That is, will the map of the genome function socially, medically, or politically as the normative profile of the human? Will it serve as a type of genetic Procrustean bed against which individuals will be measured? The issue has particular importance in genetic medicine and prenatal diagnoses where decisions are made based on the genetic profile of the fetus and the medical and social consequences—or assumptions about those consequences—of the genetic profile of the fetus.

THE PROCESS OF EMBRYOGENESIS

After the process of fertilization is completed, the zygote begins a remarkable journey of development. The nuclear contents of the egg and sperm merge and give the organism its diploid set of chromosomes in a process called syngamy. The organism now has its set of forty-six chromosomes and its genetic sex, genetic variability is established, and cleavage, or cell division, now begins.

A very important biological phenomenon characterizes this entity as it makes the journey from zygote to morula to blastomere to embryo. Although compacted, no one cell of this organism is predetermined to become a specific entity or part of a particular entity. This organism can, at this stage, twin, recombine after twinning, or—because of the totipotency of the cells—any one cell can become a whole distinct organism. The capacity resides in the organism and remains there until gastrulation or restriction occurs, around the third week of development.

> As development continues, the cells gradually lose the ability to form all types of cells that are found in the adult body. It is as if they were funneled into progressively narrower channels. The reduction of the developmental options permitted to a cell is called *restriction*. Very little is known about the mechanisms that bring about restriction, and the sequence and time course of restriction vary considerably from one species to another.[2]

This biological fact has interesting philosophical implications. While it is true that when syngamy is complete, genetic uniqueness is established, nonetheless singleness or individuality has not yet been achieved. Such singleness or individuality does not occur until the process of gastrulation or restriction is completed. Then and only then can we speak of a single individual. This leads to two important conclusions. First, genetic uniqueness is not coincident with individuality. Second is Ford's observation: "The teleological system of the blastocyst should not be identified with the ontological unity of the human individual that will develop from it."[3] This would strongly suggest that a human individual cannot be a human person until after the process of biological individuation is completed since the former is a necessary, though not sufficient, presupposition of the latter.

The purpose of this chapter is to examine the concept of individuality from a philosophical and genetic standpoint. Specifically, I will present the theory of individuality of John Duns Scotus, with particular emphasis on his notions of common nature and *haecceitas,* as a way to raise and evaluate philosophical and ethical problems in the cloning debate. I wish to use Scotus' view of the individual to respond to perceived threats to individuals and fears that nature is "so careless of the individual life," which are given contemporary shape by the genome project. I will conclude by arguing that, while prohibitions on cloning based on violations of uniqueness and individuality will not hold, other arguments against cloning can be presented.

JOHN DUNS SCOTUS' THEORY OF INDIVIDUALITY

Of the various theories developed to help explain and understand individuality, Scotus' theory of *haecceitas* is one widely commented upon and one that celebrates individuality as a positive characteristic. While Scotus certainly never considered problems such as the ones examined here, I find his ideas to be particularly helpful in illuminating several aspects of the cloning debate, as well as other ethical aspects relating to the status of the pre-embryo. This section will focus on Scotus' understanding of this issue particularly as developed in "Distinction 3," part I, questions 1–6 in the *Lectura in librum secundum Sententiarum*.[4] Other background concepts will be presented to complete his understanding of individuality.

Background Issues

Scotus' discussion of individuality, as was true of the other Scholastics of his day, is located in a discussion of the nature of the personality of angels. Wolter situates the discussion this way. Peter Lombard, whose *Sentences* were commented upon by succeeding generations of theologians and philosophers, stated that an angel had "four substantial attributes (1) a simple essence, i.e., indivisible and immaterial, (2) a distinct personality, (3) a rational nature, and (4) a free will."[5] The problem, then, was trying to reconcile the first two characteristics with the Aristotelian position that individuation comes from matter. This led to a further issue, articulated in particular by St. Thomas Aquinas, namely, that since angels are immaterial, they cannot be multiplied within the species. That is, each angel is a species in itself. The critical problem facing Scholastics of Scotus' time was that this particular teaching was condemned in 1277 by the Bishop of Paris, Étienne Tempier: that God cannot multiply individuals of the same species without matter. While this condemnation is a convenient way of refuting Thomas' opinion, for Scotus the condemnation is a challenge to find a new principle of individuation.

The other issue for Scotus is epistemological: according to the common Scholastic tradition, the mind is universal and the senses particular. What the intellect knows about a thing, therefore, "is not what is uniquely individual, but those common features or characteristics it shares with other things."[6] This raises the critical epistemological question: Can the individuality, or *haecceitas* as Scotus sometimes calls it, be immediately knowable? One response is that our simple intuitive awareness of ourselves as either an agent or as the recipient of an act implies "some primitive intuitive awareness of haecceity."[7]

Also important as a preliminary element in our discussion is Wolter's understanding of *haecceitas* in Scotus' thought.

> But what we ask is whether the proximate reason for the individuation of a material substance as such is something positive or privative (I don't mean to ask whether

"one" means merely a privation or negation or affirmation). Whether it does or not, the understanding is that a material substance has such an indivisibility that it is repugnant to it to be divided into several things each of which is like a subjective part of its whole.[8]

That is, while human nature may be divided up into individuals each of whom shares equally in human nature, an individual human cannot be so divided. A part of an individual human being is not another human being; it is only a part of an individual human being. Thus for Scotus, the key philosophical issue of individuality is indivisibility. We will see later that this is also a key biological issue and speaks directly to Scotus' philosophical concerns.[9]

Scotus' Arguments for the Principle of Individuation

Having rejected several arguments for various principles of individuality, Scotus turns to a positive development of his own arguments. First I will present a summary of his essential arguments. Then I will discuss issues such as the concept of the common nature and *haecceitas* and their relation to each other.

Individuality as a Positive Reality

Scotus presents two main arguments for his position. The first argument[10] focuses on unity and assumes that "unity is always attributed to some positive entity."[11] This would then also be true of a singularity that cannot be divided into other subjective parts—that is, a human being cannot be divided into any other human beings, only parts thereof. But such a unity neither constitutes the nature of the human being nor demonstrates why there could not be more than one human being.

The critical point is that the unity of the nature of the individual—that is, our understanding of human nature—does not explain why it is that this particular instance of human nature in this particular individual cannot be further divided into individuals of the same subjective parts. Because the nature of the individual cannot explain this, Scotus argues that there must be a positive individuating difference accounting for the impossibility of such "indivision" of the individual.

Scotus' second argument explains that the final reason why individuals of the same species differ is something primitive or radically diverse.[12] Individuals of the same species have something in common, otherwise they would not be understood to be of the same species. But they also have something by which they differ, which is the reason why they are not the same. The question is what is this basis for diversity.

> Obviously, this is not the nature, for though the nature of one is not that of the other, the two natures are identical specifically or formally. Otherwise there would be no real resemblance or agreement between the two individuals of the same species; consequently, there must be something else in each whereby they differ. Now this is not privative, but positive, not something accidental like quantity, or contingent like actual existence, as the answers to the preceding questions showed. Therefore, it must be something intrinsic, pertaining to the category of substance, that, logically speaking, contracts the indifference of the specific nature to just one unique individual.[13]

The Common Nature

Another element in Scotus' presentation of *haecceitas* is the concept of the common nature. Since his discussion of this concept is based on Avicenna's presentation, we begin there.

> For the definition of equinity is apart from the definition of universality, neither is universality contained in the definition of equinity, for equinity has a definition that does not need universality, but is that to which universality is added incidentally, hence equinity itself is nothing other that equinity, for of itself it is neither many nor one, existing in sense perceptible things or in the soul, neither it is one of these as a potency or as an actual effect, so that it was something contained intrinsically in the essence of equinity, but on this score it is only equinity.[14]

One critical element in the definition is that the common nature—"horseness" in this example—is indifferent to being universal or particular. "If it were an individual, it would be one and existent in reality. If it were a universal, it would be predicable of many and existent only in the mind."[15] The existence of the common nature as either individual or universal is accidental to it in itself. Additionally, following Park's analysis, the common nature has its own proper being that is "prior to the being in reality and the being in the mind."[16] A final point Scotus makes about the common nature disagrees with Avicenna. The position of Avicenna is that the common nature in itself has no unity. Scotus on the other hand argues that it has a unity, but a unity less than a numerical unity: "Anything whose proper unity is less than a numerical unity, is not a numerical unity; but the unity of the stone-nature is of itself less than a numerical unity; therefore the unity of the stone-nature, which stone has of itself, is not a numerical unity."[17]

Why does Scotus need to argue that the common nature has a proper unity, but one that is not, or less than, a numerical unity? If there were a numerical unity in the common nature in itself, the common nature would by definition be a single being and there would be no need for a positive individuating principle and, by implication, nominalism would be correct. Scotus rejects nominalism and is arguing for a positive individuating principle. Hence his concern to establish a certain unity in the common nature, a unity less than a numerical unity. Scotus presents his idea this way in the *Ordinatio*:

> And just as a nature is not of itself universal as it exists in the intellect, but universality is something that accrues only incidentally to this primary notion of it as an object, so also in external reality, where the nature is invested with singularity, but is not of itself limited to singularity. Rather it is naturally prior to that characteristic contracting it to this unique singularity, and insofar as it is naturally prior to what contracts it, it is not repugnant to that nature to exist without what contracts it.[18]

Another formulation of this same idea is in the *Lectura*.

> I reply that the unity in the thing is the sort of unity to which "to be universal" is not repugnant, but that there is nothing here that is formally universal, for "the universal is one in many and predicated of many." Hence, the universal according to one numerical aspect is predicated of many, because the intelligible content is numerically one that is predicated of Socrates and Plato, but this does not mean there is only one numerical being in both. The nature which is in Socrates, then, considered in itself is neither determined to be in this or in that or to be universal; nevertheless it always has one or the other of these modes of existence.[19]

As a matter of fact, the common nature is always individuated in an individual material substance, but of its nature it is indifferent to such a state of affairs. Thus we must look to something else as that which individuates the individual material substance.

Haecceitas

The term used by Scotus to point to the positive element that makes this individual be this particular individual and no other is *haecceitas*. Before we begin this section, recall that Scotus says that we cannot—at least in this life—directly experience *haecceitas*. Additionally, Wolter comments that *haecceitas* is a theoretical construct devised to explain certain experiences.

> Haecceitas *as a reality* is more difficult to comprehend because of its uniqueness, and this entire set of six questions may be regarded as a prolonged attempt on Scotus' part to describe it conceptually in negative or analogical terms like other nonempirical or hypothetical constructs. Like the quanta and quarks of theoretical physics, Scotus' "haecceity" is a rational fabrication, and like such conjectural entities

is postulated for theoretical reasons and its properties clarified through positive and negative analogies.[20]

As usual, it is easier to say what *haecceitas is* not. Thus Park argues that *haecceitas* is "neither an individual essence nor a property."[21] Neither is it matter, some accidental quality, actual existence, or some negative principle. Nor, as Park further argues, can we say of individuals "that they have the same substance. Nor can we say that they participate in the numerically identical Platonic ideal."[22]

Park situates the concept of *haecceitas* positively with two critical comments. *Haecceitas* is "the positive something that individuates the specific difference."[23] Also, as Park says, "Thus, a material substance becomes indivisible and diverse by one and the same positive entity."[24] Therefore, *haecceitas* is something positive, something that individuates, but also something that is not identical to the individual substance or common nature. And *haecceitas* accounts for both indivisibility and diversity. Let us turn now to Scotus' arguments.

What Scotus is looking to resolve is what makes the common nature individual in objects that exist in the world external to our minds.[25] One dimension of this has to do with the common nature itself. On the one hand, "though individually instantiated, it [the common nature] is conceptually indistinguishable from the nature of any other individual of the same species."[26] Yet, as the nature of that individual, the common nature "seems to be a real, extramental, substantial or per se unity that Scotus describes as 'less than specific.'"[27] Thus, although things of the same species resemble each other—because they share a common nature—they differ, according to Scotus, because of their *haecceitas*: "this positive additive that individuates an individual's nature or distinctive qualities as that individual's unique or proper 'haecceity' (haecceitas)."[28] Thus is the individual rendered incapable of being duplicated and is differentiated from every other individual.

What happens, then, in the process of individuation is that "the common nature just in itself is contracted to this individual material substance by its *haecceitas* and becomes the individuated essence."[29] Or to phrase this in a different way, "what makes a material substance an individual is a positive entity which falls within the category of substance and contracts the specific nature to this or that."[30]

How does this contraction occur? What is its basis? On the one hand, matter apparently could be the cause of such contraction of the common nature to this individual. As Scotus argued earlier, "if one could abstract 'matter' from this and that matter, and 'man' from this or that man, then matter could not pertain [to the essence of matter or man]; but this is false. . . . Hence, matter cannot be the cause of individuation, for it is a general rule that what is indifferent to several things of the same sort cannot be itself the cause of individuation."[31]

Yet as Park and Wolter argue, there is a sense in which Scotus reinterprets what Aristotle defines as matter so that what Aristotle calls matter is what Scotus calls "haecceitas."[32]

Scotus constructs his reinterpretation in this way. He argues,

> To the first argument of the preceding question when it is argued [n. 126] from V Metaphysics that "those things are numerically one whose matter is one," I reply: The Philosopher frequently—in the Metaphysics and elsewhere—takes "form" for the quiddity and "matter" for anything that contracts quiddity. (Hence he says in Bk. VIII that "forms are like numbers"—where, by "forms" he understands quiddities and definitions.) Those things are one in number, then, whose quiddity has been contracted by an entity that is one in number, and it is this he understands by "matter."[33]

The understanding of matter and the definition of it that Scotus argues for seems to be a functional one: that which constricts form is matter or that which constricts quiddity is matter. This understanding of matter is not of matter as that which one could abstract from this matter or that matter, as argued above. Such matter as could be abstracted in this fashion is common to both and is the source of neither difference nor diversity precisely because it is common to both. For Scotus, since matter is that which constricts form or quiddity, and "that which contracts form is nothing but haecceitas,"[34] then there is a sense in which Scotus understands matter to be the principle of individuation or *haecceitas*. As Wolter phrases it,

> The peculiarity of the individuating principle is that it is unique and primarily diverse; this means there is nothing in two such haecceities that is "common" and provides a basis for abstraction. Another way of putting this is to say that the only "common" feature is the relationship each unique haecceity bears to the same sort of nature, but if the two haecceities differ, so too does the relationship to these two different terms. Hence, there is no way in which one can abstract something common from what individuates. If one chooses to call this "matter"—and there is a sense, Scotus admits, that Aristotle calls "matter" whatever lies outside the essence or "form"—then one should say the same of matter as of haecceity.[35]

Therefore, we cannot look to matter as an individuation principle if such matter is common to both entities. Rather, we have to acknowledge the ultimate reality of the individual. As Wolter concludes,

> there is something positive in the category of substance in this individual that contracts or limits its specific nature to just this individual and something else in that

individual that contracts or limits its specific nature to just that individual. And it is the "thisness" in the one and the "thatness" in the other that make the two individuals of the same species or nature, primarily diverse or individual.[36]

This notion of individuality and its relation to the common nature is well summarized in an example that highlights a major theme of the next section.

God, at least, could conceivably clone any individual nature qua nature but even God could not clone its unique individuality. This implies that even in one unique individual, such as Peter the Apostle, what makes him human is less opposed to being multiplied than what makes him Peter and not his identical twin, if this be his brother Andrew, for otherwise he would not be like his twin or resemble Paul, his fellow apostle, without being either his brother or Saint Paul as such.[37]

GENETICS AND INDIVIDUALITY:
THE MORAL ISSUES

Scotus' concept of the common nature can help us think about the moral and political status of the genome. I propose that the genome, in effect, is the biological equivalent of the philosophical concept of the common nature. The Scotistic common nature is human nature indifferent to a particular manifestation. It has a unity, but not a singularity. It has a real existence, but does not exist independently. The common nature is the basis of differentiating the human species from other species. The common nature, in short, is our essential whatness, our essence as a nature, what we are born to be.

This, too, is what the genome does. The human genome is the basis on which we are human as opposed to being a member of another species. The genome is the basis on which our bodies are organized in particular ways, on which we act in certain ways, on which we think in certain ways. The genome, in short, gives us a key insight into our essential whatness.

I conclude that the common nature/genome is normative only at the species level. It is what differentiates us specifically from other members of the genus mammal. At the individual level, the common nature/genome is important insofar as it gives us an insight into our specific whatness, but this common nature has not yet been individualized, has not been expressed as this particular individual. Thus, the genome, as well as the common nature, is important for developing generalizations about the nature of human nature, for insights into how we act as a nature, what can bring us to fulfillment. But the common nature or the genome is not the end of the story, nor even the most important part of the story. What is critical is the instantiation of the common nature into this individual and how this individual actuates his or her common nature. How this will be done or resolved is the exclusive function of neither the common nature nor the genome.[38]

Thus, I think the Scotistic concept of the common nature can help us focus our attention on what unites us rather than what might divide us. The genome is the basis for our specific differentiation. It tells what divides us from others but also what unites us as a species. As such the common nature/genome reveals our essential human nature.

NATURE AND THE INDIVIDUAL

Concern for the individual is also present in modern thought. One dimension of this concern is found in the dialogue between nature and the individual in Tennyson's famous poem *In Memoriam*. While we are more familiar with the "Nature red in tooth and claw" phrase from the poem, even more interesting is a later stanza that raises the questioning of which takes priority—the type, the individual, or nothing at all.

> Are God and Nature then at strife
> That Nature lends such evil dreams?
> So careful of the type she seems,
> So careless of the single life . . .
> So careful of the type? but no.
> From scarped cliff and quarried stone
> She cries, "A thousand types are gone;
> I care for nothing, all shall go."
> O life as futile, then, as frail!
> O for the voice to soothe and bless!
> What hope of answer, or redress?
> Behind the veil, behind the veil.[39]

The unsettling thoughts suggested here are that not only does the type—or species—have priority over the individual, but that even the type may be in vain. While the latter issue may ultimately be more critical, the former topic will be considered more thoroughly.

Tennyson phrased the problem as the tension between nature's care for the preservation of the species as opposed to its indifference to the survival of the individual. Some, from the perspective of social Darwinism, would define this as the survival of the fittest. Others, from the perspective of sociobiology, would phrase this as the priority of DNA over the individual: the individual is DNA's way of making more DNA.

But no matter the phrasing, the vision is the same: the primacy of the species or, in a more contemporary phrase, the primacy of DNA. Individuals exist, to be sure, but their value is that of bearing DNA, of being the vehicle through which the next generation of DNA is replicated. This, of course, gives rise to our darkest fears: we are but means to an impersonal end. And thus the great project of the Enlightenment is dissolved in the vast sea of DNA, "so careless of the single life."

Then too there is concern about the consequence of deriving "the" human genome. Some raise concerns that a significant outcome of the Human Genome Index (HGI) will be the development of "the" profile of the human genome. The specific fear is that such a profile will be the template against which the genetic profile of each individual will be matched. This has particular significance given the development of even more sophisticated prenatal diagnostic technologies. Thus, rather than developing a map to guide us in our search for diseases and cures, the genome will become the template against which all individuals will be measured and genetic conformity will be the outcome. Such a practice could highlight uniformity rather than individuality. Again, the type takes precedence over the individual.

The position that the species takes priority over the individual is also present in Aristotelian philosophy, though this position is expressed in terms of matter and form as opposed to an evolutionary perspective. In particular, Aristotle argued that the order of nature is grounded in those orders of reality that pertain to the order of the universe. Such orders consist of species, however, not individuals.[40] For Aristotle too, the species take priority over the individual. Scotus responds to this Aristotelian perspective as follows:

> In the universe as a whole, order is mainly considered according to types or species where their inequalities or differences pertain to order. According to Augustine, however, in *The City of God* (XIX, chapter 13) "order is an arrangement of like and unlike things whereby each of them is disposed in its proper place." That is why this Agent who primarily intended the order of the universe (as the principle good, intrinsic to Himself) not only intended this inequality that is one requirement for order (among species) but also desired a parity of individuals (within the same species) which is another accompaniment of order. And individuals are intended in an unqualified sense by this First One insofar as he intended something other than himself not as an end, but as something oriented to that end. Hence to communicate his goodness, as something befitting his beauty, he produces several in each species. And in those beings which are the highest and most important, it is the individual that is primarily intended by God.[41]

Thus, for Scotus, species are not the end of creation, but rather the individuals whom God primarily intends, not as a means to an end but as ends in themselves and, as ends in themselves, are reflective of the immensity of the beauty of God. Though the species has a place—the basis of order within the cosmos—such species actually exist only insofar as matter constricts the form to eventuate in this particular individual. This individual is the actual focal point of creation and species are derived consequent to the existence of the individual. And in this vast array of individuals, Scotus argues that we catch a glimpse of the even vaster glory of the Creator.

Thus neither the species nor the genome is the measure of the individual. They are not the "gold standard" by which we reckon human worth or standing. The genome presents us with a glimpse into what Scotus would call the common nature of us humans but it is not what makes me who I am. In principle, through cloning, the genome can be replicated. We now have the technology to render the common nature truly common. But what begins the individuating process of the common nature is what Scotus describes as matter's constriction of the form (the genome) to this particular individual and what we call the process of restriction, which commits cells in the developing organism to becoming what they will only be. This process of individuation is then continued through the particular life experiences of this person. Thus, the individual is the one in whom the species receives its manifestation, fulfillment, and meaning—as well as its ultimate grounding.

CONCLUSIONS

Undoubtedly, the eventual mapping of the human genome will be a boon to science, medicine, and anthropology. This map will help us learn much of what makes us human, where to look for anomalies that cause disease, and will be of great assistance in correcting those errors. We are genuinely on the edge of a new revolution in medicine, one that will provide access to the very structure of our nature. We can literally reach inside ourselves, remove a gene or genes, and either correct or replace them. Such power is truly awe inspiring.

Yet the dangers are there as well. There is talk in the air of the new genetics inspiring a new eugenics and there is concern that the genome will be the standard by which all are evaluated. The individual seems again to be in danger of being subordinated to the "type." Additionally, new developments in behavioral genetics are building up convincing evidence for the role of genes in all manner of human behavior, from sexual preference to choice of political perspectives as well as marriage partners.

Finally, the recent cloning experiment by Drs. Jerry Hall and Robert Stillman and the brief, but lively, discussion that followed it raised once again many of the thematic issues raised by genetic engineering: power, arrogance, the technological imperative, acting before thinking, degradation of human beings, and the violation of their unique genetic structure. The experiment also invoked the values of helping infertile couples, learning more of the developmental process of pre-embryos, and developing a cure for infertility. Public and professional reaction seemed to be quite strong against the practice. And even though the experiment was cleared by the university ethics committee, Stillman and Hall have retired from the cloning business, at least for the present.

But this is not the end of cloning. Actually, it's amazing that such serious efforts have been attempted only now. Many of the technical capacities had been in place for some time and the curiosity was surely there. The major lack may have been money, for the federal government until recently supported no research on human embryos. But even if it had, cloning research might not have been the highest priority on the research agenda. But the issue is here to stay. Therefore, I will conclude by examining cloning as a way to bring together several themes that I have developed during the course of this paper.

Genetic Uniqueness vs. Individuality

One of the claims of cloning that I examine is that cloning violates individuality or the individual's right to a unique genetic identity.

First, it is important to distinguish between genetic uniqueness and individuality. A pre-embryo is genetically unique in that it is a new combination of the genes from the mother and father. But it is more precise to say that this pre-embryo represents the next genetic generation precisely because it has not yet reached the developmental stage of reduction in which the cells become irreversibly committed to forming specific body parts in a particular body. There is as yet no differential gene expression. I argue that the pre-embryo presents as the biological equivalent of Scotus' philosophical concept of the common nature. That is, because the cells of the pre-embryo have the capacity of totipotency, they are most properly designated as representing what is common to humanity. The genetic structure they possess is generic to the species but is not yet identified with a particular individual. Though the cells of the pre-embryo possess a biological, teleological unity that will eventuate into a single human being, until these cells lose the capacity for totipotency through the process of restriction and become differentially expressed, we do not have what Ford calls an "ontological individual." Such individuality is irreversible both biologically in that the part cannot become a whole human and philosophically in that this being now manifests what Scotus calls *haecceitas*: the constriction of the matter by the form to become this particular individual and no other.

In the cloning debate, much has been made of genetic uniqueness. One argument is that genetic uniqueness is established at fertilization. Given what we know about embryogenesis, a more precise way to describe this is either as the establishment of the next genetic generation or the establishment of the common nature. That is, while it is correct that the pre-embryo contains the appropriate genetic information for that organism's development, that genetic information is not morally privileged through association with a specific individual. The genetic uniqueness is association with what is common to all—human nature—not a particular individual because such an entity does not yet exist. The claim of the moral relevance of genetic uniqueness is appropriately made of the pre-embryo only after the process of restriction has occurred and we have the only individual who in fact will emerge from the constriction of the common nature to this particular individual. This is the one, all things being equal, who will become the agent of acts.

Some also argue that personhood is coincident with the formation of genetic uniqueness, which is further assumed as coincident with fertilization. In addition to the biological problems with this position that have just been described, there are also philosophical problems. One is genetic reductionism: the reduction of the person to his or her genetic structure only. That is, to identify the person with the genetic structure is to say that we are our genes only. While it is clear that our genetic structure has much to do with who we are, we are not simply the sum of our genetic code.

Second, Scotus' argument about the essentiality of incommunicability as the essence of personhood is useful here. What the pre-embryo precisely lacks is incommunicability, for it is biologically indifferent to singleness until after restriction occurs. Any of its individual cells until that time can be a whole other being; whereas after restriction, in that individual a liver cell will be only a liver cell, a heart cell only a heart cell. Individuation means that a single being cannot be divided into a whole other; rather it can be divided only into parts. Thus after restriction there is an incommunicability of the individual. Thus begins biologically what Scotus calls the "ultimate solitude" of the individual's existence.

But this biological dimension of incommunicability is not a full presentation of the reality of the incommunicable essence of the person. I further argue that the developing embryo resulting from this process of biological individuation is what Scotus would call a nature: an entity in which "the potency of itself is determined to act, so that it cannot fail to act when not impeded from without."[42] A nature is essentially the reason a being acts as it does or is the principle of activity by which a being seeks and actualizes its own fulfillment. To act according to one's nature is to seek the good of one's nature, what Scotus calls acting according to the *affectio commodi*. That is to say, the being set in motion by the process of individuation is one that essentially acts out its nature. To act according to the *affectio commodi* or nature is to act according to the genetic instructions given the individual during biological development. One's good is set by one's nature and this nature is set by one's genes.

But to act on the basis of one's genetic instruction does not mean to act on the basis of one's genetic instruction only. Scotus describes another action in which we engage: an act of seeking, for example, the good of another or the love of someone for his or her own sake. Scotus calls this the *affectio justitiae,* the capacity to transcend nature and go beyond what our nature prescribes as our individual good. This capacity is the source of true liberty and is a "freedom from nature and a freedom for values."[43] Scotus highlights this by identifying one's intention in acting as a key element in evaluating the morality of an action.

Personal incommunicability, as distinct from but not contrary to biological incommunicability, is expressed through the free commitment of one's self to be a good beyond, but not contrary to, one's nature. It is the commitment of the self to a good for the good's own sake. It is the act of love that is so taken by the good that is loved that the individual wishes this good to be shared by others. This represents the supreme moment of the coincidence of personhood and individualization for in this act of transcendence of my nature I achieve myself in the fullest sense. Or as Gerard Manley Hopkins phrases it in the poem "As Kingfishers Catch Fire":

> Each mortal thing does one thing and the same:
> Deals out that being indoors each one dwells;
> Selves—goes its self; *myself* it speaks and spells,
> Crying *What I do is me: for that I came.*[44]

And in doing this, we also achieve what Scotus described as the fullness of his incarnational and religious vision of the ultimate significance of the human individual. For in so acting we become who we are to become, for I act, to continue Hopkins' thought,

> in God's eye what in God's eye he is—
> Christ. For Christ plays in ten thousand places,
> Lovely in limbs, and lovely in eyes not his
> To the Father though the features of men's faces.[45]

This is the act that can be actualized only by myself and I bear the responsibility for it. Neither the motivation nor the consequences of a true act of freedom—what Scotus calls the *affectio justitiae*—can be attributed to or communicated to another. Thus the ultimate solitude that Scotus ascribes to the core of personhood is not an atomistic individualism that separates us from one another. Rather, by so acting, we transcend our own nature and reach goods that can be experienced with others and that can become the basis of a community. In so acting we do not lose our own moral identity or responsibility; rather, we find the grounds of community.

These ideas, through which Hopkins gives existential perspective to Scotus' perspective, help in thinking about so-called identical twins, whether these occur because of a natural cleavage of the egg or because of cloning. What is identical about these individuals is their genotype and frequently much of their phenotype as well. But what is not identical is their individuality. Thus while they may be, for all practical purposes, genetically interchangeable, they are not individually interchangeable. In each of these individuals there has been a contraction of their common nature to form an individual who can never be replicated and whose moral acts constitute a unique moral agent. The priority again is on individuality, not genetic uniqueness.

Second, we can complement Scotus' thought by Hopkins' more existential expression of these ideas to help us think about the relation between genotype and action. I would characterize Scotus' vision of individuality as a state of being; Hopkins' as a state of becoming. Neither can exist without the other. For Scotus, the process of individuation is accomplished by the constriction of the form by matter. While this process is a passive one, the result is active in that this individuated being is now set on a course of self-realization. As previously noted, this is similar to the equally passive process of restriction, which accomplishes biological individuation and sets a single life in motion. For Hopkins, the process of individuation is accomplished by finding one's pitch, those personal acts of self-transcendence through which we express our deepest selves.

> Each mortal thing does one thing and the same:
> Deals out that being indoors each one dwells;
> Selves—goes its self; myself it speaks and spells,
> Crying *What I do is me: for that I came.*

Specific Ethical Issues

What, then, are we to think of efforts to replicate a human, either through dividing the cells of the pre-embryo and placing them in an artificial medium or through organism cloning via nuclear transplantation? First, dividing the cells of the pre-embryo into separate entities. What one has with the pre-embryo is a teleologically united cluster of cells that have the capacity to become a distinct or ontological individual. The pre-embryo is neither all of humanity nor a particular human, but is the common nature out of which a particular human can develop.

Therefore, to divide the four, eight, or sixteen cells of the pre-embryo into separate cells is not, in the memorably inaccurate phrasing of Germain Grisez, "splitting themselves in half."[46] Rather, it is to divide the whole organism into its parts that themselves can become wholes. To do so is not to divide an ontological individual or to violate that entity's distinct individuality. While living, a bearer of the human genome, distinct from mother and father, and the next genetic generation, such features of the pre-embryo do not form the basis of a claim of an absolute value for this entity because there is as yet no subject of such a claim. There is no individual.

Second, cloning. Organism cloning, as distinct from gene and cell cloning, takes the nucleus of an adult cell and puts it in the enucleated cell of another organism. The purpose is to replicate genetically the adult organism from which the nucleus came. The key to cloning is that while each adult cell contains all the DNA necessary for the development of an entire organism, not all of that DNA is expressed. Such differential gene expression makes possible the development of the individual body parts and organs. The technical key to the success of cloning is to discover whether these unexpressed genes in the adult cell can be turned on and develop a genetically identical organism.

The common argument against cloning is that it violates the genetic uniqueness of the pre-embryo. This claim of moral standing based on genetic uniqueness in the pre-embryo cannot be sustained for there is no subject of whom the claim can be made, as previously argued. Additionally, even if cloning of humans were to succeed, what is replicated is the genetic structure, not the individual. No one claims that genetically identical twins violate each other's right to genetic individuality by virtue of bearing the same genetic structure. That is because, I argue, the more critical moral claim is that of individuality, which is biologically secured only after restriction. Genetic uniqueness and its relation to identity is important for questions of lineage, but it is not the totality of individuality.

How does one evaluate the morality of acts performed upon the pre-embryo? I suggest an examination of the object, the intention and the circumstances of the act, particularly the circumstances of the end, the way the act is performed, the likely success of the act, and the circumstance of place.[47]

With respect to the object, the pre-embryo, these entities have a premoral value in that they are living, bear the human genome, and have a biological teleology directed to the moral category of personhood. However, since there is no individual subject of whom a claim can be made, there can be no violation of individuality or personhood. This premoral value must be judged in the light of other premoral and moral goods such as the benefits to come from research on these entities and the good of assisting in reproduction. I conclude that such goods outweigh the claims of protection of the pre-embryo and that research, including division of the cells of the pre-embryo and experiments to discover the mechanisms to turn unexpressed genes on, can be done on the human pre-embryo.

Another example has to do with one of the scenarios mentioned in cloning: having replacements on hand in the event that one would need a new organ. The intention of such an act is to reduce this individual to a means to an end. Though the pre-embryo as such may not be mistreated in the technical process of cloning, the individual who comes from this pre-embryo will be by virtue of the fact that he or she is valued for his or her parts only and not the whole of his or her being. Thus, a consideration of the intention as well as the end leads one to the conclusion that this purpose is morally prohibited.

Considerations of the likely success of the act of cloning are difficult to calculate, for one genuinely does not know the full outcome or range of consequences that may follow the first experiment. This suggests that one consider the intentions very carefully as well as the end at which one aims. If the purpose of the cloning is to learn more of early cell development to aid in IVF, one could accept a lower level of success because the purpose is narrow and focused on internal development of the cells. Experiments to attempt to turn on unexpressed genes could also be justified even though the lack of success may be low. The end of the experiment is focused on internal mechanisms of the gene. However, experiments that seek to apply such knowledge would have to be very carefully examined in light of the end and intention.

I would interpret the circumstance of place to address the question of the priority of such research in relation to other priorities in health care. Because such research is so expensive and applicable to only a narrow range of cases, a strong argument can be made against such research. If one broadens the argument to understanding the mechanisms of gene expression, then the range of application may be much broader—for example, a better understanding of the immune system—and a different moral argument can be made. What is critical is that the criterion of the circumstance of place makes us look to the setting of the research and its location in the full range of health-care services as an appropriate source for moral evaluation of the act we wish to undertake.

Therefore, I argue that individuality takes moral precedence over genetic uniqueness and is the key to the ethical analysis of research on the pre-embryo. Though I am factually the only one who bears my genetic identity, in principle, genetic identity is not unique. Genetic identity can be replicated either in vivo through a natural cleavage of the pre-embryo into genetic twins or in vitro through division of the cells of the pre-embryo or through organismic cloning (though that is not yet technically possible). Genetic identity is significant because it constitutes the establishment of my "bodyliness," my human nature, and for tracing my lineage. But more significant is individuality both in the sense of indivisibleness and in the sense of the subject of moral acts. It is only that "I" who cannot be divided into parts, who can personalize that genetic structure, and who can transcend that genetic structure in an act of self-commitment. The absence of such individuality in the pre-embryo provides a key justification for the lack of its absolute protection just as the presence of such individuality is a significant feature of its moral evaluation.

ENDNOTES

This chapter was written with the support of "Theological Questions Raised by the Human Genome Initiative" sponsored by the Center for Theology and the Natural Sciences at the Graduate Theological Union, Berkeley, Calif., National Institutes of Health Grant No. GNM 1 R01 HG00487–01.

1. "The Human Genome Project," *Los Alamos Science* 20 (1992): 333. In this definition, the term *eukarote* refers to species in which cell division occurs in specific ways: one-celled organisms reproduce asexually or multicellular organisms increase and replace dead cells. The cell division occurs through mitosis in which the daughter cells are genetically identical to the mother cell. *Autosome* is another term for all chromosomes in eukarotic species other than the sex chromosomes.

2. Bruce M. Carlson, *Patten's Foundations of Embryology*, 5th ed. (New York: McGraw-Hill, 1988), 23.

3. Norman M. Ford, *When Did I Begin? Conception of the Human Individual in History, Philosophy, and Science* (Cambridge: Cambridge University Press, 1988), 158.

4. In this chapter I rely on Allan Wolter's Latin text and English translation entitled *Duns Scotus' Early Oxford Lecture on Individuation*. This is available from Fr. Wolter, in a desktop edition, at Old Mission, 2201 Laguna St. Santa Barbara, CA 93105.

5. Wolter, *Duns Scotus' Early Oxford Lecture*, x.

6. Wolter, *Duns Scotus' Early Oxford Lecture*, xi.

7. Wolter, *Duns Scotus' Early Oxford Lecture*, xvi.

8. Duns Scotus, *Lectura*, book II, d. 3, q. 2, n. 42, quoted from Wolter, *Duns Scotus' Early Oxford Lecture*, 23.

9. Woosuk Park, "Haecceitas and the Bare Particular: A Study of Duns Scotus' Theory of Individuation," PhD diss., SUNY, Buffalo, 1988. This dissertation is a particularly cogent presentation of Scotus' theory and has been extremely helpful in understanding Scotus' theory.

10. Scotus' text for this argument is, "My first point then is to show that the specific nature is constricted to this singularity by something positive. All unity follows upon some

entity—and just as 'one' in general follows upon 'being' in general, so analogously with what is special. Hence the unity characteristic of singularity, which excludes any sort of division, will have some analogous entity as its base. But such unity does not stem from the entity of the nature. For, as was shown above [nn. 9–25], the unity of nature is less than the singularity that is numerical unity. That is why the unity characteristic of nature can stand in opposition to this [numerical] unity and is not a sufficient reason for such. Hence this must stem formally from some extra entity besides what is essential to the specific entity. This unity then does not follow from the specific entity. Nevertheless that entity [or haecceity] from which it does stem, forms *a per se* unity with the specific nature, because the individual—as was proved above [nn. 65, 72–76, 87, 91–93]—is *a per se* unity and not through unity of another genus [such as that of quantity]. It follows then that the specific nature is determined to be this individual by something positive." *Lectura,* d. 3, q. 6, a. 166.

11. Wolter, "Individuation Theory," 90.

12. Scotus' text for this argument is, "Furthermore, things that differ are 'other-same things'; but Socrates and Plato differ, hence there must be something whereby they differ, the ultimate basis of their difference. But the nature in the one and the other is not primarily the cause of their difference, but their agreement. Though the nature in one is not the nature in the other, nature and nature are not that whereby the two differ primarily, but that whereby they agree (for they do not differ just of themselves—otherwise there would be no real agreement between them), hence there must be something else whereby they differ. But this is not quantity, nor existence, nor a negation, as was established in the preceding questions [nn. 153–163]; therefore it must be something positive in the category of substance, contracting the specific nature." *Lectura,* d. 3, q. 6, a. 167.

13. Wolter, "Individuation Theory," 90.

14. Avicenna, *Metaphysics,* V, Ch. 1, quoted in Wolter, "Individuation Theory," 72; Park, "Haecceitas," 152.

15. Park, "Haecceitas," 152.

16. Park, "Haecceitas," 152.

17. *Lectura,* d. 3, q. 1, a. 9.

18. *Ordinatio,* n. 34, quoted in Wolter, "Individuation Theory," 83; Park, "Haecceitas," 105.

19. *Lectura,* d. 3, q. 1, a. 34.

20. Wolter, *Duns Scotus' Early Oxford Lecture,* xv.

21. Park, "Haecceitas," 9.

22. Park, "Haecceitas," 105.

23. Park, "Haecceitas," 13.

24. Park, "Haecceitas," 36.

25. The relevant text from Scotus is, "If you ask me: What is this 'individuating entity' from which the individual difference is taken? Is it matter or form or the composite? I give you this answer. Every quidditative entity—be it partial or total—of any sort, is of itself indifferent 'as a quidditative entity' to this entity and that entity, so that as a quidditative entity it is naturally prior to this entity as just this. Now just as, in this natural priority, it does not pertain to it to be this, neither is it repugnant to its essential nature to be other than just this. And as the composite does not include qua nature its entity whereby it is

formally this, so neither does its matter qua nature include its entity whereby it is this matter, nor does its form qua nature include its entity whereby it is this form.

"This [individuating] entity therefore is not the matter or the form or the composite insofar as each of these is a 'nature,'—but it is the ultimate reality of the being [i.e., the ens] that is the matter or that is the form or that is the composite; so that whatever is common and nevertheless determinable, no matter how much it is only one real thing [i.e., una res], we can still distinguish further several formally distinct realities, of which this formally is not that; and this is formally the entity of singularity and this is formally the entity of a nature. Nor can these two realities ever be two distinct real things, in the way the two realities might be from which the genus is taken and that from which the difference is taken [from which the two realities the specific reality as a whole is taken],—but in the same real thing there are always formally distinct realities [be they in the same real part of the same real whole." *Ordinatio*, 87–88, quoted in Wolter, "Individuation Theory," 93–94.

26. Wolter, *Duns Scotus' Early Oxford Lecture*, xiii.

27. Wolter, *Duns Scotus' Early Oxford Lecture*, xiii.

28. Wolter, *Duns Scotus' Early Oxford Lecture*, xiii.

29. Park, "Haecceitas," 94.

30. Park, "Haecceitas," 197.

31. *Lectura*, d. 3, q. 5, a. 133.

32. Park, "Haecceitas," 94.

33. *Lectura*, d. 3, q. 6, a. 189.

34. Park, "Haecceitas," 95.

35. Allan B. Wolter, "Scotus' Theory of Individuation," in *Individuation in Scholasticism*, edited by Jorge J. E. Garcia, forthcoming.

36. Wolter, "Scotus' Theory of Individuation."

37. Allan B. Wolter, "Scotus' Individuation Theory," in *The Philosophical Theology of John Duns Scotus*, edited by Marilyn McCord Adams, 68–97 (Ithaca, NY: Cornell University Press, 1990), 76.

38. The one place where the analogy between common nature and genome breaks down is the area of sexuality, defined by the presence of the X or Y chromosome. Here, I think the concept of the common nature will be *more inclusive* since one will understand the genome as either a male or female genome. But even here I think the concept of a common nature is helpful because it looks to what is common and does not seek to establish social differentiation based on genetic differentiation.

39. Alfred Lord Tennyson, *In Memoriam*, LV, LVI.

40. *Ordinatio* II, d. 3, p. 1, q. 7, a. 221.

41. *Ordinatio* II, d. 3, p. 1, q. 7, a. 251. Italics in Fr. Wolter's translation.

42. *Quaestiones in Metaphysicam* I, Q. 15, a. 2, quoted in Allan B. Wolter, *Duns Scotus on the Will and Morality* (Washington, D.C.: Catholic University of America Press, 1986), 151

43. Allan B. Wolter, "Native Freedom of the Will as a Key to the Ethics of Scotus," in *The Philosophical Theology of John Dims Scotus,* edited by Marilyn McCord Adams (New York: Columbia University Press, 1990), 152.

44. In Gerard Manley Hopkins, *The Oxford Authors*, edited by Catherine Phillips (Oxford: Oxford University Press, 1986), 129.

45. In Gerard Manley Hopkins, *The Oxford Authors*, 129.

46. *Time* (November 8, 1993): 69.

47. Here, I am explicitly using the ethics method of John Duns Scotus, a fuller account of which can be found in *Theological Studies* 53 (1993): 272–93.

8

Reproductive Technologies: Ethical and Religious Issues

Thomas A. Shannon

This chapter discusses several ethical dimensions of assisted reproduction (AR). First, it identifies general ethical issues that have not been fully evaluated, primarily because of the way the field of assisted reproduction developed. Second, I argue that while Roman Catholicism has a fairly developed and clear teaching about assisted reproduction and that while some of this teaching has a value beyond the boundaries of this religion, ultimately the teaching lacks credibility because of use of a problematic understanding of natural law. The teaching is overly physicalist or biological in its development of norms, and this narrowness of interpretation impedes Catholicism from responding constructively to historical changes in marriage and in the family. Finally, I develop aspects of Roman Catholic social ethics that could contribute to a discussion of assisted reproduction, particularly within the discussion of health insurance. Here, I move beyond a traditional understanding of natural law but remain within the general context of Roman Catholic social teaching. While criticizing many aspects of traditional Roman Catholic teaching, I want to argue that there are, nonetheless, resources within this tradition that are both constructive and useful in evaluating this important, developing branch of reproductive medicine.

ASSISTED REPRODUCTION: AN OVERVIEW

The birth of Louise Brown in England in 1978 was a reproductive revolution as profound as the introduction of artificial contraceptives in the 1950s. For several years, Patrick Steptoe and Robert Edwards had been doing experiments on in vitro fertilization (IVF) with varying degrees of success. However, the main lines of the technique were established, and the outcome seemed to depend as much on luck as technique. Everything came together, though, in the birth of Louise Brown, and reproduction was never the same.

After this beginning, the use of this technology spread rapidly, first in England, Australia, and the United States and now around the world. Although it was far from established as successful, the technology moved immediately to the clinic. In the early decades of AR, few data were collected and few, if any, controlled studies were performed. Thus the details of AR were learned and gathered in a rather random fashion, remaining primarily within the particular clinic, since increased success gave the clinic a financial advantage. Fortunately, the technology itself and the various means of manipulating sperm, egg, and preimplantation embryo do not appear to be harmful to these entities. Nor does the technology appear to cause harm to the children born of the technology. The critical issue, though, is that we have learned this from clinical practice, not from carefully designed research protocols.

Because of the rapid move from experimental procedure to clinical practice, few, if any, regulatory standards were in place. There were no requirements for any type of board certification or for any particular training in human reproduction or obstetrics, with the possible exception of assisting at the birth itself. (Midwives, for example, need certification by the state, as well as those in the field of ob/gyn before they can assist at birth.) The same was true of the clinics themselves. These were essentially private enterprises and were not regulated either by the state or the medical establishment. Who was entitled to do what and based on what training and credentials was simply unclear. The alleged training standard of "see one, do one, teach one" appeared to be normative, not stereotypical.

As attention focused on the growing field and as the practice spread more widely, a core procedure of egg retrieval, fertilization, incubation, and implantation became established. This was helped by the publication of articles in professional journals, the establishment of several journals devoted to AR, new training programs at medical schools, and the development of guidelines by professional medical societies. More attention thus was paid to the biology of reproduction and the technologies used to assist in reproduction. Now, almost twenty years after Louise Brown's birth, AR is an accepted part of standard medical practice, some dimensions of which are now covered by many insurance plans.

But critical issues still remain. While AR is widely available in both hospitals and private clinics, access to it is still restricted, primarily by costs, with fees for a single IVF cycle ranging from $8,000 to $10,000. Although AR is covered by some insurance plans, what the plans cover varies widely. Some will pay for infertility workups; others will also pay for one or two cycles of in vitro fertilization. Still other plans will pay for some procedures and not others. Even if insurance pays for some parts of the procedure, there will be many out-of-pocket expenses, such as travel costs, hotel stays, and time off from work. And while costs are coming down, prices vary dramatically from clinic to clinic. Hardly anyone becomes pregnant on the first cycle, so cycles will be repeated and often new technologies are used. One is quickly beyond one's insurance coverage. Thus accessibility to the technology is limited both by insurance limits and one's disposable income.

Some clinics prorate the costs of IVF, refunding many costs if no child is born. For example, Pacific Fertility Center, with branches in Los Angeles, San Francisco, and Sacramento, recently took out a half page ad in the *New York Times*.[1] For a set fee, the client receives a single cycle of IVF with either her eggs or a donor's eggs and, if she does not get pregnant on this try will have all the remaining frozen embryos implanted. If the client does not carry a pregnancy for at least twelve weeks, she receives a 90 percent refund. Pacific Fertility Center also offers a variety of other financial options: a single cycle for customary fees, shared IVF egg donor programs so that two couples can split the fees, a plan for women forty-three years of age and younger that allows up to three IVF cycles for a single fee, and discounts of up to 35 percent for couples demonstrating financial need. There is also a pro bono grant program that provides free IVF services.[2]

A 1983 study, focusing on the first five years of IVF programs in Britain, Australia, and the United States, showed that while success rates of various AR technologies were increasing, they were still low. Steptoe and Edwards had reported an early success rate of 2 percent per embryo transfer; several years later this rate had risen to 9 percent per laparoscopy. Other groups in Australia and the United States report rates up to 20 percent.[3] Notice, though, two different measures of calculation of success rates: per embryo transfer and per laparoscopy. Such lack of standardization makes accuracy of results difficult. Also, the definition of success is not clear. One can be pregnant chemically in that a rise in hormones can be measured, or one can be pregnant clinically in that the embryo has actually implanted. Neither of these necessarily results in a live birth. Nor is a pregnancy of twelve weeks, which is criterion for success, a necessary predictor of a live birth.

A recent story in the *New York Times* gave the success rate of various IVF clinics in that metropolitan area, defining success as a live birth. The rates for women under the age of thirty-nine ranged from a low of 9.3 percent through about 20 percent at four clinics, to a high of 34 percent at one clinic.[4] In general, though, of the 267 clinics that report their data to the Society for

Assisted Reproductive Technology, the professional association for individuals involved in IVF, the success rate is 21.2 percent per IVF cycle.[5]

GENERAL ETHICAL ISSUES

The costs associated with IVF raise several ethical issues. Rebate programs, at first flush, sound like a good idea. But some describe this as "at best an eye-catching marketing gimmick, and at worse a breach of medical ethics." An American Medical Association task force argued, "Such publicized guarantees manipulate and unfairly attract patients."[6] For example, Pacific Fertility Center charges $7,725 for its basic, single IVF cycle, while its rebate plan costs $12,500 and up. The plan looks good if one does not become pregnant on the first try, but there is a much more rigorous screening program for people to enter the rebate program, based on one's age and the nature of fertility problems. The desperation for a child may cause individuals to overlook costs or not to do a careful examination of costs or entrance criteria to various rebate plans. It is true that doctors in such programs may do more to enhance the odds of a pregnancy and that the plans can save a couple some money. But they can also lose money if they do not examine all of the fine print; for example, there is no rebate if there is a pregnancy loss after the twelfth week.

The discussion of success rates of IVF procedures also raises ethical issues. I have already noted the problems associated with the lack of common definitions of success as well as of pregnancy, and the choice of one standard over another can greatly increase one's success rate. And this leads to a second problem: the use of such success rates as the basis for advertising, which leads to an increase in clientele and, in turn, to greater income for clinics. IVF clinics appear to be the "only branch of medicine doing success-rate advertising on this scale."[7] Five clinics have had to change advertising claims because of Federal Trade Commission interventions. While most people know to be at least moderately suspicious of advertising claims, these appeals are being made to a rather large and also desperate and vulnerable audience. While such individuals should not be prevented from attempting to have a child, clinics can be held to a strict disclosure standard for both success rates and the basis of their calculations.

A third ethical problem is related to the so-called older woman seeking IVF. Success rates for women forty and older drop by a half to three-quarters of the average rate; these women therefore need very specific information on success rates. Moreover, an increase in the number of women over forty seeking IVF has given rise to a market in eggs from younger women. Some of these come from younger women who successfully underwent IVF and did not need all the eggs that were harvested. Others come from egg donor programs that pay women several thousand dollars to undergo egg retrieval. Such eggs are now part of the advertising campaign. For example, in the January 13, 1997, issue of the *New Yorker*, the Genetics and IVF Institute in Fairfax, Virginia, advertised the availability of almost one hundred fully screened donors. While it is true that men have sold their sperm for decades for this purpose, the procedures for egg retrieval are dramatically different and expose the donor to the possibility of both short- and long-term health risks.

The Roman Catholic Ethical Perspective: "Donum Vitae"

In this section, I want to turn to a different, and perhaps unlikely, source for an evaluation of some ethical aspects of AR: the 1987 Instruction from the Congregation for the Doctrine of the Faith, "Donum Vitae" (DV). This source is unlikely because it prohibits almost every procedure in the area of AR. While I will eventually argue for the rejection of the core of DV's natural law argument, there are perspectives in this document that are helpful in evaluating the cultural context in which AR occurs as well as the culture of the clinics themselves. I will identify DV's opposition to AR and then turn to a discussion of its positive contributions.

The core argument is a reverse application of the traditional ethical argument used to prohibit artificial contraception. The argument is a classic natural law perspective that says, in the case of contraception, that to separate artificially the act of intercourse from its inherent biological reproductive teleology is to separate what God intended to be united. To separate the unitive and procreative dimensions is to violate the natural integrity of the total act of intercourse. When applied to assisted reproduction, the identical argument is used, but only in reverse. That is, to attain egg and sperm and to unite them in a petri dish and then to implant the zygote is artificially to break apart the inherent unity of the act of intercourse. Or to use the words of DV: "The Church's teaching on marriage and human procreation affirms the 'inseparable connection, willed by God and unable to be broken by man on his own initiative, between the two meanings of the conjugal act: the unitive meaning and the procreative meaning.'"[8]

Citing "Humanae Vitae," the congregation goes on to say that "it is never permitted to separate these different aspects to such a degree as positively to exclude either the procreative intention or the conjugal relation."[9] Finally, the congregation identifies the key ethical flaw in both artificial contraception and artificial conception: "Contraception deliberately deprives the conjugal act of its openness to procreation and in this way brings about a voluntary dissociation of the ends of marriage. Homologous artificial fertilization, in seeking a procreation which is not the fruit of a specific act of conjugal union, objectively effects an analogous separation of the goods of marriage."[10]

Essentially, the argument of DV met the same fate as that of its predecessor and source, "Humanae Vitae." The majority of commentators, Catholic and non-Catholic alike, reject the primacy given to a biological structure over the personal dimension of the act of married intercourse. This overly biological reading of natural law fits uneasily with the ethical standard suggested in the Vatican II document "Gaudium et Spes," which suggests that the moral norm is to be "the nature of the human person and his acts."[11] Many would argue that the key to moral analysis is whether the marriage as a whole is open to procreation, not whether an individual act is. And even here, the tradition notes exceptions. Beginning with "Casti Conntibi" and continuing through "Humanae Vitae," valid reasons for avoiding conception (without the use of artificial contraception, of course) included the health of the mother and the need to care for the welfare and education of one's current family. And much earlier Thomas Aquinas noted that reproduction was an obligation that fell on the species, not on any particular individual.

There is an irony in the moral analysis within DV: within the context of a marriage, two individuals are attempting to have a child. That is the object and intent of everything done within the context of AR. DV focuses only on the physical integrity of the act of sexual intercourse and ignores "the fact that husband and wife are seeking to become father and mother,"[12] which of course is what the tradition says is a goal of marriage. Why the physical integrity of the act should take moral priority over the intention of the husband and wife to become mother and father through the use of their own genetic material is both unexplained and unclear.

While the core argument of DV may be misplaced or wrong, the document does raise other features that can be helpful in thinking about the development and practice of AR. For example, DV recognizes that, thanks to scientific and medical progress, we have many more effective therapeutic resources available to us. But the document also notes that we "can acquire new powers, with unforeseeable consequences, over human life at its very beginning and in its first stages."[13] While DV uses this to argue for the prohibition of almost all reproductive technologies, that is not its only application. Research protocols do include the consideration of consequences, and therapeutic interventions are monitored for problems. But typically the focus is whether the intervention or procedure solves the problem. This occurs because our culture is results oriented: We want to solve the problem and we want to solve it now—or yesterday. Only when unforeseen or unintended consequences occur does the focus shift. As I have noted, very little research was done on IVF in humans before various procedures were put into widespread clinical application. Fortunately, the outcomes did not prove to be problematic with respect to the well-being of the children born of these processes and, generally speaking, with respect to the well-being of the women using the procedures. But that may be a matter of luck.

Nor should AR be used as a precedent for rapid clinical application of the next technology to be developed. We have a strong bias in this country to act and to refrain from critiques of people's actions. DV notes that we are faced with the "temptation to go beyond the limits of a reasonable dominion over nature."[14] The congregation is not arguing that we should not intervene in nature or seek therapeutic relief. Rather, it speaks to the dangers of overreach and of not thinking carefully before we act.

DV also notes that values cannot come exclusively from the science or technology itself: "It would on the one hand be illusory to claim that scientific research and its application are morally neutral; on the other hand one cannot derive criteria for guidance from mere technical efficiency, from research's possible usefulness to some at the expense of others or, worse still, from prevailing ideologies."[15]

Science and scientific research are not neutral activities. They are engaged in to achieve certain ends, and these ends are based on particular values. We need to examine why this particular line of research, why this particular project, why this application. And in answering these questions, we may learn that there are competing values: for example, service to the patient versus income stream. Certainly, individuals involved in IVF want to provide their patients with the best service possible. However, infertility is approximately a $350-million-a-year business. Competition for clients is keen. There is also competition between clinics to recruit successful physicians, who must then achieve even higher success to justify their salaries. In this context, primacy is not necessarily given to a patient's best interest. We need to go beyond the science of IVF and the values it bears to provide an appropriate evaluation of the practice.

Additionally, the congregation argues that "an intervention on the human body affects not only the tissues, the organs and their functions, but also involves the person himself on different levels."[16] Later, it approvingly quotes Pope John Paul II: "Thus, in and through the body, one touches the person himself in his concrete reality."[17] This points to several critical issues in contemporary medicine and particularly in assisted reproduction.

One is the tendency of modern medicine to objectify the body,[18] which began with the Cartesian perspective that the body was a machine. The Enlightenment tradition consolidated this perspective by focusing on the person as the essential self with the body as an external element, a machinelike addition. This reintroduced a Platonic dualism into philosophy that had been to a large extent overcome by Christianity's insistence on the unity of the person and the subjectivity of the body. For Christianity, it is only the living unity, a substantial union of body and soul, that is the person.

The important point here is that modern medicine has a philosophical perspective built into it. Ironically, that perspective has helped bring about enormous advances in modern medicine. Surgery, organ transplantation, the many visualization technologies, genetic engineering, and AR all rely, to some degree, on seeing the body as an object, as a composite of interchangeable parts or the sum of its parts. The problem occurs when we forget that this perspective has an embedded ideology that leads us to see ourselves in one dimension only: as object. Of course, one comes to the physician because of a problem and the desire to have it solved. But the problem exists within a person and may also raise a host of personal or psychosomatic issues. The particular problem can be solved technically, but the personal issues may remain.

For example, a man may discover that he has a low sperm count and that is the reason for the infertility. While a single sperm may be implanted in the egg and fertilization accomplished, he may feel inadequate, and such inadequacy may in fact be heightened by the continual presence of the child. Or the various tests and procedures for IVF may become routinized, and less attention paid to the woman who experiences these procedures and whose anxiety may be increasing as she gets deeper into the process. The procedures are not neutral somatic experiences. They are done in the context of biological abnormalities and a cultural context that disapproves of childlessness. If, additionally, they are done in isolation from the person's hopes, fears, and expectations, the person can be harmed even though the treatment was successful.

Particularly with IVF, there is the assumption that to cure the disease, repair the damage, or to circumvent the problem is to heal the person. The various technologies of AR, when successful, resolve childlessness but not infertility. Will the infertility that caused the childlessness still be a problem for the individual thus afflicted, as I noted above in the case of a man with low sperm count? Will the use of donor sperm or donor egg have an effect on the individuals or the couple? Or will the joy of the child remove any such difficulties? The fact that a pregnancy has been achieved does not necessarily resolve the totality of the problems associated with infertility: issues of identity, psychosocial integration, and, perhaps, feelings of inadequacy because of infertility.

An analogy is frequently made between individuals who achieve pregnancy through AR and those who have an ongoing condition such as diabetes, depression, or visual impairment. The symptoms of these chronic conditions may be resolved, but the underlying problem is not. Though insulin corrects the blood sugar and drugs may lift the depression, their very use and presence are daily reminders of one's problem. A decline in the ability to focus one's eyes for reading is a normal consequence of aging and is easily correctable by a trip to the local drugstore; nonetheless, the fact of our new and daily dependency on these glasses is a constant reminder of our aging. While some may take this in stride, for others it may be a major developmental crisis.

Thus the larger issue is the perception of the self and how that is related to the outcome of the treatment. For some, achieving a pregnancy and live birth may be enough. For others, the resulting child is a source of joy, but one's inability to do this without technical assistance may be a constant source of frustration. Infertility, even though resolvable, may be a severe blow to one's self-esteem. My point here is not to argue against the use of AR, but to remind us that we continuously need to think of the totality of the person, not just the biological functioning or the technical elements of a solution. If the main focus is on the techniques, if the biology becomes the center of attention, then IVF becomes much more production than reproduction. If the couple and their needs are kept to the foreground as much as possible, then the couple has a context in which to base and understand all the procedures that they will undergo. A great many of the procedures in which they will participate are very impersonal—and that is the way they must be. But if they can be made part of a larger process, grounded in the couple's relationship and their desire for a family, then some of the depersonalization can be softened and the impersonality of the procedures humanized. Even obtaining sperm, obviously not a high-tech procedure in most cases, can be very depersonalizing and difficult if thought of as a procedure and not within a personal context. Even having one's partner present or involved in the process maintains the presence and reality of a relationship. This affirms the procreative dimension much more than being sent to a room to "obtain a sample."

The couple using IVF is essentially doing what another couple is doing without IVF: cooperating in the creation of a new being from their love and their bodies. From a moral perspective, there is no difference between IVF and physical intercourse. The psychological difference, which has moral overtones, is that given the conditions under which IVF occurs there is a danger of depersonalization, of stressing the means over the end. What is critical here is the context in which IVF is done and keeping one's attention on the couple, their relationship, and their desire for a family. While this will not lessen all the tension, eliminate the pain, or resolve all the frustrations that come with IVF, the couple will at least have a critical moral center in which to understand what they are doing.

Finally, we need to consider the language of assisted reproduction. This term describes the procedure correctly. But there is a critical nuance between reproduction and procreation. Reproduction is a language of manufacture; it is a language of commodification. Procreation is the language of persons and personal engagement. Our language can shape our thinking, and if we use terms that connote objectification we may begin to think in terms of objectification. Of course, all the acts performed in AR are objectifications of the body or body parts. I am not arguing that such a process renders the acts unethical or invests them with a deep ethical flaw. But there is a tension between the technological procedures and language of IVF and its personal outcome. The former can make us forget the latter as well as serve to restructure our thinking because of the language we use to describe the process. The language and the techniques of IVF can help us forget that to touch the patient is to touch the person.

Mining the Resources

Let me conclude by reflecting on some broader issues related to Roman Catholicism, social ethics, and issues of public policy. I will not necessarily be arguing for a normative position on AR; Roman Catholicism has such a position, and I disagree with elements of it, as noted above. Rather, I will excavate the fundamental weaknesses of the official sexual ethic of Roman Catholicism and show why its social ethics are a better resource for responding to assisted reproduction. My aim is not to present a comprehensive or substantive position on AR, but to mine Catholic ethics for principles that are critical in this public policy debate.

NATURAL LAW

The premise of "Donum Vitae," as well as that of "Humanae Vitae," is natural law traditionally understood. Priority is given to biological processes and procedures in understanding the morality of sexual acts. Such a priority is essentially rejected by a majority of contemporary Catholic theologians and ethicists. In "Humanae Vitae" the moral grounding of the argument against artificial contraception is the inseparable connection between intercourse and conception. So too with "Donum Vitae." As previously noted, such an interpretation rejects or at least diminishes the moral significance of any intentionality on the part of the couple—for example, to have a child as a part of their marriage—and posits the sufficiency of the physical integrity of the biological act as determinate for the moral evaluation of their actions. In this perspective the goal of a family—at least a traditional part of the understanding of marriage—is held hostage to biology.

The priority of the physical over the personal is deeply imbedded in the modern ecclesiastical tradition. In his book *Love and Responsibility,* written while John Paul II was still Cardinal Karol Wojtyla, we find an example of this framework for the moral evaluation of human acts. The order of nature has its origin in God, "since it rests directly on the essences (or natures) of existing creatures, from which arise all dependencies, relationships and connections between them."[19] Thus the order of nature grounds morality. Or, as John Paul again states it, "But before and above all else man's conscience, his immediate guide in all his doings, must be in harmony with the law of nature. When it is, man is just towards the Creator."[20]

The clear message here is that moral integrity consists in discovering the metaphysical order embedded in the biological order and then conforming ourselves to both. Thus, not only does the natural law perspective as represented here call for caution and a sense of limits but also mandates a genuine nonintervention in the biological order. This overly biological view of natural law in turn shapes the Roman Catholic understanding of marriage. The primary focus is on the physical integrity of sexual relations between the couple, rather than how a couple might achieve a family within the context of their marriage or how marriage might contribute to the social good.

In spite of the efforts of the current pope to maintain this tradition, a slight, but significant, shift had already occurred. The Second Vatican Council took major strides forward in the theology of marriage by approving Paul VI's teaching that the procreative and unitive ends of intercourse were coequal, though morally inseparable. This again spoke to the issue of natural law. The council proposed, for example, this as the norm of human activity: "That in accord with the divine plan and will, it should harmonize with the genuine good of the human race, and allow men as individuals and as members of society to pursue their total vocation and fulfill it."[21] This was further specified by the assertion that by the very fact of being created, "All things are endowed with their own stability, truth, goodness, proper laws, and order."[22] The council walked a fine line here, arguing for the integrity of the created order but not that created things are independent of God or that "man can use them without any reference to the Creator."[23] It vacillated between a less biological and a more personalistic understanding of natural law, suggesting that while physical reality is important, one also needs to look at the good of humanity and one's vocation in that context.

This tension was not resolved, as was shown clearly when "Gaudium et Spes" discussed human reproduction. "Therefore when there is a question of harmonizing conjugal love with the responsible transmission of life, the moral aspect of any procedure does not depend solely on sincere intentions or on an evaluation of motives. It must be determined by objective standards."[24]

But the text goes on to say that these standards must be "based on the nature of the human person and his acts."[25] This part of the criterion, while rooted in the tradition, opened the way to a consideration of the person that incorporates more than the biology of his or her acts. But even this opening could not overcome the biologized understanding of natural law as the continuing standard for marital morality.

Given the tension that remained in the documents of Vatican II and the continued assertion of the definitive (some say infallible) character of "Humanae Vitae," it is no wonder that the priority of the physical over the personal is almost unconsciously assumed as correct. Such an assumption, however, neglects to account for almost thirty years of continuous critique of this position by leading Catholic theologians and ethicists. These critiques focus on whether to define the object of morality as one's intentions or the physical object. Do impersonal structures take precedence over personal acts? Can the goal of a family, which is a major element in the theology of marriage, be frustrated because of malfunctioning biology? The critique continues to recognize the importance of the biological dimension of the person. What it does differently is to argue that the biological should not be understood as a physiological process that is morally normative, but rather as the person's mode of presence in the world, a dynamic and developing reality, a body-self. Through this incarnational presence we are both present to and bound to the world, society, community, and the dynamic of history.

The continued focus on the biological skews the official teaching on marriage by focusing mainly on the sexual—understood mainly but not exclusively as a biological reality—rather than the personal or social-ethical dimension. Traditionally, however, the goods of marriage are defined in terms of sacramentality, family, and personal fulfillment—a formulation going back to Augustine. The focus on sacramentality looks to the presence of grace, expressed and experienced through the mutual love of the partners, and to the indissolubility of a valid marriage.

In the current code of canon law, marriage has been redefined as a covenant, not a contract. Covenant is the biblical term used to describe the love between God and Israel, which was extended to the relations between the people of the nation. This makes it possible to reconceptualize marriage within a more dynamic context, a more interpersonal framework, and to emphasize the graced dimension of all aspects of marriage, including the sexual. Thus, while much attention is focused on the indissolubility of marriage as a feature of its sacramentality, there is also a critical opening to develop a much more dynamic theology of marriage based on the covenantal union of persons.

Because the concept of covenant extends to the relation between the members of the community, it also carries with it a social dimension. Marriage can model the virtues needed to keep the community together, it can show the service needed to ensure a harmonious community, it can present a constructive use of sexuality, and so on. The roles of marriage in community become constitutive elements of marriage, not just afterthoughts.

Family remains a key issue for Catholics, as indeed it does for growing numbers of individuals and groups within society. A hallmark of traditional Roman Catholic social teaching about the family was that it was the cornerstone and basis of social life. And so it was in pre-Industrial Revolution Western countries. However, after the Industrial Revolution, socialization as well as the production of goods, services, and foods were transferred outside the family. Thus, the family changed from the cornerstone of society to one institution among many.

The response of the Catholic Church was to try to hold on to its tradition as long as possible, losing many opportunities to construct a teaching that both respected the tradition and responded to changing times. Thus, the tradition called for a living wage, but this was defined in terms of what the father of the family should be paid, assuming that the wife/mother would stay with the children. In something of a gesture to contemporary society, "Humanae Vitae" spoke of responsible parenthood—but only within the context of the traditional meaning of natural law.

The consequences of affirming the tradition in spite of a changing social world were twofold. First, the opportunity to address the positive dimension of the new social reality—as well as to critique its shortcomings—was missed. Calls for social reform, such as the emphasis on the living wage, were essentially strategies to restore the family to its status before the Industrial Revolution. Second, the changing role of women was not constructively addressed. Equality between men and women, even in current papal teaching, is defined metaphysically, not in terms of social roles and social conditions. The teaching that was developed was paternalistic; it sought to maintain women's role as the heart of the family and to protect them from the dangers of the outside world. Teaching about the family, then, has focused on the ethics of reproduction, rather than on creatively developing a theology of the family in the modern world. Encyclicals on women have been written and theologies of marriage and the family have been developed, but these have been done within the traditional context and with the traditional concepts. The argument aims to restore the past rather than to construct the future.

"Humanae Vitae" did provide some seeds of renewal by officially recognizing that the unitive end of marriage is coequal with the procreative end. Nonetheless, coequality of the unitive and procreative still means coequality, and this puts a burden on Catholic couples who discover they are infertile. These couples are told that a family is the fulfillment of marriage but are given few ways to achieve that. Thus, they may feel abandoned by the church at a time when they need the church most. Certainly adoption is an option, and many couples choose it. But the desire for a child of their own creation testifies to the embodied reality of marriage and to their relation with each other. While pregnancy through IVF may be one step removed from pregnancy through physical intercourse, adoption is yet another step removed. Thus, for the infertile Catholic couple, the reaching on the coequality of the procreative and unitive dimension of intercourse returns in a paradoxical way: given the depth of the unity in their marriage, a couple wishes to affirm the procreative dimension. But they are physically unable to do this and are told by the church that they are also morally unable to have children of their bodies through artificial means. Thus, the very positive teaching on the place of children in marriage frustrates this couple because they are not morally able to avail themselves of alternative means to this end.

Finally, the church's emphasis on childbearing, intensified by the pronatalist assumptions of American society, inhibits the couple from considering infertility anything other than a loss. Again, a tie to Catholic social ethics might be useful here in helping to remind the couple, as well as the church, that there are other forms of generativity and fruitfulness within the community. While the pain of the loss from infertility will remain, the opportunity to consider these others forms of generativity through a life of service to others might help transform that pain.

ROMAN CATHOLIC SOCIAL ETHICS AND REPRODUCTIVE ISSUES

Over the past century, Roman Catholicism has amassed a rather comprehensive corpus of social teachings in areas such as wage justice, human dignity, human rights, economic justice, justice in the conduct of war, civil rights, and capital punishment. These teachings have had a major impact on American society in a way that the sexual ethic has not: recall the substantive discussions and indeed reactions of the federal government both to "The Challenge of Peace" and "Economic Justice for All." To some extent, these teachings are built upon the edifice of natural law, particularly in the earlier encyclicals of Leo XIII and Pius XI. But human dignity and rights, based in the nature of the person rather than in biological nature, have played an increasingly critical role, particularly since John XIII's "Pacem in Terris." This trend continued, and in Vatican II the document "Gaudium et Spes" identified the person and his or her acts as a legitimate source of morality.

The first and most critical difference between Catholicism's social and sexual ethic is that the sexual ethic, based on the inviolability of biological structure, admits *no exceptions*. Thus, contraception is always wrong; IVF is always wrong. Social ethics are open to exceptions or compromise because they are based on obligations inherent in the relations of persons and institutions. Killing is wrong, except when in self-defense or when ordered by the state as in war or capital punishment. A living wage is mandatory but must be calculated with respect to a variety of social and economic circumstances. One way to explain this is to argue that in the field of social ethics, things are more complicated than with sexual ethics. The economic situation of a country is a complex phenomenon; foreign policy involves a host of difficult interactions. To consider these dimensions is not moral relativism, but an acknowledgment that complex situations require complex analysis.

But I would also argue that with regard to sexual ethics, things are not as simple as the tradition would suggest. For example, the decision of whether or not to have a child is a complex one. One or both prospective parents may have a history of genetic disease in their family. The woman may have a medical condition that could compromise her own health during pregnancy. The couple may have debts from their education that they wish to deal with. Or a couple may identify social service as a priority for their marriage. Recognizing that consequences and circumstances have a role in sexual ethics (unfortunately a forgotten part of the Catholic tradition) would go a long way in helping individuals think through in a responsible manner critical decisions they need to make. It would also have the merit of keeping such individuals in contact with the church and its teachings. While there will surely be actions that Catholicism will always prohibit, this approach would provide a more open mode of analysis and a more nuanced argument in that it appeals to a broader normative framework. It would remain faithful to the best instincts of the tradition but would also appreciate the moral dimensions of the dynamic social situation in which we find ourselves.

Roman Catholic social ethics can also make an enormous contribution to the question of health care in this country. Services for various reproductive technologies are but a subset of a much larger question of what services are covered by insurance and the even larger question of who is insured. Currently most people are insured through private payments, employment, or government programs such as Medicare or Medicaid. But there are large numbers of individuals who do not fit into these frameworks or who have inadequate coverage. A strong argument for universal coverage can be made from Roman Catholic sources: it is a basic matter of justice to citizens; it is in the best interests of the country as a whole; it is a long-term investment in a healthier population; it is an expression of care for the marginalized. Roman Catholic social ethics can argue strongly that the current system is unjust because so many are uninsured or underinsured, because benefits are distributed in favor of the wealthy or those fortunate enough to have employment, and because prevention is not adequately addressed.

If coverage is a justice question for Catholic social ethics, so too is financing such coverage. Roman Catholic social ethics could make a strong argument for federal funding of such programs, and for a variety of other funding sources. One could argue, as did Pius XI, that the government should provide insurance only until individuals are able to do so for themselves. It could also be argued that insurance is no longer what it was at the time of Pius XI and now should be provided by the state. Wherever one wishes to enter the coverage and funding debate, there are many ethical issues that Roman Catholicism could constructively address.

The more engaging question, given some sort of universal care, is what to include in the basic benefits package. Few would have trouble with a basic package oriented to prevention, with provisions for routine physicals, vaccinations, prenatal care, well-baby care, dietary advice, and so forth. Such interventions are relatively inexpensive and have long-term benefits. The problem comes when we move beyond these interventions to others, such as expensive diagnostic and screening technologies, organ transplants, kidney dialysis, and assisted reproduction. Procedures like these are in fact provided for by many insurance programs obtained through employment.

How ought reproductive technologies to fare within a system of universal coverage? This question is made difficult because of several unarticulated assumptions on health care held by most Americans: the funding barrel has no bottom; since I have insurance, I'm entitled to everything; quality health care means as much as possible for as long as possible. Catholic social ethics would seriously challenge all of these assumptions. And such a challenge will not be warmly received, as we saw during the disastrous debate over health care in 1993.

Roman Catholic ethics could argue, on the basis of justice and the common good, that access to AR should not be part of a basic package of universal health coverage. First, the shift from the traditional understanding of natural law to a more historically grounded understanding of the person would argue that biological procreation need not have a place of privilege in a marriage. Also, if marriage is no longer a contract that gives partners access to each other's bodies but a covenantal relationship, procreation becomes one among many goods of marriage, not necessarily the defining good. Marriage as a covenant has a more dynamic relation to society; in this context, we could recall the traditional teaching that reproduction is a species obligation, not an individual one. Thus, from a contemporary theology of natural law and of marriage, one can reasonably argue that reproduction is not essential to the integrity of a marriage. And if so, justice claims to including access to assisted reproduction in a basic health-care package are weakened.

A second relevant principle is the traditional Catholic concept of the common good. Here one would focus on individual rights in relation to the good of society as well as to the good of the individual. At its best, the concept of the common good is a way to mediate what society and the individual owe each other. One of the strong implications is that, while everybody should be able to participate in social life and to achieve their potential, everybody is not entitled to everything. The concept of the common good would prioritize prevention over cure or, in the case of assisted reproduction, over compensation for a problematic biological condition. It could, in justice, also restrict access to expensive, low-success, high-risk, nonvalidated therapies. Artificial reproduction is certainly expensive and has a relatively low success rate. Having a family historically has been important for individuals and has been strongly encouraged by the Catholic Church along with other religious organizations. Nonetheless, rethinking health insurance will force us to ask how central to individual fulfillment and desire, and how critical to the common good, is having a child of one's own body and partner. Is the provision of basic benefits to all not more important than ensuring that a small group has its reproductive desires fulfilled?

One solution, of course, would be to devise an insurance system so that individuals can, after receiving a basic package, buy other features such as coverage for artificial reproduction. Such a combination of private and public plans would certainly give the wealthy a major advantage. But if it were not totally inaccessible to the less wealthy, it would not be inherently unjust. From the perspective of Catholic social ethics, the key issue would be to ensure that the poor had access to services covered by the basic package. The question of access to other health-care options, however, would continue to be welcomed in the context of much larger questions of economic justice within the society.

As I have shown, Roman Catholicism can engage in a very critical public policy debate over AR without making any reference to its sexual ethic, which prohibits AR as unnatural. The more critical Catholic arguments would focus on the relative importance of biological childbearing, funding for research into artificial reproduction, access to reproductive clinics, the place of artificial reproduction in relation to other health-care services, and the status and role of children within our society. Catholicism has a vast treasury of social teachings that can be brought to bear on these and other questions, if it lets go of the traditional sexual ethic and develops a moral theology in dialogue with the past, but appreciative of contemporary issues and perspectives.

ENDNOTES

I want to thank in a very particular way Kathleen Sands for twice reading this manuscript with a very critical and constructive eye. Her comments have been helpful not only with respect to the organization of the overall argument, but also in terms of pushing the thrust of the argument forward. I am extremely grateful for her editorial and collegial assistance.

1. *New York Times*, October 18, 1996, B21.

2. *New York Times*, October 18, 1996, B21.

3. Clifford Grobstein, Michael Flower, and John Mendeloff, "External Human Fertilization: An Evaluation of Policy," *Science* 222 (October 14, 1983): 127.

4. Trip Gabriel, "High-Tech Pregnancies Test Hope's Limit," *New York Times*, January 7, 1995, A10.

5. Gabriel, "High-Tech Pregnancies," A11.

6. Ann Wozencraft, "It's a Baby, or It's Your Money Back," *New York Times*, August 25, 1996, B1.

7. Gabriel, "High-Tech Pregnancies," A11.

8. "Donum Vitae," 11, B-4. The citation can also be found in Thomas A. Shannon and Lisa S. Cahill, *Religion and Artificial Reproduction* (New York: Crossroad, 1988), 161.

9. "Donum Vitae," 11, B-4.

10. "Donum Vitae," 11, B-4.

11. "Gaudium et Spes," para. 51. The document can be found in David O'Brien and Thomas A. Shannon, *Catholic Social Thought: The Documentary History* (New York: Orbis Books, 1992), 200.

12. I am indebted to James Keenan for this insight. See his "Moral Horizons in Health Care: Reproductive Technologies and Catholic Identity," in *Infertility: A Crossroad of Faith, Medicine and Technology*, edited by K. Wm. Wildes (Netherlands: Kluwer Academic), 53–71, but especially see 61–62.

13. "Donum Vitae," introduction, I. Also see Shannon and Cahill, *Religion and Artificial Reproduction*, 1431.

14. "Donum Vitae," introduction, I. Also see Shannon and Cahill, *Religion and Artificial Reproduction*, 141.

15. "Donum Vitae," introduction, I, 2. Also see Shannon and Cahill, *Religion and Artificial Reproduction*, 143.

16. "Donum Vitae," introduction, I, 3. Also see Shannon and Cahill, *Religion and Artificial Reproduction*, 144.

17. "Donum Vitae," introduction, I, 3. Also see Shannon and Cahill, *Religion and Artificial Reproduction*, 144.

18. For an excellent overview of this perspective, see James F. Keenan, "Christian Per-

spectives on the Human Body," *Theological Studies* 55 (1994): 33o–46. His work illuminated several of my perspectives on this topic.

19. Karol Wojtyla, *Love and Responsibility*, trans. H. T. Willetts (New York: Farrar, Straus, and Giroux, 1981), 246.

20. Wojtyla, *Love and Responsibility*, 247. Italics in original.

21. "Gaudium et Spes," 209.

22. "Gaudium et Spes," 209.

23. "Gaudium et Spes," 209.

24. "Gaudium et Spes," 229.

25. "Gaudium et Spes," 229.

9

Theological Parameters: Catholic Doctrine on Abortion in a Pluralist Society

James J. Walter

No issue since the Vietnam conflict, or maybe since Prohibition,[1] has so plagued the American moral conscience as has abortion. The 1973 Supreme Court ruling on *Roe* v. *Wade* has plunged this country into what seems to be an endless—and nearly hopeless—polarization of extreme positions such that the American public has begun to lose confidence that any moral middle ground can be found. Many in society are numbed by the frequent revision of abortion laws at the federal and state levels, congressional proposals to prevent legal constraints on abortion,[2] Republican executive attempts to establish "gag rules," and the latter's recent reversal by President Clinton. We are told in nearly every survey that a majority of the American people believes that the Supreme Court went too far when it granted a Fourteenth Amendment right to an abortion. The abortion of 1.6 million fetuses each year becomes even more complex and debatable when public funds are used to finance these medical procedures.

Politicians have hardly been immune to the machinations of this debate. Not only have they been forced to state publicly their personal views, but in many cases their positions on abortion have become the litmus test for election. Possibly no group in society dreams more of the day when this controversy will go away than those running for public office. The situation is further complicated for those politicians who are Catholic. The legacy of the 1984 presidential election campaign still lingers. The intramural debate between John Cardinal O'Connor, the archbishop of New York, and Governor

Mario Cuomo and Congresswoman Geraldine Ferraro, the Democratic candidate for vice president, poignantly illustrates the additional pressures that Catholic politicians face.[3]

In an address at Georgetown University, William Byron, the outgoing president of the Catholic University of America, claimed that academics concerned with the protection of human life have much work to do. He argued that it is the academic's responsibility to clarify the philosophical foundations of the abortion issue and to provide those in public office with the reasoned arguments necessary to move this debate to higher ground.[4] To meet Fr. Byron's challenge, I offer my own reflections as a Catholic ethicist on the theological parameters that determine the Catholic Church's position on abortion.

The purposes of this chapter are both theological and practical. They are theological because I discuss the theological beliefs and value judgments that underlie the official church's moral position on abortion. I concentrate primarily on the official teachings of the Catholic Church, that is, the teachings from the authoritative magisterium. Consequently, I do not focus much attention on the theological perspectives and critiques offered by many contemporary Catholic theologians. In addition, my intent is not to discuss directly the *morality* of abortion; others have done this elsewhere.[5] Although the church's moral position on abortion is not solely based on religious views, an argument that I develop, theological beliefs about who God is and how God acts in the world nonetheless lie behind and influence the Catholic moral position.

My purpose is also practical in that I seek to help all politicians, but in particular those who are Catholic, to understand better the Catholic position on abortion and, in light of this understanding, to help them better negotiate the abortion controversy in a pluralist society. To this end, I highlight and briefly analyze some background issues related to abortion, for example, views of the human person and community, that become neuralgic points between the church's position and those positions embraced by our contemporary pluralist society.

Before I proceed, though, a few definitions of the terms in the title of this chapter are necessary. "Theology" is a discipline that reflects on religious experience and religious texts in order to understand. Theology is not faith itself, nor is it doctrine. Theological reflection proceeds from faith, and its object is an interpretation of the meaning of faith in a culture. As St. Anselm of Canterbury defined theology after the turn of the first millennium, it is *fides quaerens intellectum*, faith seeking understanding. "Doctrine" or teaching, on the other hand, is one moment in faith's attempt to say what is the case about reality, and thus doctrine establishes the common beliefs of a church about what is true, real, and valuable.[6] However, only a few doctrines are considered irreformable or infallible (dogmas) in the Catholic tradition, while most others possess various levels of authoritative but noninfallible weight.

Similar to its root meaning in mathematics, I use the word *parameter* to signify "a constant or a variable" that determines the Catholic Church's moral position on abortion. Actually, there are several theological parameters that come together in a complex form to make up the church's teaching. I show that there are several theological and moral beliefs that constitute the *substance* of the Catholic position on abortion. These basic affirmations and value judgments about God, humans, and the world go to the very core of the tradition, and they are what have been explicitly taught or implied in various doctrines. They are the "constants"; they neither can nor should change if the church is to remain faithful to its own tradition.

On the other hand, basic beliefs are always further interpreted and applied in detail to concrete situations and circumstances of human life. Although these further interpretations and applications may take regular form, appear over a long period of time, and even find themselves somehow articulated in doctrines, they do not have the same status in the tradition as the basic beliefs and value judgments.[7] As important and necessary as they may be, interpretations-applications are "variables," that is, by nature they are open to change or reformulation.[8] Such a claim should not be construed to imply that every further interpretation must necessarily be changed; rather, the claim simply implies that a development of doctrine on concrete moral issues within the Catholic Church is indeed possible.

I am aware that what I have called basic beliefs and value judgments (constants) are themselves interpretations. However, I would argue that they differ from interpretations-applications (variables). The latter are either second-level interpretations or applications of basic beliefs about God, humans, and the world. For example, I may hold to the basic theological belief that God's presence and power are not only transcendent to but also immanent in the world. Thus, I may believe that God is related to or acts immanently in the world (constant), but then I may interpret *how* God acts in the world by holding the further belief that God possesses certain rights to act in areas of human life analogous to how human agents possess rights to act in the world (variable). On the basis of this second-level interpretation—God is another actor in the world with certain rights to act—I might infer or somehow derive a moral principle, which itself is a further interpretation, that embodies my understanding about how God acts immanently in the world. For example, I might infer the moral principle that human agents may never directly kill an innocent person from my theological belief that only divine activity possesses legitimate power, dominion, and rights over the life and death of innocent persons. Finally, I may apply the moral principle to a concrete instance of human behavior (e.g., abortion) and prohibit the action on the basis of my theological interpretations. As I argue, the second-level interpretation that God acts in the world with certain rights—that is, in a way similar to how human agents act—is open to change or reinterpretation. It should be obvious that any strict application of a second-level interpretation to a moral issue would also be variable in the sense that I am using the term here.

I show that there are four theological parameters that function in the magisterium's position on abortion: anthropological, ethical, value, and legal. In each parameter there are both constants and variables, as difficult as it may be to distinguish these two in practice. If true dialogue is to go forward between Catholic and other positions on abortion in society, then anyone thoughtfully engaged in this dialogue must take notice of what is the substance and what is an interpretation-application of the tradition.

Finally, there is the term *pluralist*. By pluralist I mean that there are multiple and competing views and convictions about the nature of persons, society, morality, and so forth that function at the public level in society. A priori, none of these views is considered true, and de facto none commands universal public acceptance. In fact, each view must compete in the public arena for attention, and persuasion is the vehicle by which any one of these views is accepted. Not only is secular society pluralist in this country, but there is a certain plurality of positions within and between the various Christian churches on concrete issues such as abortion.[9] Consequently, one of my practical purposes is to concentrate on those points of convergence and divergence—points of agreement and disagreement—between the Catholic tradition and society's pluralist position on abortion. Throughout the chapter, I hope to offer politicians some horizons and perspectives on the interaction of the Catholic position within a pluralist society.

BRIEF SUMMARY OF THE CATHOLIC CHURCH'S MORAL TEACHING ON ABORTION

My intention in this section is to present a concise summary of the Catholic magisterium's moral position on abortion. I am interested neither in debating this moral position nor in establishing its validity; rather, I am interested only in stating what this position is, in assessing the status and authoritative weight of the teachings that proclaim the position, and in analyzing the various sources that the magisterium draws on in formulating its position.

Moral Position

Historically, the Christian tradition in general has approached the abortion issue with great respect for all human life. Though there is very little explicit evidence from the Hebrew and Christian scriptures that would warrant an absolute prohibition of abortion,[10] it is clear from many texts that every life is valued because of its relation to God's creative activity (e.g., Gen. 4:1; Job 31:15; Isa. 44:24; Jer. 1:5). Very early in the Christian era, however, we begin to find many writers condemning abortion—for example, the author of the *Didache*, Tertullian, Jerome, and Augustine. Surely, these early Christian authors not only wanted to distance the Christian community from the pagan practices of abortion and infanticide but also to call the members of this community to imitate the love that God has for all human life, especially for innocent human life. Despite the centuries-long debate over when the human soul is infused into the body (animation), and thus exactly when the fetus becomes a person, the Catholic tradition has consistently condemned abortion from the time of conception as a grave sin, even though the penalties for aborting an animated fetus were greater than those for aborting an unanimated one.[11]

The deep respect for and the protection of all human life have come down through the centuries to be formulated into a moral norm that has been proclaimed often by the modern magisterium. The moral norm as we find it formulated in many recent documents can be succinctly stated as: all direct killing of innocent human life either as a means or as an end is morally wrong. I leave to another section the discussion of what precisely constitutes *direct* killing as a means or as an end and why these acts are absolutely prohibited on theological and ethical grounds. What is important here is the tradition's evaluation of both the moral status (value) of all unborn life and the claims that this life makes on us. At the outset, it is important to note that the Catholic tradition has never taught any definite philosophical position on when the human soul is infused, and thus when the fetus becomes a *person*.[12] Nonetheless, it is the case that the tradition has viewed all unborn life as "innocent," and it has stated in the recent "Instruction on Respect for Human Life" that from the moment of conception the life that is present at all stages of development must be treated *as a person*.[13] In other words, although the tradition has not definitively defined when nascent life becomes a person, all human life from the moment of conception must be treated and respected as the *moral equivalent* of a person. No matter at which stage of development, the unborn life is granted an identical ethical value,[14] and it must "be respected in an absolute way."[15] Consequently, all unborn life makes a moral claim on us to respect its fundamental right to life.[16]

Status and Authoritative Weight of the Teachings

Teachings on the respect for human life at all its stages and on the corresponding presumption against taking human life are long-standing, authoritatively proclaimed by the church, and consistently expressed in both papal and conciliar texts. This set of doctrines is certainly central to the core of the Catholic Christian tradition. They state not only that life itself is truly a fundamental value but also what moral attitudes and dispositions we should have toward life.

On the other hand, a question arises about the status and authoritative weight of a second set of teachings. These doctrinal claims are concerned with the probability of the human soul (animation) being present from the time of conception, the teaching in the "Instruction" that all unborn life is the moral equivalent of a person, and the teaching that all direct abortions are morally wrong. Concerning the last of these doctrines at least, some of the recent documents that I have briefly surveyed claim that this teaching has not changed and is unchangeable.[17] It would take me too far afield to discuss all the ramifications of a claim such as this,[18] but I would state succinctly that none of these teachings has the same status as the first set mentioned above. Nor does any of them constitute the core of the Catholic tradition. They are either second-level interpretations or applications—and thus variable parameters—that attempt to make concrete the more general and central attitudes and value judgments taught in the first set of doctrines, that is, constant parameters. Consequently, the weight of the second set of teachings is not as substantial as those in the first set.[19]

Sources of the Moral Position: Reason and Revelation

One of the distinguishing characteristics of the Roman Catholic tradition is the way that it uses the resources of both reason and revelation in approaching moral issues. Its basic conviction is that in the moral order it is neither reason alone nor faith alone that discovers the truth. Rather, it is reason *and* faith; better stated, it is reason informed by faith. Because the basic values of the moral life are available to all people of goodwill and knowable through rational insight and reflection, the conclusions reached on specific issues as abortion are not *logically* dependent on Christian religious beliefs.[20] Consequently, one of the more common misperceptions in the public debate over abortion is that the Catholic Church has sought to impose a specifically religious morality on society. Though the Catholic position is nourished and supported by religious resources, the condemnation of all direct abortions is not established exclusively on the basis of these resources.

Historically, the Catholic tradition has relied on Thomas Aquinas's theory of natural law as a way of formulating its position on the ability of reason to discern objective morality. Although Aquinas's synthesis is a second-level interpretation, and therefore variable, what is central to the Catholic tradition are its claims that humans are intelligent, that reality is intelligible, and that reality, when grasped by intelligence, imposes on the person an objective moral obligation. The commitment of the tradition to the position that morality is both objective and available to reason is one basis for why all recent magisterial documents on morality, even those specifically devoted to abortion, include a separate section on rational (i.e., natural law) arguments against certain actions.[21]

The claims that objective morality is available to human insight, however, do not make the resources of faith irrelevant to moral decision making. As the "Pastoral Constitution on the Church in the Modern World" ("Gaudium et Spes") asserted, "For faith throws a new light on everything, manifests God's design for man's total vocation, and thus directs the mind to solutions which are fully human" (11). The resources of explicit faith and revelation enable us to know more clearly and fully the nature of human persons and their worth, but they do not bypass what reason has arrived at, nor do they add new content in terms of general values and obligations to the moral life.[22] Because the Catholic tradition does not hold to an exclusively religious position on abortion, any charge that the church is merely imposing a religious morality on others in society is false. Consequently, Catholics, whether they are speaking as citizens or as politicians, should not cast the tradition's position in purely religious terms. Dialogue between the magisterium's position on abortion and other positions in society is possible based on rational reflection and moral argument.

THEOLOGICAL PARAMETERS

I would like to turn now to the four theological parameters that lie behind and determine to a great extent the official church's moral position on abortion. The parameters are theological in the sense that they all imply basic beliefs and value judgments about God, humanity, and the world. These beliefs and value judgments are also interrelated. For example, the sacredness of human life, which is a basic judgment about the value of human life, is an implication of Christian convictions about who God is. The theological interpretation of how God is related to and acts in human history—that is, a theology of divine providence—underlies the church's view of human authority over the taking of human life, especially innocent life. As I have stated above, some elements within each of these parameters are constants because they constitute the substance of the tradition, and some elements in each are variables because they are second-level interpretations or applications of more fundamental and basic perspectives. While analyzing each parameter, I briefly compare its contents with what I understand to be the dominant societal views on the respective issues. By "societal views" I mean the beliefs and positions that appear to operate at the public or social level, albeit these positions may not necessarily operate at or even inform the more personal or private level of people's lives. My purpose here is to locate points of agreement and disagreement between the two perspectives so that an informed discussion of the morality of abortion might proceed toward a more intelligent and comprehensive public policy.

Anthropological Parameter

This parameter is concerned with the tradition's basic beliefs about who the human person is, the general condition or situation of humanity as a whole, and the value accorded to human life. These beliefs, as I have already indicated, are intimately related to and rely on theological beliefs and convictions about who God is and how the divine relates to the created order.

There are several theological doctrines that come to bear on this parameter. The doctrine of creation is a coherent combination of basic affirmations about the created nature of all that is, that there is a divine creator whose presence is both transcendent to but also immanent in this creation, that humankind is created in the image and likeness of the divine other, and that humans are essentially free creatures who share responsibility in the unfolding nature of God's creative act. This doctrine also affirms the fundamental unity of the human body and spirit, and it professes that true humanity is found only in human community.

The doctrines of the fall, of the covenantal relationship between humanity and God, of the incarnation of Jesus Christ, of redemption, and of God's call to an ultimate future (eschatology) also contribute to and fill out the tradition's theological anthropology. Though all humanity is fallen due to human fault and continues to be prone to sin, the imperfection and sin that now infect our personal and social lives are neither all-pervasive nor ultimately victorious. All humanity is called again into a covenantal relation with God, and this covenant reaches its fulfillment in the incarnation of Jesus the Christ. This man, who is both fully human and fully divine, took upon himself all human malice by freely accepting the cross. The redemption of all humanity, which was wrought through the death and resurrection of Jesus, not only heals us but it becomes the primary symbol of God's call for all to participate in the fullness of the divine future. God's eschatological future, which contains the fullness of all the created order and human history, is already partially present here and now in the preaching of the good news and in the personal and social relations that we create with one another.[23]

The theological convictions about the nature, situation, and future of humanity both entail and generate basic value judgments about human life in general and about innocent human life in particular. Though these value judgments are deeply informed and supported by the scriptures and a doctrinal tradition, the Catholic Church has consistently argued that the values themselves are available to rational human insight and reflection. Based on the privileged insight into the nature of true humanity, the resources of faith do enable Christians to articulate human values more clearly. However, religious resources themselves are not the origin of these values, that is, human values are neither divinely revealed nor in principle discoverable only by believers.

The most fundamental value judgment that applies to the discussion of abortion is concerned with the dignity and sanctity of each human life. The Catholic tradition has consistently affirmed this value judgment, as has the Christian tradition in general. The inherent and equal value of each human life is inferred from the beliefs that we are created in the image of God, redeemed by Jesus, and called to a future destiny with God. What is noteworthy here is that the value judgment itself is based not on one Christian doctrine alone but on a series of doctrines, namely, creation, incarnation-redemption, and eschatology.[24] What is also noteworthy is that the theological or doctrinal grounding of this value judgment has not precluded the Catholic tradition from arguing that the value of human life can also be founded on humanist or rational grounds.[25]

Historically, a further specification of this general value judgment has been made to apply to *innocent* human life. In this case, all innocent life is valued as absolutely inviolable.[26] Because all nascent life is classified in this category, the fetus's life possesses this inviolable status. Now, two further interpretations have been added to this value judgment that fill out the Catholic position on abortion. The first interpretation, which I have already noted above, is that human life from the moment of conception must be respected and treated *as a person*.[27] This means that the fetus, like every other person, must be treated as possessing the fundamental right to life. The second interpretation, which is formulated as a moral principle, is that fetal life may never be directly taken, just as no other *innocent person's life* may be directly taken either as a means or as an end. As I show later, the latter interpretation-principle is most often justified by reference to the theological affirmation that God alone is the lord of life and death.[28] What is both interesting and important here, however, is that this theological justification is used only when innocent life is at stake. I am not aware of any other instance of killing in which this theological affirmation is used to prohibit a deadly deed, for example, in cases of capital punishment, self-defense, and just war.

One further set of issues must be examined briefly before proceeding to a description and analysis of the anthropology that appears to predominate in U.S. secular society. These issues are concerned with the tradition's evaluations of the role of human freedom and choice, on the one hand, and of the responsible use of modern technology, on the other. These two evaluations are interconnected in the abortion debate, and both are determined to a large extent by the church's theological anthropology and by a specific, but revisable, interpretation of divine providence.

First, the level of freedom that I am addressing is the capacity to choose. In the Catholic tradition, freedom is only the presupposition or the *conditio sine qua non* for an action to enter into the moral order; the fact that a person has freely chosen to do something does not in itself make an action moral or immoral. As I show below, this is important because some people in society hold to the view that the freedom to choose is not only an absolute value but that it alone is what makes actions right or wrong.

Second, a more problematic issue arises when one places human freedom in the context of modern technology and its application to issues of life and death. To rephrase the problem in terms of a question, one might ask—as the Catholic tradition has repeatedly done since the beginning of this century— should issues concerned with the beginnings of human life and with death be subjected to human choice and the application of technology?[29] In other words, do humans have the right to use technology over the origin and destiny of the human person? This is an important question because, as David Thomasma has rightly noted,[30] the responsible use of technology is the nub of the ethical problem with abortion.

In general, the Catholic Church has evaluated the development and application of technology as at least ambiguous. Particularly in this century, one of the central concerns of the church has been to protect the dignity and sanctity of the human person against the onslaught of burgeoning technology. Science and technology must be constantly evaluated in light of the fundamental criteria of the moral law, that is, according to whether they are in the service of the human person.[31]

Has God shared divine power with humanity to intervene into the very processes of the generation of human life or to take life? This is a complex question, and it would require a more detailed analysis than I can provide here. However, the tradition's answer to the question is in the negative, at least as far as *innocent* human life is concerned. In the abortion debate, when humans use their freedom to employ technology in such a way as to directly take innocent life, they act from the lack of a legitimate right (*ex defectu juris in agente*), and their actions are judged to be intrinsically immoral. The theological position on divine providence adopted by the church has been that God, as the lord of life and death, has decided to withhold from humanity the power over, and thus the right to kill, innocent human life. However, God has delegated to certain members of the human community (e.g., government officials or soldiers) the right to kill noninnocent human life. Thus, within the Catholic Church there is more at stake in the abortion debate than merely the *moral* issue of directly killing innocent life. It also involves the *theological* issue of the life and death of the innocent being subject to human choice and technology within the context of a specific second-level interpretation of divine providence.[32] The obvious theological question that must be raised here is whether God has really reserved divine power over the life and death of the innocent, or whether, similar to all other areas of human choice, God has shared even this power with humanity so that the fate of the unborn is truly subject to *free* but *responsible* human choice.[33]

If we turn now to an analysis of the dominant anthropological views of U.S. society, what we find is a different interpretation of the nature of the human person and of human freedom and technology than that found in the Catholic tradition. The value judgments that flow from this secular anthropology are sometimes at variance with the church's judgments on several key issues.

Robert Bellah and his colleagues have appropriately described the dominant anthropology in the United States as individualism. They borrow a quotation from Alexis de Tocqueville to define individualism as "a calm and considered feeling which disposes each citizen to isolate himself from the mass of his fellows and withdraw into the circle of family and friends; with this little society formed to his taste, he gladly leaves the greater society to look after itself."[34] Further refined, individualism becomes ontological in that citizens believe "that the individual has a primary reality whereas society is a second-order, derived or artificial construct."[35] Lying at the very core of modern American culture, individualism has increasingly pursued individual rights and personal autonomy in contrast to the biblical view of the essential sociality and interrelatedness of the human family.[36] The liberal secular view does exalt the value of human dignity, and in this regard it would agree with the Catholic tradition. However, this liberal ethos interprets human dignity and its sacredness in an individualist and rights-oriented way. Consequently, the emphasis on protecting the individual's right to privacy generates the normative value judgment that, "[A]nything that would violate our right to think for ourselves, judge for ourselves, make our own decisions, live our lives as we see fit, is not only morally wrong, it is sacrilegious."[37] In assessing this perspective, Richard McCormick has accurately stated that "The good life—and eventually the morally right and wrong—is irreducibly pluralistic, because it is tied to individual preferences, which are precisely individual."[38] The result is that genuine public discussion of complex moral issues such as abortion is thwarted, and so each person retreats into his or her own moral world where individual preferences hold sway. In this private world, morality becomes a matter of personal taste about which there can be little or no rational, public argument.

Joseph Tamney and his coauthors have argued that the defense of legalized abortion is rooted in individualism.[39] In attempting to increase the zone of privacy, American society has pursued the libertarian desire to limit the role of government.[40] In this sense, liberal society cherishes the Enlightenment stress on freedom *from* external constraint and authority.[41] Whereas the Catholic perspective has sought to place limits on the exercise of human freedom in its interpretation of divine providence, individualism has steadily fought to extend the role of freedom to include control over one's body and the fate of unborn life. In this sense, liberal society cherishes the modern technological emphasis on the freedom *to* control and to have dominion over the self and world. Freedom to choose is not merely the necessary condition for an action to be assessed morally, as it is in the Catholic tradition; freedom to choose alone is both necessary and sufficient in itself to make an action morally right.[42] The result is that individual freedom, understood now as autonomy and enshrined legally in the constitutional doctrine on privacy, not only is viewed by many as the central value at stake in the debate over abortion, but, as we shall see later, it trumps every other value in situations of conflict between maternal and fetal lives.[43]

As inveterate pragmatists, U.S. citizens place a high value on technology and its application to solve human problems. Their imaginations and feelings are so shaped by technology that they view the world through what Daniel Callahan has called the "power plasticity" model of reality.[44] The world and we are malleable, and the answer to both personal and social problems is to intervene with increasing technology. It is not difficult to conclude from this view of reality that technology creates its own morality based on human control and the imposition of free human choice. The development and use of technology in modern medicine, especially in the emergence of neonatal medicine, embryology, and genetics, now control the very way that the whole abortion debate is framed.[45] Even the establishment of the time of viability by the Supreme Court in 1973 was itself controlled both by the general inability of medicine to care for fetuses whose gestational age was less than twenty-eight weeks and by the techniques available to determine genetic defects.

This brief review of the two different anthropologies and the value judgments that flow immediately from each of them was constructed to highlight some of the neuralgic points between the Catholic tradition and society's position on abortion. Failure to attend to the radical differences that endure at this level of the debate will inevitably continue the gridlock that we experience today. Though it is important to focus analyses at the *moral* level of this debate where questions of rightness and wrongness of abortion must be discussed, I have attempted to show that these analyses rely on deeper and more profound *anthropological* and *theological* analyses and basic value judgments that undergird and inform the moral level.

Ethical Parameter

The second theological parameter that informs the Catholic position on abortion is ethical. The magisterial condemnation of all direct abortions is a complex normative judgment, and it is based on two distinct sources: one is an ethics that connects sex and procreation, and the other is an ethics of killing the innocent.[46] The tradition has argued that the conclusions of both ethics are grounded in a natural-law theory of morality, and so it is assumed by the magisterium that these normative judgments are in principle open to the ethical insight of all people of goodwill. Despite this assumption, however, many in society intensely disagree with the Catholic position on these two ethics. It is possible that only a minority of people in the United States believe that there is a necessary or essential link between sexual relations and procreation. Furthermore, one of the most disputed issues in the abortion debate among feminists and others who support a pro-choice stance concerns the value or innocence of the fetus. Consequently, the official Catholic position on the value of nascent life has been repeatedly rejected in favor of the value of the woman's right to choose.

The Ethics of Sex and Procreation

The substance of the Catholic position on sex is that human sexuality is created by God and therefore constitutes a basic human good. It is a great gift from God by which humans share in the creative activity of the divine. Sexuality is neither divine nor is it demonic, but it can be turned to the service of God's kingdom.[47] The fact that Jesus took on all of human nature, including sexuality, testifies to the essential goodness of human sexuality. When this view of sexuality was made more concrete in the fourth and fifth centuries to counteract negative evaluations of the body and of procreation espoused by various factions, St. Augustine formulated second-level interpretations to protect the biblical and Christian view. These interpretations described human sexuality as created by God solely for the sake of procreation.

In the thirteenth century, Thomas Aquinas undertook the task of constructing a systematic and theological theory of natural law in which he argued that God had placed the sexual inclination in humans, just as God had done in the animal kingdom, for the sake of reproducing the species.[48] Noteworthy here is how Thomas interpreted God's creative intentions vis-à-vis human sexuality. He believed that some divine purposes for humanity are embodied in the nature of biological acts, for example, sexual intercourse. Since God is the author of nature, to act against the divine purposes in nature was a direct affront against God. Aquinas defined the natural law as a participation of God's eternal law in a rational creature. At the level of the natural law that pertains to procreation, he argued that all humans absolutely know what the Creator had intended when they engage in sexual intercourse.[49] The Thomistic positions on the natural law and on the ethics of sexuality were frequently adopted by subsequent theologians and popes.[50] Later, another second-level interpretation developed concerning the inseparable link between the unitive and procreative aspects of sexual intercourse. The application of this interpretation, which was formulated into a moral principle, prescribed that *each and every act* of marital sexual intercourse must be both an expression of love (unitive significance) *and* open to procreation.[51]

The import of this ethic of sex for our purposes is that all direct abortions sever what was willed by God as an inseparable link between sexual activity and procreation. Consequently, on the basis of this ethic the magisterium would condemn any action that intentionally terminates a pregnancy. Though the ethic is based on a theological understanding of natural law and thus God's purposes for humanity, again the tradition has consistently argued that the moral judgments that flow from this theory are available to all people.

The Ethics of Killing the Innocent

The second ethic that applies to abortion in the Catholic tradition is the ethics of killing the innocent. Here, we enter into the very heart of the magisterium's moral and theological position on abortion. It is also here that we encounter the absolute or exceptionless rule prohibiting all direct killing of the innocent either as a means or as an end. Theologically, the magisterium's interpretations of divine providence, the divine-human relation, the nature and scope of God's dominion and authority over life and death, and the significance of redemptive suffering are the background to this ethic.

The Catholic Christian position has consistently understood human life to be a great and fundamental good, and consequently it has constantly taught the presumption against the taking of all human life. It seems to me that both this value judgment and the presumption against taking life make up the substance of the tradition.[52] On the other hand, the tradition has developed second-level interpretations to deal with conflict situations. Thus, the church has morally permitted the taking of human life, for example, in self-defense, just war, and capital punishment. The theological defense of this position is that God has delegated to humans the authority and responsibility in some circumstances to take noninnocent life, and the ethical rationale of the position can be traced back to a moral judgment about what would occur if all killing were forbidden. Theologically and ethically, the problematic issue in general is the killing of any innocent human life, but more specifically it is the *direct* killing of innocent life. Because the tradition morally permits the *indirect* killing of the innocent, it is erroneous to say that the Catholic Church absolutely prohibits *all* abortions. In approaching this complex and problematic area in the Catholic tradition, it might be best first to define what "innocent" means and then to indicate briefly how the magisterium determines the directness or indirectness of killing through a discussion of the principle of double effect.

Though historically the term is not absolutely clear,[53] "innocent" has been used to place a limit on the prohibition against killing to instances where no material injustice was involved.[54] When Aquinas discussed the case of killing the innocent, he prohibited such taking of life because the righteous person does nothing to harm the community or the common good of society.[55] Thus, the innocence of a person seems to be morally determined on the basis of the absence of injustice being perpetrated on another person or on the community. Because the tradition has argued that the fetus in no way perpetrates any kind of injustice on either society or on the mother, even if it threatens maternal life by developing in an extrauterine site, the Catholic Church judges all fetal life to be innocent life and thus inviolable from direct attack.

Notwithstanding its inviolability from direct assault, the fetus's life can be taken in certain circumstances of conflict. To understand how and why exceptions are made to the taking of innocent life, we must turn to a discussion of the principle of double effect.[56] This moral principle, which itself is a second-level interpretation of the conditions under which the presumption against killing can be limited, was established to deal with actions that produce more than one effect in conflict situations. It presumes that one effect of the action is good and that the other is evil, and then it seeks to determine if the *action* can be performed in such a way that the evil effect—for example, death of the innocent—is not traced back to the will or intention of the agent. The principle is not applicable to just any action that produces two effects, one good and the other evil; it applies only to a certain class of actions whose evil *effect* is already judged to be *morally* evil.[57] In the issue of abortion, the actions that produce a morally evil effect are those performed from a lack of a legitimate right on the part of the human agent (*ex defectu juris in agente*). For these actions to be morally performed, and thus for the evil effect to be tolerated or permitted, all four conditions of the principle of double effect must be fulfilled. If the conditions are fulfilled, then the deadly act against the innocent is considered an indirect act of killing. On the contrary, a violation of any of the four conditions presumes that the agent intended the death of the innocent either as a means or as an end, and thus the action is prohibited absolutely.

The following are the four conditions of the principle of double effect:

1. The action, considered by itself and independently of its effects, must not be morally evil;
2. The evil effect must not be the means of producing the good effect;
3. The evil effect is sincerely not intended, but merely tolerated; and,
4. There must be a proportionate reason for performing the action, in spite of its evil consequences.[58]

In the twentieth century, the tradition has applied this principle to the potentially fatal cases of ectopic pregnancy and of a pregnant but cancerous uterus. Recently, the principle has been applied to instances of maternal hemorrhage during pregnancy and of all extrauterine pregnancies.[59] Surgical measures to save the mother's life are permitted in these situations even when fetal death is certain because the physician's action is aimed at curing a life-threatening condition of the woman. The mother's life is preserved by such actions without procuring the death of the fetus as the means to this end. If the medical procedure has only one effect—that is, the death of the fetus—or if it produces the good effect through or by means of the fetus's death, then the tradition assumes that the physician intended or wanted to kill innocent life. In the latter cases, the action is judged to be a direct abortion, and it is absolutely prohibited in every situation of conflict.

The ethics of killing the innocent, as interpreted and applied through the principle of double effect, is in fact a moral construct that is derived or inferred from a specifically theological interpretation of God's providence. The recent "Instruction on Respect for Human Life" has increasingly convinced me that the magisterium has adopted a rather anthropomorphic image of God in its theological interpretation of God's dominion and lordship over the life and death of the innocent.[60] This image construes God anthropomorphically by implying that the divine acts in the world in ways that are similar to how human agents act.[61] In other words, when God providentially acts in the world, the divine possesses certain rights and has a specific "place" in which to act. For example, one of the central reasons why the "Instruction" condemns the voluntary destruction of human embryos in *in vitro* fertilization is because "By acting in this way the researcher usurps the *place of God*; and, even though he may be unaware of this, he sets himself up as the master of the destiny of others inasmuch as he arbitrarily chooses whom he will allow to live and whom he will send to death and kills defenseless human beings."[62]

Not only does this image portray God as having a place to act, but it depicts the divine as possessing specific rights that belong exclusively to the divinity. The "Instruction" states, "Human life is sacred because from its beginning it involves 'the creative action of God,' and it remains forever in a special relationship with the Creator, who is its sole end. God alone is the Lord of life from its beginning until its end: No one can in any circumstances claim for himself the right to destroy directly an innocent human being."[63] What is implied in this quotation is the narrowing of the prohibition against direct killing to innocent life. In other situations of conflict, the tradition permits the killing of human life, and this is justified on the basis that God has delegated to certain members of the human community the right to kill. As Jan Jans has argued, "If to speak of delegation, therefore, is to have any sense, it can only mean that God possesses certain categorical rights, which normally belong to Him exclusively, but which under circumstances can be delegated to humans."[64] On the other hand, God has not delegated to any member of the human community the divine right to directly kill innocent life, and thus God remains the sovereign over the life and death of the innocent. Consequently, it seems that the wrongfulness of directly killing a fetus is not derived from the intention of causing death; it is morally wrong on the theological grounds that God has not authorized such killing.[65] To act without divine authorization is to act from the lack of a legitimate right, and such actions are judged to be intrinsically morally wrong.[66] Because the indirect killing of the innocent does not violate God's sovereignty,[67] it can be licitly performed to save the life of another, the pregnant woman.[68]

One final issue remains to be discussed briefly at this point. The theological interpretation of God's dominion entails a theological corollary in the Catholic tradition. This corollary is concerned with an interpretation of the meaning and relevance of redemptive suffering. The tradition has taught that suffering is part of the human condition, but it is multiplied and made worse by sin. In most cases suffering ought to be relieved by human efforts, but in some situations it can and must be accepted redemptively. It seems that this is the substance of the Catholic tradition. However, when suffering can and should be alleviated, and when it must be redemptively endured, are determined not on theological grounds but on the basis of moral criteria. How the tradition determines when suffering is to be tolerated is dependent on a second-level interpretation that is itself open to reformulation.

When their actions conform to the moral law, human agents are considered to be cocreators with God. As cocreators they have the moral obligation and responsibility to relieve human suffering. On the other hand, when an action is judged to be immoral (e.g., on the basis of the principle of double effect), one's moral obligation is both to acknowledge God's sovereignty and to accept the suffering that results from obeying the moral law.[69] In the latter situation, humans are not considered to be cocreators with God in the relief of suffering; rather, they are creatures who must submit themselves to God's sovereign will and join their suffering to Christ's cross. The suffering that results from avoiding an immoral act such as the direct abortion of innocent life is not meaningless, and it is not without redemption. Thus, this interpretation of suffering is used as the theological justification for actions already judged to be right on moral grounds, and it is the theological warrant for prohibiting actions previously judged to be morally wrong.[70]

Value Parameter: Scale of Values and Reasons to Justify Abortion

The third theological parameter is concerned with a number of issues related to the concrete values at stake in the abortion question. The primary issue in the abortion debate revolves around the value that is or should be accorded to the fetus. In other words, the core issue is the evaluation or moral status of nascent life. However, there are always other important values involved in any decision to abort fetal life, for example, the welfare of pregnant women, the freedom of women to determine their reproductive futures, and the interests of others such as the father, family, and community.[71] When two or more of these values conflict, which one takes precedence over the others? This question, then, asks whether there is a scale or hierarchy of values that comes into play in conflict situations such that values higher in the scale must be preserved at the expense of values lower in the hierarchy. Because values are used as reasons to justify or not to justify abortion, this issue is obviously concerned with the reasons considered morally sufficient to defend one's choice about abortion. Since all these issues rely on some explicit or implied moral theory about the nature and epistemological status of values, I begin by briefly describing the moral theory adopted by the Catholic tradition.

The substance of the Catholic position on the moral theory of values and of the rightness and wrongness of actions can be described as moral realism. Values are objectively real, and they are capable of being grasped through human reason and experience. Rightness and wrongness of actions are objective judgments, and some views of what constitutes the good life are plainly superior to others.[72] This theory has historically been conveyed through a second-level interpretation called natural-law morality. One rendition of this natural-law morality—a rendition that appears to be adopted by the modern magisterium—purports that there exists a hierarchical order of values and goods such that there can be no true conflict of rights and obligations. As Josef Fuchs once claimed about the abortion issue,

> There exists indeed *an order* of goods and values, of commands and demands through the very nature of things, so that there can be no true conflict of rights but at most an apparent conflict. The two obligations concerning a pathological birth, to preserve the life of the mother and not to kill the child, only seem to contradict one another. There is in fact no commandment to save the mother at all costs. There is only an obligation to save her in a morally permissible way and such a way is not envisaged in stating this given situation. Consequently only one obligation remains: to save the mother without attempting to kill the child.[73]

This interpretation of the objective and fixed order of values and obligations is clearly the backdrop for the Catholic position on abortion.

As I have already stated, the Catholic tradition holds that all nascent life from the moment of conception is to be considered objectively valuable. The fetus possesses the objective right to life, which society must respect, and it must be treated as a person. As innocent, the fetus's life may never be taken as a means to a further value or as an end in itself. Though recent statements from the magisterium do recognize that there are difficulties when the value of innocent life comes into apparent conflict with other values in the situation, nonetheless the magisterium denies that these values can ever justify the direct killing of the fetus. As the *Declaration on Abortion* states,

> Divine law and natural reason, therefore, exclude all right to the direct killing of an innocent man. However, if the reasons given to justify an abortion were always manifestly evil and valueless the problem would not be so dramatic. The gravity of the problem comes from the fact that in certain cases, perhaps in quite a considerable number of cases by denying abortion one endangers important values to which it is normal to attach great value, and which may sometimes even seem to have priority. We do not deny these very great difficulties. It may be a serious question of health, sometimes of life or death, for the mother; it may be the burden represented by an additional child, especially if there are good reasons to fear that the child will be abnormal or retarded; it may be the importance attributed in different classes of society to considerations of honor or dishonor, of loss of social standing, and so forth. We proclaim only that none of these reasons can ever objectively confer the right to dispose of another's life, even when that life is only beginning.[74]

As this quotation makes clear, the magisterium denies that any value, as serious as it may be, can justify a direct abortion. Though one might offer genuinely important reasons for directly killing the fetus, these reasons can only make the abortion in some circumstances a lesser evil; the reasons themselves can never justify the act.[75]

It is frequently claimed by many in the abortion debate that, in arguing its position, the Catholic tradition denies the freedom of the woman. Several recent documents have addressed this claim,[76] even if the reply may appear less than satisfactory to many. The position espoused in these documents is that personal freedom must always begin by recognizing and respecting human relationships and justice.[77] Because a direct attack on nascent life violates its right to life, a woman's freedom to choose another value at the expense of the fetus's life would violate justice and her natural relationship to the fetus. Thus, the woman's right to self-determination is not denied; rather, her right is placed within a hierarchy of rights that is both objective and fixed. Even in an indirect abortion, which is considered morally permissible under the principle of double effect, only the necessity to save the life of the mother can be used as a moral reason for indirectly aborting the fetus.[78]

When the Catholic position on this parameter is compared with the prochoice position in secular society, several areas of disagreement become poignantly apparent. Pollsters continue to tell us that many U.S. citizens would personally permit direct abortions only in situations of rape, incest, or where the mother's life is endangered. However, less than 2 percent of the twenty-seven million abortions in this country have been performed for one or other of the above reasons; the vast majority of the fetuses were aborted as a form of birth control. At a public level, then, the right of the woman to autonomy continues to hold sway in the public mind. Perhaps Robert Bellah and his associates are correct that freedom "is the most resonant, deeply held American value,"[79] and so Americans appear to be publicly resistant to limitations on this value.

Though many U.S. citizens are not pro-choice at a personal level of morality, a certain moral agnosticism appears to pervade public life and morality. Pro-choice advocates in particular seem to hold to moral agnosticism as a moral theory, and this position is opposed to the Catholic position on value. In moral agnosticism one does not believe that there is any objectivity to values, or at least one has little confidence that values can be known. As David Carlin Jr. describes this position,

Thus there can be no agreement as to what constitutes the good life for human beings. Every person's individual view of the good life is just as valid as every other person's. If you and I differ in our moral views, there is no way either of us can prove the other wrong; all we can do is tolerate our mutual differences. But if there is no science of the good life and no inner light to reveal it to me, how do I find my values and my moral code? I choose; I simply choose; there is no alternative. In the world of the moral agnostic, choice is the essential action and tolerance the supreme virtue.[80]

There is also in the United States a popular morality or structure of moral thinking that is utilitarian.[81] Rightness and wrongness are determined solely on the basis of the results of actions. Because utilitarianism denies the intrinsic rightness or wrongness of actions and because it tends to view the person functionally, it too clashes with the Catholic position on the objective moral assessment of acts and on the intrinsic value placed on persons.

The evaluation of fetal life in the above perspectives differs substantially from the Catholic tradition. Some view the fetus as living but disposable tissue; others evaluate the fetus as making some moral claims on us, but these claims are overridden by either maternal or familial concerns.[82] In the first view, the fetus makes no moral claims on us whatsoever, at least not until the legally established point of viability. A feminist pro-choice position adopts this perspective, although some forms of this position maintain that the value of the fetus is really contingent on the pregnant woman's bestowal of humanhood.[83] In the second view, there is some recognition of the value of fetal life, but the scale of values does not necessarily favor the fetus. In a 1987 survey, the following reasons and percentages were given by abortion patients. Three-quarters of the respondents said that a baby would interfere with work, school, or other responsibilities; two-thirds said that they could not afford a child; and one-half replied that they did not want to be a single parent or that they had problems in their relationship with husband or partner.[84] The clear implication of this survey is that a variety of personal, familial, or economic values can and do override the value of fetal life, but the most important singular value seems to be the freedom of women to choose. There is little doubt, then, why the Supreme Court legally enshrined this value in its extension of the Fourteenth Amendment right to privacy to include the freedom of women to choose an abortion.

Richard McCormick has proposed two different sets of rules to guide the public discussion of this debate and to help mediate the differences between the Catholic and societal positions.[85] Unfortunately, his efforts to find a mediating position have not been met with much success. In one way, given the opposing philosophical theories of value that are at work on each side, it is quite understandable, albeit distressing, that there is a lack of public support for discussion that attempts to appreciate the worth in each position.

Legal Parameter: Relationship between Civil Law and Morality

The final parameter is concerned with the Catholic Church's theological position on the relationship between civil law and morality. Broader issues lie behind this discussion, for example, the general relation between religion and society and the relationship between church and state, but I restrict my analysis to the narrower topic. We need to pursue briefly why the church is involved in the public debate over abortion and how the tradition views the function of law in society. Historically, the Catholic tradition has focused on the legal and public implications of issues of conscience, although other Christian denominations have focused more on the moral limits of law and public policy.[86] In addition, the Catholic tradition has generally feared that the use of law primarily to protect the freedom of individuals could lead to moral anarchy, and such anarchy would hardly be conducive to making abortion unnecessary.[87]

Let me begin with what I take to be the substance of the Catholic tradition. If procured abortion is categorized as a religious issue and not as a moral one, then the controversy is immediately transposed into a debate about religious freedom. The consequence of this categorization is that pro-choice constituents will and do claim that one group cannot impose its religious beliefs and morality on others in a pluralist society.[88] As I have argued above, though, the Catholic tradition does not consider abortion to be solely a religious issue. Abortion is essentially a moral issue, and the natural-law arguments designed to arrive at the church's conclusion are considered to be intelligible to others on rational grounds. Thus in the church's view, its doctrinal position on abortion does not result in the imposition of a specifically religious morality on society but rather represents a reasoned argument that can be accepted by many.[89] In addition, the substance of the tradition has contended that civil law and morality are objectively related to one another, and therefore human laws cannot be decided by mere judicial positivism, by simple expediency, or irrespective of moral criteria.

There are both theological and moral reasons why the church is involved in the public debate over abortion. The theological reasons are related to the tradition's various ways of relating civil law and morality,[90] and the moral reasons are concerned with both the rights of nascent life and justice in society.

The tradition has employed two distinct theological approaches to the relation between civil law and Christian morality.[91] Before the Second Vatican Council, the standard interpretation of this relationship was that civil law applied the natural law to the changing and particular cultural circumstances of different societies by promulgating the conclusions of the natural law directly or by specifying what the natural law had left undetermined. Though civil law was not identified with the natural moral law, nevertheless a very close relation was fashioned between the two. In this view, civil law is concerned with what is necessary for the common good, and it may tolerate moral evil to avoid greater evil in society. Just laws never violate the true freedom of citizens, but anything that is contrary to the natural law will ultimately produce bad consequences.[92] Thus, in this first interpretation, the moral reason why the church is involved in the abortion debate is because procured abortions violate the natural law by directing killing the innocent. As a result, this view frequently imposed obligations on civil authorities, especially on those who were Catholic, to pass various laws against procured abortions to protect the life of the innocent.

An alternative interpretation was adopted at Vatican II.[93] This approach makes a distinction between the secular and sacred orders of human life, and also between society and the state. In the latter distinction the state is viewed as playing a limited role in society because the purposes of the state are neither the same as nor coextensive with society's purposes. The state has the responsibility for the public order—that is, the orders of peace, justice, and public morality, which is only one aspect of the common good of society. The primary role and function of civil law in issues of *private* morality—actions that have little effect on others—was formulated by Vatican II as, "For the rest, the usages of society are to be the usages of freedom in their full range. These require that the freedom of man be respected as far as possible, and curtailed only when and insofar as necessary."[94] However, in matters of *public* morality—actions that have a greater impact on others in society—the state has the responsibility to protect the rights of individuals by serving the order of justice. The state can intervene through the passing of civil laws to limit the freedom of individuals when the rights of innocent people are being violated.[95] However, many would argue that even the intervention of the state through law can be limited by the criterion of feasibility. Within a pluralist society where people disagree on moral issues, the state must prudentially consider the practicality and feasibility of a law before enacting it to restrict people's freedom. Clearly, the ethos of a pluralist society would concur much more with this interpretation than with the one adopted before Vatican II.

Because the church maintains that the fetus must be respected and treated as a person who possesses the right to life, it argues that the state must intervene to protect the fetus's right by limiting a woman's freedom to choose a direct abortion. In fact, this value judgment about the status of the fetus forms one of the bases for the moral reason why the church is involved in the public

debate over abortion. More specifically, because the moral rights of the innocent are violated in direct abortions, and thus the order of justice is thereby
transgressed, not only the state but also the church must be involved to find
ways to prevent these actions.[96] The unanswered question raised by many in
society about this second perspective, though, is whether any law that
restricts a woman's freedom to a procured abortion can meet the test of the
criteria of practicality and feasibility in a pluralist society. Many people of
goodwill do not share the tradition's value judgment that fetal life is the moral
equivalent of a person with legal rights, and this fact is a source of tremendous divergence between the ecclesial and societal positions. It is certainly
possible that one could accept the church's second approach to the relation
between civil law and public morality but deny that the fetus has any moral
status at conception. Consequently, if the fetus has little or no moral status at
conception or somewhere else along the gestational continuum, then killing
the fetus for the sake of other values would neither violate anyone's rights
nor vitiate the orders of justice and public morality. I do think that most in
society would accept the second formulation of the civil law–public morality
relation, so the divergence between the two views continues to revolve around
the moral status of fetal life.

Though the Catholic tradition has officially adopted the second theological
approach to the relation between civil law and morality, several recent official
documents on sexual and medical ethics have continued to use the first
approach. For example, in the *Declaration on Abortion* the Congregation for
the Doctrine of the Faith (CDF) states, "It is true that civil law cannot expect
to cover the whole field of morality or to punish all faults. No one expects it
to do so. It must often tolerate what is in fact a lesser evil, in order to avoid
a greater one."[97] This is the basic assumption of the first approach in that it
assumes that the function of civil law is to apply the natural law.[98] Later in
the document it is stated that

> The law is not obliged to sanction everything, but it cannot act contrary to a law
> which is deeper and more majestic than any human law: the natural law engraved in
> men's hearts by the Creator as a norm which reason clarifies and strives to formulate
> properly, and which one must always struggle to understand better, but which it is
> always wrong to contradict.[99]

It is obvious here that the congregation holds to the first approach in which
civil law must respect the natural law, and thus these human laws should not
be contrary to God's moral law.

In conclusion, as long as one accepts the tradition's value judgment on the
fetus's moral status, one *could* argue in either interpretation of the relation

between civil law and public morality for a legal restraint on a woman's freedom to choose a procured abortion. However, the fact that official documents vacillate between two distinct theological interpretations has compromised the church's efforts in its public arguments against direct abortion. This is especially true in a pluralist society that values individual freedom and restrains legal intervention as much as U.S. society does. It is equally true in a legal environment in which the country's highest court has subscribed to a constitutional doctrine that appears at face value to be a form of judicial positivism. As the Supreme Court has recently stated, this doctrine holds that "where reasonable people disagree the government can adopt one position or the other."[100]

CONCLUSION

My intention in this chapter has been to locate and analyze some of the theological parameters that underlie the Catholic tradition's moral position on abortion. As we have seen, the Catholic position is rather complex, and so any reductionist or simplistic caricature of its moral position should be resisted in public debate. There are indeed several points of serious disagreement between the Catholic tradition and that of our secular society. Much of this disagreement revolves around the issues of anthropology, the moral status of the fetus, the meaning of sex and its relation to procreation, moral theory, and how one resolves conflicts between values. To deal with these differences, though, it is most important not to focus simply on the conclusions that a tradition or a society can reasonably articulate and passionately support. My purpose here is not to underrate the significance of conclusions to moral issues; conclusions are significant, and they can result in immense political and moral consequences. However, behind people's moral conclusions to very complex questions there always exist fundamental beliefs about and basic value judgments on a host of issues. It is one's positions on these more essential issues—for example, anthropology, and the nature and hierarchy of values—that determine conclusions. Informed discussion will not proceed to a more reasonable and just public policy on abortion until greater efforts are focused at these deeper and more enduring levels of the abortion debate. William Byron was indeed correct to remark that intellectuals *and* politicians have much work to do to accomplish this task.

When politicians engage the Catholic position on abortion within our pluralist society, it is helpful to recall that not everything found in this moral position is part of the substance of the tradition. Second-level interpretations and applications have historically been articulated in the tradition to specify and to make concrete what is held to be true and valuable at a more fundamental level. As I indicated at the beginning, to call these parameters "variable" does not *necessarily* imply that they must change. However, I have used this language to indicate where perspectives and horizons for future discussion and possible change might exist on the Catholic side of the debate. I would likewise assume that there are "variable" parameters in society's position that provide the opportunities for future discussion and change.

To a great extent, the church's position is theologically controlled by a certain "variable" interpretation of how God relates to humanity and to the created order. In turn, this rather anthropomorphic interpretation of divine providence influences a number of other important interpretations and value judgments, for example, the immorality of directly killing the innocent, and the relationship between civil law and morality. If we were to understand that God operates most appropriately in the world through the exercise of free human activity, then we would realize that in fact we are the ones who are truly responsible for the decisions over life and death.

Despite potential abuse, such an interpretation would not make morality less objective, nor would it make us into gods. At the least, this view would morally and politically require us to create social and economic conditions that would make decisions for procured abortions far less likely.[101] In addition, it would require all of us to cooperate responsibly in fashioning a more reasonable and just public policy on abortion. To be sure, such a policy must meet the criteria of practicality and feasibility in a pluralist society, and it must accept the fact that people of goodwill can and will disagree. However, the policy can no longer be based on either moral agnosticism or on legal positivism. To reject both of these positions does not leave us with only one other option as the basis for public policy, namely, the existence of a concrete moral order that is already-out-there-to-be-looked-at-and-respected. We do have another option, and this realist position holds that values are indeed objective and that we must create both moral and legal orders based on these values. Values will conflict in a finite and less-than-perfect world, and so we must responsibly choose which values we can and will preserve. Reasonable and objective criteria should guide our choices, and our attitudes should be to preserve as many values as possible in conflict situations. This implies that the resolution of value conflicts at the level of public policy cannot be decided by always preferring one of the values *regardless of the circumstances*—for example, freedom of the woman to choose or the value of fetal life, or by denying the very existence of one of the values at stake. To settle this complex issue in either of those two ways is to abdicate the moral and political responsibilities that are truly ours to take up as God's gift and challenge.

ENDNOTES

1. David R. Carlin Jr. argues that the debate over abortion promises to be the deepest and most intense moral controversy since Prohibition or slavery. See his "The New/Old Abortion Battle: Taking Up Where We Left Off," *Commonweal* 118 (September 13, 1991): 505.

2. Congress is currently debating H.R. 25, the so-called Freedom of Choice Act, that would prohibit states from legislating abortion restrictions. For a response to this bill from the director of planning and information in the National Conference of Catholic Bishops (NCCB), see Helen Alvare, "Testimony Opposing 'Freedom of Choice Act,'" *Origins* 21 (April 2, 1992): 692–96.

3. For a brief history and analysis of this intramural debate during the 1984 presidential campaign, see Richard P. McBrien, *Caesar's Coin: Religion and Politics in America* (New York: Macmillan, 1987), 135–68. For Mario Cuomo's lecture that he delivered at the University of Notre Dame on September 13, 1984, see his "Religious Belief and Public Morality: A Catholic Governor's Perspective," in *Abortion and Catholicism: The American Debate*, edited by Patricia Beattie Jung and Thomas A. Shannon (New York: Crossroad, 1988), 202–16.

4. William Byron, "Abortion Debate: How Intellectuals and Moral Leaders Can Help Politicians," *Origins* 22 (June 18, 1992): 81, 83–87.

5. The literature discussing the morality of abortion is voluminous. For a brief sample of the literature dealing with the Catholic moral position, see Jung and Shannon, *Abortion and Catholicism*; Susan T. Nicholson, *Abortion and the Roman Catholic Church* (Knoxville, Tenn.: Religious Ethics, 1978); Germain Grisez, *Abortion: The Myths, the Realities, and the Arguments* (New York: Corpus Books, 1970); Edward Batchelor Jr., ed., *Abortion: The Moral Issues* (New York: Pilgrim Press, 1982); and John Connery, *Abortion: The Development of the Roman Catholic Perspective* (Chicago, Ill.: Loyola University Press, 1977).

6. Stephen Happel and James J. Walter, *Conversion and Discipleship: A Christian Foundation for Ethics and Doctrine* (Philadelphia: Fortress Press, 1986), 125–26.

7. There is a hierarchy of truths or doctrines in the Catholic tradition. As the Second Vatican Council maintained in its *Decree on Ecumenism* (*Unitatis Redintegratio*), "When comparing doctrines, they [Catholic theologians] should remember that in Catholic teaching there exists an order or 'hierarchy' of truths, since they vary in their relationship to the foundation of the Christian faith." See Walter M. Abbott, ed., *The Documents of Vatican II* (New York: America Press, 1966), 354.

8. The distinction that I am making between substance (constant) and interpretation-application (variable) is similar to the one that Richard McCormick has made between a principle and a formulation-application. See Richard A. McCormick, *The Critical Calling: Reflections on Moral Dilemmas since Vatican II* (Washington, D.C.: Georgetown University Press, 1989), 147–53.

9. For a concise summary of the many positions on abortion among Christian denominations and non-Christian religions, see the Park Ridge Center Report, *Abortion, Religion, and the State Legislator after Webster: A Guide for the 1990s* (Chicago, Ill.: Park Ridge Center, 1990), 12–16. In addition, for a concise description of the various moral positions on abortion within the American Jewish communities, see Scott Aaron, "The Choice in

'Choose Life': American Judaism and Abortion," *Commonweal* 119 (February 28, 1992): 15–18.

10. There is only one reference in the Hebrew scriptures that deals explicitly with the issue of abortion (Exodus 21:22–23), and it seems that this text is concerned primarily with meting out a penalty for a man who strikes a pregnant woman and causes her to miscarry her fetus.

11. See Connery, *Abortion*, 105–224; and the Sacred Congregation for the Doctrine of the Faith (CDF), *Declaration on Abortion* (Washington, D.C.: USCC, 1974), 7.

12. *Declaration on Abortion*, footnote 19; the Sacred Congregation for the Doctrine of the Faith, "Instruction on Respect for Human Life in Its Origin and on the Dignity of Procreation," I, 1, in *Origins* 16 (March 19, 1987): 701; and Connery, *Abortion*, 212. Over the past several decades, several contemporary Catholic theologians and physicians have argued that hominization is not possible until after developmental, and not merely biological, individualization has occurred around the fourteenth day after fertilization. For a sample of the literature arguing this position, see Andre E. Hellegers, "Fetal Development," *Theological Studies* 31(1970): 3–9; Charles E. Curran, "Abortion: Law and Morality in Contemporary Catholic Theology," *Jurist* 33 (Spring 1973): 162–83; Gabriel Pastrana, "Personhood and the Beginning of Human Life," *Thomist* 41 (April 1977): 247–94; Norman Ford, "When Does Human Life Begin? Science, Government, Church," *Pacifica* 1 (1988): 298–327; Thomas A. Shannon and Allan B. Wolter, "Reflections on the Moral Status of the Pre-Embryo," *Theological Studies* 51 (December 1990): 603–26; and Richard A. McCormick, "Who or What Is the Preembryo?" *Kennedy Institute of Ethics Journal* 1 (March 1991): 1–15. For a recent article that strongly opposes this position, see William E. May, "The Moral Status of the Embryo," *Linacre Quarterly* 59 (November 1992): 76–83.

13. The phrases "respected as a person" or "treated as a person" occur several times in the "Instruction." For example, see part I, 1 (pp. 701–2 in the *Origins* edition).

14. "Instruction," foreword (p. 699 in *Origins* edition).

15. "Instruction," introduction, 5 (p. 701 in the *Origins* edition).

16. *Declaration on Abortion*, 11.

17. *Declaration on Abortion*, 7; and "Instruction," I, 1 (p. 701 of the *Origins* edition). Both documents are either quoting or paraphrasing a remark made by Paul VI in one of his speeches entitled *Salutiamo con paterna effusione*, which was delivered on December 9, 1972.

18. In the Dogmatic Constitution on the Church (*Lumen Gentium*) at the Second Vatican Council it is stated that even noninfallible teachings impose on Catholics an obligation of "religious submission (obsequium religiosum) of will and of mind." See Abbott, *The Documents of Vatican II*, 48. To say the least, the precise meaning of "religious submission" has been heatedly debated by contemporary theologians and canonists.

19. There is a hierarchy of authority in official Catholic documents. The fact that all the documents on abortion reviewed thus far have come from a Roman congregation indicates that these teachings do not possess the same weight and authority as those from a pope or a council. The intent of most of these documents is to recall or to clarify teachings, not to proclaim new teaching.

20. As the *Declaration on Abortion* states, "Respect for human life is not just a Christian obligation. Human reason is sufficient to impose it on the basis of the analysis of what

a human person is and should be." This position has been regularly stated by Cardinal Bernardin in his various speeches on the "consistent ethic of life." For a collection of his speeches, see Thomas G. Fuechtmann, ed., *Consistent Ethic of Life* (Kansas City, Mo.: Sheed and Ward, 1988). For a more detailed discussion of reason's ability to reach conclusions on abortion, see the commentary in *Ethics and the Search for Christian Unity: Two Statements by the Roman Catholic/Presbyterian-Reformed Consultation* (Washington, D.C.: USCC, 1981), 8, 17–18.

21. For example, Paul VI devoted several paragraphs of his encyclical on birth control ("Humanae Vitae," 10–12) to natural-law arguments against all artificial means of regulating births. The CDF also devoted the entire third part of its document on abortion (*Declaration on Abortion*, 8–13) to a consideration of the immorality of procured abortion *in the light of reason*. Similar claims and arguments are made in the CDF's document on sexual morality. See the *Declaration on Certain Questions Concerning Sexual Ethics* (Washington, D.C.: USCC, 1976), 3.

22. Though I would argue that this claim is central to the Catholic position, nonetheless it is a claim that has been hotly debated among contemporary theologians. For a collection of recent essays on the issue of whether Christian faith adds new content to the moral life, see Charles E. Curran and Richard A. McCormick, eds., *Readings in Moral No. 2: The Distinctiveness of Christian Ethics* (New York: Paulist Press, 1980).

23. For a more comprehensive account of the tradition's theological anthropology, see *The Pastoral Constitution on the Church in the Modern World* (*Gaudium et Spes*), part I, in Abbott, *The Documents of Vatican II*, 209–48.

24. For example, see Abbott, *The Documents,* 29; and the "Instruction on Respect for Human Life," introduction, 5 (p. 701 of the *Origins* edition).

25. See the *Declaration on Abortion*, 8; and the NCCB's *Documentation on Abortion and the Right to Life II* (Washington, D.C.: USCC, 1976), 24. David Thomasma has recently argued that the inherent and equal value of all human beings can be grounded on philosophical and political views of the human person. See David C. Thomasma, *Human Life in the Balance* (Louisville, Ky.: Westminster/John Knox Press, 1990), chaps. 6 and 7.

26. For example, see the "Instruction on the Respect for Human Life," introduction, 5 (p. 701 of the *Origins* edition).

27. Paul VI did not formulate the status of the fetus in exactly these terms, but he did describe nascent life as *une personne en devenir* (a person in the process of becoming). See Pope Paul VI, "Pourquois l'église ne peut accepter l'avortement," *Documentation catholique* 70 (1973): 4–5.

28. For example, see the "Instruction on the Respect for Human Life," introduction, 5 (p. 701 of the *Origins* edition).

29. This question has been consistently asked whenever a new technology has been developed and then applied to life and death issues. For example, Paul VI raised this question in his encyclical on artificial birth control ("Humanae Vitae," 2–3), and the CDF raised the same query with regard to modern reproductive technologies in its "Instruction on Respect for Human Life," introduction, 1, and II, B-5 (pp. 699 and 707 respectively in the *Origins* edition).

30. Thomasma, *Human Life in the Balance*, 147.

31. For example, see the "Instruction on Respect for Human Life," introduction, 2 (p. 699 in the *Origins* edition).

32. Denis O'Callaghan has pointed out that traditional Catholic morality made exceptions to moral principle—for example, no killing of the innocent—"where these depended on chance occurrence of circumstances rather than on free human choice." Thus, the tradition made exceptions precisely because "the occurrence of the exception was determined by factors of chance outside human control." When O'Callaghan applied his point to the issue of abortion, he argued that in cases of tubal pregnancies the tradition "accepted what is in principle an abortion because it posed no threat to the general position." In other words, the "tubal pregnancy is a rare chance occurrence, an occurrence which is independent of human choice and so does not lay the way open to abuse." See Denis O'Callaghan, "Moral Principle and Exception," *Furrow* 22 (November, 1971): 686–96, especially 694. In my opinion, as long as the tradition was assured that the deadly deed against innocent life was not subject to human choice but was due only to factors outside human control, the right of God to be the lord over life and death was protected against human striving to usurp God's providential power.

33. For a more extensive discussion of how different views of human freedom and technology play an important role in the religious debate on abortion, see John Badertscher, "Religious Dimensions of the Abortion Debate," *Studies in Religion* 6 (1976–1977): 177–83. Charles E. Curran has recently argued that "the Catholic tradition in moral theology in the past and also today does not and should not appeal to divine providence in any way to change, alter, or attenuate human responsibility and actions in this world." See his *The Living Tradition of Catholic Moral Theology* (Notre Dame, Ind.: University of Notre Dame Press, 1992), 213. I agree with the general substance of Curran's argument, but I think that there is one exception where his assessment of the tradition does not apply, viz, when the tradition attempts to resolve conflict situations in which the death of an innocent person is a foreseen consequence.

34. Robert N. Bellah et al., *Habits of the Heart: Individualism and Commitment in American Life* (San Francisco: Harper & Row, 1986), 37.

35. Bellah et al., *Habits of the Heart*, 334.

36. For an excellent contrast between liberalism and communitarianism as ways of interpreting the human condition, see David Hollenbach, "Liberalism, Communitarianism, and the Bishop's Pastoral Letter on the Economy," in D. M. Yeager, ed., *The Annual of the Society of Christian Ethics* (Washington, D.C.: Georgetown University Press, 1987), 19–40.

37. Bellah et al., *Habits of the Heart*, 142.

38. McCormick, *The Critical Calling*, 220. In a section below ("Value Parameter"), I argue that in many cases the moral theory of rightness and wrongness that lies behind this individualist perspective is moral agnosticism.

39. Joseph B. Tamney, Stephen D. Johnson, and Ronald Burton, "The Abortion Controversy: Conflicting Beliefs and Values in Society," *Journal for the Scientific Study of Religion* 31 (March, 1992): 32–46.

40. Tamney, Johnson, and Burton, "The Abortion Controversy," 33.

41. Bellah and his coauthors also note that Americans place a high value on being free *from* any type of external limitation. See Bellah et al., *Habits of the Heart*, 25.

42. For a critique of this view of morality as exclusively a matter of human agency and freedom, see Sidney Callahan, "Abortion and the Sexual Agenda: A Case for Pro-life Feminism," in Jung and Shannon, *Abortion and Catholicism*, 133–34.

43. For an interesting analysis of the anthropology adopted by the Supreme Court in the *Roe* v. *Wade* decision, see Edward McGlynn Gaffney, "Law and Theology: A Dialogue on the Abortion Decisions," *Jurist* 33 (1973): 134–52, especially 142–50.

44. Daniel Callahan, "Living with the New Biology," *Center Magazine* 5 (1972): 4–12.

45. Daniel Callahan, "How Technology Is Reframing the Abortion Debate," *Hastings Center Report* 16 (February, 1986): 33–42.

46. This is the thesis of Susan Teft Nicholson's monograph on the ethics of abortion within the Catholic tradition. See her *Abortion and the Roman Catholic Church.*

47. James P. Hanigan, *What Are They Saying about Sexual Morality?* (Ramsey, N.J.: Paulist Press, 1982), 12.

48. St. Thomas Aquinas, *Summa Theologiae, I–II*, q. 94, art. 2.

49. For a more comprehensive study of both St. Augustine's and St. Thomas's positions on the nature of human sexuality and its relation to procreation, see Louis Janssens, *Mariage et Fécondité: De* Casti Connubii *à* Gaudium et Spes (Paris: Editions J. Duculot, Gembloux, 1967), especially 13–61.

50. Both Pius XI in his encyclical *Casti Connubii* (1930) and Paul VI in his encyclical *Humanae Vitae* (1968) accepted Thomas's natural-law position on the link between sexuality and procreation.

51. For example, see Paul VI, *Humanae Vitae,* 12; and CDF, "Instruction on Respect for Human Life," II, B-4 (p. 705 in the *Origins* edition).

52. Richard McCormick also holds this conclusion. See his *The Critical Calling,* 150.

53. See Lisa Cahill, "A 'Natural Law' Reconsideration of Euthanasia," *Linacre Quarterly* 44 (1977): 47–63.

54. McCormick, *The Critical Calling,* p. 226.

55. Aquinas, *Summa Theologiae, II–II,* q. 64, a. 6.

56. Despite the fact that the premises of this principle can be found in Aquinas' *Summa Theologiae, II-II*, q. 64, a. 7, the conditions of the principle date from the sixteenth and seventeenth centuries. The precise formulation that is used today dates from the mid-nineteenth-century manual *Compendium Theologiae Moralis* by Jean Pierre Gury. For a historical study of the principle, see Joseph T. Mangan, "An Historical Analysis of the Principle of Double Effect," *Theological Studies* 10 (1949): 41–61. Over the past several decades the validity of the principle of double effect has been contested. For a collection of essays that assess this principle, see Charles E. Curran and Richard A. McCormick, eds., *Readings in Moral Theology No. 1: Moral Norms and Catholic Tradition* (New York: Paulist Press, 1979).

57. The Catholic tradition has recognized that there are different kinds of evil. Some evils are natural (e.g., tornadoes), some are physical evils (e.g., amputation of a limb), but other evils enter into the moral order and thus are assessed as moral evil. The crucial issue is on which grounds does the effect of an action enter into the moral order and thus become subject to a negative moral evaluation. I argue that the grounds are principally, though not only, theological in nature.

58. Gerald Kelly, *Medico-Moral Problems* (St. Louis, Mo.: Catholic Hospital Association, 1958), 13–14.

59. See the *Ethical and Religious Directives for Catholic Health Facilities* (Washington, D.C.: USCC, 1971), 13–17.

60. Jan Jans also draws this same conclusion in his assessment of the 1987 "Instruction." See his "God or Man? Normative Theology in the Instruction *Donum Vitae*," *Louvain Studies* 17 (Spring 1992): 48–64.

61. See Josef Fuchs, *Christian Morality: The Word Becomes Flesh* (Washington, D.C.: Georgetown University Press, 1987), 40–44, 71–73.

62. "Instruction on Respect for Human Life," I, 5 (p. 703 in the *Origins* edition). Emphasis mine.

63. "Instruction on Respect for Human Life," introduction, 5 (p. 699 in the *Origins* edition).

64. Jans, "God or Man?" 58.

65. See Bruno Schüller, "The Double Effect in Catholic Thought: A Reevaluation," in *Doing Evil to Achieve Good: Moral Choice in Conflict Situations*, edited by Richard McCormick and Paul Ramsey (Chicago, Ill.: Loyola University Press, 1978), 189.

66. See Josef Fuchs, *Christian Ethics in a Secular Arena* (Washington, D.C.: Georgetown University Press, 1984), 78–80, 102–4.

67. David F. Kelly, *The Emergence of Roman Catholic Medical Ethics in North America: An Historical—Methodological—Bibliographical Study* (New York: Edwin Mellen Press, 1979), 275.

68. An alternative to this anthropomorphic interpretation of how God relates to humanity and to the world is to construe God as the transcendent other who immanently acts through free human activity. In this image, God is neither another actor in the world alongside human agents, nor does God possess certain categorical rights, some of which are delegated and some of which are exclusively reserved to the divine. For a further discussion of this image of God, see Happel and Walter, *Conversion and Discipleship*, 89.

69. See Kelly, *The Emergence of Roman Catholic Medical Ethics in North America*, 276. A clear example of this reasoning is found in the "Instruction on Respect for Human Life," II, 8 (p. 708 in the *Origins* edition). Also, see the *Declaration on Abortion*, 24, where heroism is called for to remain faithful to the requirements of the moral law; and *Declaration on Abortion*, 27, where redemptive suffering is the theological consequence of remaining faithful.

70. For an analysis of how the liberal ethos in society views sacrifice and suffering, see Lisa Sowle Cahill, "Abortion, Autonomy, and Community," in Jung and Shannon, *Abortion and Catholicism*, 91–92.

71. For a brief discussion of some of these values, see Lisa Sowle Cahill, "Abortion," in *The Westminster Dictionary of Christian Ethics*, edited by James F. Childress and John Macquarrie, 1–5 (Philadelphia: Westminster Press, 1986).

72. For a further discussion of moral realism in relation to the abortion issue, see Carlin, "The New/Old Abortion Battle," 505.

73. Josef Fuchs, *Natural Law: A Theological Investigation* (New York: Sheed and Ward, 1965), 131. Emphasis in the original. It is doubtful that Fuchs himself any longer holds to such a position.

74. *Declaration on Abortion*, 14.

75. See the commentary in the document containing the joint statement on abortion by the Roman Catholic/Presbyterian-Reformed consultation, *Ethics and the Search for Christian Unity*, 18.

76. For example, see the *Declaration on Abortion*, 15.

77. See the NCCB's *Documentation on Abortion and the Right to Life II*, 11. Also, see the *Declaration on Abortion*, 20, where the CDF clearly states that "One cannot invoke freedom of thought to destroy this life" [fetal life].

78. See the commentary in the joint statement by the Roman Catholic/Presbyterian-Reformed consultation, *Ethics and the Search for Christian Unity*, 19.

79. Bellah et al., *Habits of the Heart*, 23.

80. Carlin, "The New/Old Abortion Battle," 505.

81. Richard A. McCormick, *How Brave a New World? Dilemmas in Bioethics* (Washington, D.C.: Georgetown University Press, 1981), 204.

82. McCormick, *How Brave a New World?* 191.

83. For an analysis and critique of this perspective, see S. Callahan, "Abortion and the Sexual Agenda," 134.

84. *Chicago Tribune*, July 5, 1992, sec. 4, p. 1.

85. Richard A. McCormick, "Rules for Abortion Debate," *America* 139 (1978): 26–30; and Richard A. McCormick, "Abortion: The Unexplored Middle Ground," *Second Opinion* 10 (March, 1989): 41–50.

86. See the commentary in the joint statement by the Roman Catholic/Presbyterian-Reformed consultation, *Ethics and the Search for Christian Unity*, 3–4.

87. Roman Catholic/Presbyterian-Reformed consultation, *Ethics and the Search for Christian Unity*, 21–22.

88. McBrien, *Caesar's Coin*, 167.

89. This is the consistent claim by Cardinal Joseph Bernardin in his many speeches on the "consistent ethic of life." See Fuechtmann, *Consistent Ethic of Life*.

90. To pursue adequately all the theological reasons, it would be necessary to discuss in some depth what the church understands its general mission to the world to be. This ecclesiological parameter is beyond the immediate scope of the chapter. For a recent article that describes how ecclesiology shapes Catholic public policy on abortion, see J. Bryan Hehir, "Policy Arguments in a Public Church: Catholic Social Ethics and Bioethics," *Journal of Medicine and Philosophy* 17 (June 1992): 347–64.

91. Charles E. Curran has succinctly summarized these two approaches in his *Ongoing Revision: Studies in Moral Theology* (Notre Dame, Ind.: Fides, 1975), 107–43. The standard and most formative scholarship done in this area remains the work written by John Courtney Murray. For example, see Murray's *We Hold These Truths: Catholic Reflections on the American Proposition* (New York: Sheed and Ward, 1960) and *The Problem of Religious Freedom* (Westminster, Md.: Newman Press, 1965).

92. Curran, *Ongoing Revision*, 121–22.

93. See the "Declaration on Religious Freedom (Dignitatis Humanae)," in Abbott, *The Documents of Vatican II*, 675–700.

94. "Declaration on Religious Freedom (Dignitatis Humanae)," 7, in Abbott, *The Documents of Vatican II*, 687.

95. "Declaration on Religious Freedom (Dignitatis Humanae)," in Abbott, *The Documents of Vatican II*, 686–87, and n. 20.

96. This moral argument was used by Archbishop John R. Roach and Cardinal Terence Cooke in their testimony before Congress. See their "Testimony in Support of the Hatch Amendment," in Jung and Shannon, *Abortion and Catholicism*, 29–30. Also, see Cardinal Joseph Bernardin's statement on abortion in the NCCB's *Documentation on Abortion and the Right to Life II*, 38.

97. *Declaration on Abortion*, 20. For a similar argument, see the "Instruction on Respect for Human Life," III (p. 709 in the *Origins* edition).

98. Curran, *Ongoing Revision*, 137. Also see Richard M. Gula, *Reason Informed by Faith: Foundations of Catholic Morality* (Mahwah, N.J.: Paulist Press, 1989), 254–55.

99. *Declaration on Abortion*, 21. For a similar argument, see Paul VI's encyclical on birth control *Humanae Vitae*, 23. This kind of reasoning also appears to be the rationale used in the revised version of the document on discrimination against homosexuals by the Congregation for the Doctrine of the Faith. See "Responding to Legislative Proposals on Discrimination against Homosexuals," *Origins* 22 (August 6, 1992): 173–77.

100. See the Supreme Court's ruling on the Pennsylvania Abortion Control Act, part I, in *Origins* 22 (July 9, 1992): 116.

101. Bishop Untener's pastoral letter to Catholics in Saginaw, Michigan, who are contemplating an abortion decision is one of the most compassionate and far-reaching proposals for change of social conditions that I have read. See Bishop Untener, "Those Struggling with Abortion Decision," *Origins* 21 (January 16, 1992): 516.

III

ISSUES CONCERNED WITH GENETIC MEDICINE
AND THE CARE OF ILL PATIENTS

10

Perspectives on Medical Ethics:
Biotechnology and Genetic Medicine

James J. Walter

STATE OF THE QUESTION

When the Second Vatican Council opened on October 11, 1962, Francis Crick and James Watson had discovered the double helical structure of the DNA (deoxyribonucleic acid) molecule only nine years earlier, in 1953. The classical genetics of Gregor Mendel (ca. 1884)—the Austrian monk who had discovered the laws of heredity by working with garden peas—were beginning to give way to the study and application of the new molecular genetics. In 1962, there was no biotechnology as we currently know it; that area of biology and technology did not begin to develop until almost a decade later. Medical ethics at that time was still basically restricted to the study and application of traditional deontological rules to the physician-patient relationship. The new interdisciplinary field of bioethics, which would supersede but incorporate standard medical ethics into itself, would not develop into an academic discipline for approximately another decade in the United States. This new area of scholarly study, generally understood as the systematic study of the moral dimensions of the life sciences and health care,[1] would evolve partially in response to both the new genetics and biotechnology.

The two areas that this chapter will study are contemporary medical genetics and biotechnology. They are certainly related to one another, as we shall see, and each has had a rapid period of development since the 1970s. Medical genetics is "the aspect of human genetics that is concerned with the relation between heredity and disease."[2] Though the categories of the field overlap, many would consider the following list to comprise medical genetics: diagnosis of genetic disease (e.g., preimplantation diagnosis, prenatal diagnosis, population screening); eugenics as the elimination of disease-related traits (e.g., through selective mating, sterilization); gene therapy on either body cells or germ cells; genetic enhancement of body or germ cells; patenting human gene sequences or techniques of genetic control; embryo research; cloning; and genetic testing on controlled groups.[3]

Biotechnology, on the other hand, involves any technique that uses living organisms to make or modify products, to improve plants or animals, or to develop microorganisms for specific uses.[4] It involves using biology to discover, develop, manufacture, market, and sell products and services. Many of the applications of biotechnology will be used in the health-care arena, and this is where the linkage to medical genetics is made. As an industry, biotechnology was first developed by about ten to twenty venture-backed companies that were involved in pharmaceuticals.[5] Controversies over biotechnology and its applications to plants, animals, and humans began to arise in the mid-1970s due to the powerful techniques that allowed dramatically increased control over the design of living organisms.[6]

What are some of the developments in medical genetics and biotechnology—along with the ethical reflection that has accompanied them—that have occurred since the 1970s? Surely, recombinant DNA (rDNA) research that was developed in the mid-1970s is a watershed for much of the work that is being done today in both medical genetics and biotechnology. Known as gene splicing, recombinant DNA research is a procedure whereby segments of genetic material from one organism are transferred to another organism or species. The basis of the technique lies in the use of special enzymes (restriction enzymes) that split DNA strands wherever certain sequences of nucleotides occur. These procedures have led to the production of vaccines against a number of diseases and the introduction of certain substances as insulin, interferon, and growth hormone. The pharmaceuticals developed from this technique have substantially improved patient outcome and quality of life, but many have also questioned the wisdom of "playing God" with the very molecules that make up all life.[7] In 1976, the National Institutes of Health established the Recombinant DNA Advisory Committee (RAC) to study and evaluate various clinical proposals to use this new scientific technique.

In the last twenty years, scientists have discovered that DNA is virtually interchangeable among animals, plants, bacteria, and humans. Consequently, biotechnology has been extended to plants and animals where the DNA from one animal or plant is spliced into the genetic material of another. I will focus briefly on the area of plant bioengineering only as an example.

Most of the plant genetic engineering projects that are in progress globally fall under one of the following three types: 1) engineering for improved crop production and quality (e.g., herbicide or pest resistance); 2) engineering for improved health (e.g., edible vaccines for the prevention of diseases); and 3) biopharming or the engineering of plants for alternative nonfood uses (e.g., rather than building expensive factories we might be able simply to grow the chemicals needed for the making of plastics, detergents, and construction materials). In the last case, within the next ten years it is possible that 10 percent of the U.S. corn acres will be devoted to this type of bioengineering.[8] Some of these projects involve the insertion of animal genes into plants to create what are called transgenic plants. For example, the DNA Plant Technology Corporation in New Jersey added a gene from the Arctic flounder to make a tomato frost-resistant. In addition, corn and tobacco plants have been engineered to accept human genes as part of their DNA in order to make drugs to fight cancer and osteoporosis.

There have been mixed reactions to these biotechnologies around the world. In the United States, where people tend to be pragmatic and more willing to take risks with the environment, it seems that the biotech companies are moving forward with great speed to produce these transgenic plants. Things may be moving forward even more rapidly in China where, in 1986, Chinese scientists were already aggressively pushing for governmental efforts to bioengineer plants to feed their 1.2 billion people. On the other hand, in Europe the situation has been much different. The United Kingdom and Germany have staged many protests against the introduction of these genetically altered foods into their countries, but the Swiss, after many protests, voted decisively in June 1998 to reject a proposal to outlaw the production and patenting of genetically modified plants, ostensibly because they did not want to surrender Swiss leadership in biotechnology.

In October 1990, the publicly funded Human Genome Project was launched in the United States at an estimated cost of $3 billion. Its aim was to map and sequence all the genetic material of the human person. The project ended approximately five years early in June 2000, and a rough map was unveiled in February 2001. We now know that the human person possesses far fewer genes than previously thought—instead of 80,000 to 100,000 genes, we have 30,000 to 40,000 (and maybe as few as 26,000). The knowledge that we have gained from this scientific endeavor, and the biotechnologies that will be developed, will truly revolutionize clinical medicine over the next twenty to thirty years. Cancer treatments will soon be developed to treat the specific DNA of the patient, personalized pharmaceuticals will be created and marketed by the pharmaceutical industry, and physicians will be able to splice out defective sequences of genes and replace them with proper ones.

Now, the newest scientific venture is concerned with the proteome, or the mapping of all the human proteins coded by genes. Enormous ethical, social, and legal problems are already being raised about the medical genetics and the proteomics that will be developed out of these efforts by big science. How will we be able to protect the confidentiality of this genetic information? Should we use the new technology involved in gene therapy and apply it to enhancing ourselves? Who owns the rights to the genes and their sequences once they are discovered? Who will have fair access to the new biotechnologies that will be developed? Will we discriminate on the basis of genetic makeup, such that we will deny health insurance or employment to those who possess certain genetic traits or defects? The U.S. Department of Energy has established the Ethical, Legal, and Social Issues Program (ELSI) to study many of these issues, but the questions seem almost endless. Religious groups wonder about the wisdom of "playing God" with DNA,[9] and they are forced many times to rethink their traditional doctrines of creation, divine providence, and redemption.[10]

The final areas that we will briefly review where medical genetics and biotechnology come together to present us with great potential opportunities but also with tremendous ethical questions are human cloning and stem cell research. Once Dolly the sheep was successfully cloned by Ian Wilmut in Scotland, the expectation by some has been that we could or should do the same with humans. Wilmut succeeded by taking a body (somatic) cell that contained all the genetic material to make an exact duplicate of the donor sheep and inserted it into an egg whose own nuclear DNA had been destroyed. Once the full complement of nuclear DNA from the body cell was fused with the egg by using a small electrical charge, the fertilized ovum began to divide and grow. The National Bioethics Advisory Commission (NBAC) was asked to study the scientific and ethical dimensions of human cloning and to make recommendations to the president of the United States and Congress. NBAC recommended against the application of this technology to humans on the basis of its lack of safety.[11]

But one does not have to use this technology to duplicate a whole human person; one could use it with stem cell research to grow organs or tissues for a wide range of diseases (e.g., Alzheimer's disease, Parkinson's disease, and so forth). Pluripotent stem cells exist as very special cells in the early embryo (ES cells) or in the primordial reproductive cells of the developing fetus (EG cells). Since they have the capacity to become almost any of the 210 cell lines in the mature human body, many believe that the retrieval and differentiation of these special cells could benefit hundreds of thousands of patients. However, to retrieve these cells one must destroy the early embryo or retrieve them from aborted fetuses, and either of these procedures presents great ethical problems for some in our society, especially if the research is funded by public monies. Once again, President Clinton asked NBAC to study the scientific, ethical, and religious issues related to this technology. The commission's report was complex, but it did recommend the public funding of the derivation and use of pluripotent stem cells from both embryos remaining after infertility treatments in vitro fertilization (IVF) labs and from cadaveric fetal tissue.[12]

If one did pursue this course, the technology could be combined with human cloning for therapeutic purposes. In this case, the scientist would take a body cell from a patient, extract the nuclear DNA from his or her somatic cell, and insert its nucleus into a human egg whose own nucleus has been destroyed. Once fused, the fertilized egg would be allowed to develop to the four-to-six-cell stage and then the pluripotent stem cells would be removed, destroying the embryo in the process. Then the stem cells would be differentiated into the tissue needed by the patient (e.g., spinal cord tissue or brain tissue). Since the tissue would have been cloned from the patient's own body cells, there would no need for special drugs to suppress the patient's immune system after the transplant. Many believe that there is great promise in this new technology when combined with medical genetics, but others question the morality of such procedures that rely on the taking of one life to save another.

CURRAN'S CONTRIBUTIONS TO MEDICAL GENETICS AND BIOTECHNOLOGY

This section will develop in four parts. First, a broad overview of Charles E. Curran's writings in the general field of bioethics or medical ethics will be presented. Since Curran has been one of the most influential U.S. Catholic moral theologians in the second part of the twentieth century, a study of his writings on bioethics would be very instructive. The second part will narrow the discussion by briefly presenting his moral positions specifically on genetic medicine and biotechnology. In the third section, I will analyze what I and others have judged Professor Curran's theological, philosophical, and ethical contributions to be on the topics of genetics and biotechnology. Finally, a brief critical assessment of Curran's writings will be undertaken on the topics under consideration.

Overview of Curran's Writings in Medical Ethics

Approximately six months after the Kennedy Institute of Ethics at Georgetown University opened its doors on July 1, 1971, Charles Curran took a sabbatical leave from the Catholic University of America and went to the Institute as a Fellow to complete a book on the writings of Paul Ramsey, a Protestant theologian at Princeton who had already written on issues in medicine and ethics.[13] One of Curran's doctoral dissertations had been in the area of medical ethics,[14] and he had already published several additional essays in the field before going to the institute. Though he would not consider himself a "bioethicist" as such, Curran was certainly one of the original group of theological ethicists[15] who had begun to dedicate at least some of their scholarly research to the new field of bioethics in the late 1960s and early 1970s.

More than one-tenth of all Curran's published works have been in the general field of medical ethics. He has contributed substantially to the areas of medical genetics and biotechnology, as we shall see, but he has also written on many of the bioethical topics that were confronting society since the 1970s. He is probably best known for his many essays on birth control, especially in light of the Catholic tradition.[16] However, his essays have also analyzed issues ranging from abortion[17] and assisted reproductive technologies[18] at the beginnings of life, to topics of experimentation on human subjects[19] and the right to health care[20] in the middle of life, to care for the dying[21] and euthanasia[22] at the end of life. Despite the fact that bioethics has not been one of the central areas of Curran's research, it is clear that he has made some important and lasting contributions to the general field.

Overview of Curran's Writings on Medical Genetics and Biotechnology

A substantial portion of Charles Curran's publications in the field of bioethics has been dedicated to the two areas under consideration. One reason for his focus on these topics has to do with the proposals that were coming from noted geneticists, for example, H. J. Muller, a Nobel Prize winner from the University of Indiana. Curran is interested in these proposals because they contained recommendations about how to overcome the deficiencies of the human genetic code through the implementation of eugenic measures. Perhaps more importantly, the field of medical genetics was beginning to expand enormously in the 1960s, and the biotechnology industry was establishing itself and its research and development programs in the 1970s after the introduction of recombinant DNA technology. An ethical voice amidst these scientific and technological developments was needed, especially a voice that could also address the deep religious and anthropological questions that lay beneath the ethical surface. Yet, from Curran's own perspective, writing on these topics gave him the opportunity to place contemporary science and technology in a critical dialogue with his own theological tradition of Roman

Catholicism in order to challenge the methodological and anthropological assumptions of both.[23] As we shall see later, this latter strategy has been one of the distinctive marks of Curran's contributions to bioethics.

Curran recognized early in the development of medical genetics and biotechnology that science had the possibility of improving the human condition around the world. Deleterious genes in the gene pool could be eliminated and new genes could be added to improve not only individuals but also the human species. Curran saw these as potential pluses. However, he recognized that a scientific mentality could become so predominant that trust in science and technology, and their emphasis on power over the human and nonhuman world, could negate the possible gains. A careful analysis and critique were called for, and Curran was prepared to bring to bear his theological and ethical talents on these topics.

In the area of medical genetics, Curran consistently recognized that there are three issues at stake. First, there is eugenics, or the selection and recombination of genes already existing in the human gene pool. This issue can be further divided into negative and positive eugenics. Whereas negative eugenics aims at removing deleterious genes from the gene pool, positive eugenics attempts to improve the genes already existing in the gene pool.[24] There are three possible technological procedures that eugenics can use: artificial insemination with sperm that have been stored, in vitro fertilization and embryo transfer to a womb, and the cloning of human beings.[25]

The second issue in medical genetics for Curran is called genetic engineering, genetic surgery, algeny, or transformationist eugenics as distinct from selectionist eugenics. The aim of genetic engineering is to change the genes in such a way as to either eliminate a certain defective gene (negative) or to improve the genotype (positive).[26] When he wrote many of his early essays in this area, he noted that medical science does not have the ability to perform what is now called "human gene transfer"—that is, the process of using restriction enzymes to open the DNA molecule, splice out a defective gene or splice in a new gene sequence and then, using another enzyme (ligase), close the molecule. The Human Genome Project (1990–2000) had not even been conceived when Curran wrote on eugenics in the late 1960s and early 1970s, so his understandings of the real possibilities of this technology for therapy or enhancement purposes may have been somewhat understated.

The third issue is concerned with euphenics, which for Curran is somewhere between eugenics and euthenics, or environmental engineering. It aims at the control and regulation of the phenotype rather than the genotype, and it would involve all efforts at controlling gene expression in the human without changing the genotype.[27]

What are Curran's moral conclusions on the application of these genetic technologies to the human? On the issue of negative eugenics, he is in favor of supporting voluntary efforts to use genetic counseling for couples who are carriers of deleterious genes. More scientific experimentation must go forward, but such experimentation must respect human dignity and not totally subordinate the individual to the goals of scientific advancement.[28] On the issue of positive eugenic interventions, Curran has taken a rather negative stance. He does not believe that we have enough knowledge or wisdom for such undertakings,[29] and he argues strongly against the use of assisted reproductive technologies, for example, in vitro fertilization and embryo transfer, to achieve eugenic ends.[30] Though the technique of cloning mammals (somatic cell nuclear transplant cloning) used by Ian Wilmut was not yet developed when Curran wrote his essays, he does note that, if human cloning were ever available, it would create enormous problems.[31] On the issue of gene splicing, Curran takes a relatively positive, though cautious, position on this medical technology. He believes that constant oversight and vigilance are needed, but he does not hold that such interventions necessarily open a Pandora's box or are acts of "playing God."[32]

Curran has focused a good deal of his scholarly analysis in the area of bioethics on the proper role of biotechnology in human life. He understands all technology, including biotechnology, as "applied science by which human beings are able to control and influence human existence."[33] The issue of control is important here, because there is always the tendency in the application of technology to manipulate not only the nonhuman world but also the human person. A process of discernment must be in place to distinguish the proper from the improper forms of control over the world and self, and Curran will frequently look from within his theological tradition to discover this process.

Curran establishes a general framework for understanding and evaluating technology—especially biomedical technology—from the perspective of theological ethics in the Catholic tradition. He develops three theses from this framework. First, we must be open to the data of science and the possibilities of technology. He gives two reasons to support this thesis. The first reason for a basic openness to biotechnology stems from an acceptance of the goodness of human reason and the belief that religious faith and reason can never contradict one another. The second reason comes from the theological recognition of the goodness of the natural and of the human. The Catholic tradition has insisted on the compatibility between grace and nature.[34]

The second thesis for Curran is essentially historical. It recognizes that the Catholic theological tradition has not always lived up to its theoretical affirmations about biotechnology and science. History is replete with examples of where the Catholic Church has been suspicious or even hostile to science—for example, the Galileo case.

The third thesis focuses on the limitations of science and biotechnology and argues that they must always be in the service of the human. There is not an identity between the human and the scientific or technological, and thus three limitations arise on the use and application of science and technology. Because there is not an identity between the human and technology, Curran argues that sometimes we must simply say no to what science and technology can offer us. The second source of limitation comes from the limitation inherent to any one particular science or technology. There are other sciences (e.g., psychology, sociology) that can add insight into the human; and so a total focus on what basic science or technology can offer is inappropriate. The final source of limitation comes from the different opinions within any one particular empirical science or applied technology. These differences of opinion for Curran are clear signs that the nature of the human is complex and that no one position can possibly capture the entirety of what it means to be human.[35]

Curran's moral position on the development and application of biotechnology is rather consistent throughout his writings. First, he holds that biotechnology is an essential good, though it is only a limited good that cannot be identified with the totally human.[36] Second, all medical technology, including biotechnology, must be used in the service of the human and in terms of truly human progress in overcoming disease and improving the length and quality of human life.[37] Truly human progress and technological progress are not the same; in fact, they may even be opposed to one another on certain occasions. However, whenever human and technological progress do coincide, Curran argues that we can view technology as positively related to God's final kingdom.[38] Third, he notes that there may be points of conflict between the scientific/technological worldview and the one espoused by Christianity. When the former focuses on effects and performances and values success and results, then conflict will exist with the Christian understandings of reality and the nature of the person. For Christianity, the value of the person is not primarily determined by what he or she does or can do. Rather, value is seen in terms of what God has first done for us.[39] Finally, Curran argues that there is a constant danger in biotechnology to give such great attention to comparatively esoteric procedures that many times basic medical care tends to be neglected. Justice and the right to health care become important moral considerations in this context. For forty-four million people under the age of sixty-five in the United States who have no health insurance, this judgment on biotechnology is particularly poignant. In the end, Curran seeks some kind of fair and equitable balance between the needs to develop and apply new biotechnologies and the medical needs of people in our society.

Curran's Contributions to Medical Genetics and Biotechnology

Charles Curran's contributions to the areas of medical genetics and biotechnology are major, and his writings have had an enduring effect on the way in which Catholic ethicists now approach these and other topics in bioethics. The focus throughout his scholarly essays is to place medical science and biotechnology in a dialogical conversation with both his own religious tradition and with the ways in which that tradition has approached bioethical topics in the past. Consequently, I would proffer that Curran's most incisive and lasting contributions are not primarily in his concrete investigations and in the particular moral recommendations that he offers on the two topics under consideration. These are important and certainly worthy of careful consideration. However, the lasting contributions that he makes can be analyzed under three categories: 1) theological-anthropological issues, 2) philosophical issues, and 3) ethical issues.

When the field of bioethics was coming into existence in the United States in the mid-1960s, many of the founders of this discipline were originally trained in the theological sciences. As they began to tackle the two major concerns of the time—experimentation on humans and the dramatic development of scientific knowledge and technology—most of them brought their theological anthropology to bear on the issues. Maybe more than others, Curran is convinced that a fully articulated theological anthropology is necessary to meet the challenges of the modern era. However, he does not believe that one formulates a view of the human and then simply applies it from the top down to the contemporary questions of medical genetics and biotechnology. Rather, he argues that the very questions posed by biomedicine help to form his understanding of theological anthropology, and thus a dialogical relation must exist between the two areas.[40]

As he carries on this dialogue over a number of years, Curran formulates his theological anthropology in terms of a Christian stance. For him, stance or the horizon of meaning forms the way a person interprets reality and structures his or her understanding of the world and reality. Stance is logically the first and primary consideration in any methodology, and hence its importance in the analysis of any concrete issue in bioethics.[41] Curran formulates his stance by reference to the fivefold Christian mysteries: creation, sin, incarnation, redemption, and resurrection destiny. Each one of these mysteries is informed by the questions of biomedical science and technology, and each mystery in turn plays an important part in critiquing science and technology. One example will be helpful to demonstrate how this dialogical structure operates in Curran's writings on bioethical issues, especially those concerned with medical genetics and biotechnology.

Contemporary developments in genetics and biotechnology raise important questions about the control that humans should have over all creation, but especially the control they should have over themselves and their genetic future. Modern science also adopts a concept of the universe as unfinished and evolving. Now, from a theological perspective, different views of creation and of the special place that humans have in creation need to be sorted out. If creation is entirely completed by the divine and the human serves the principal role of conserving and preserving what the divine has already accomplished, then human control over the genetic future of humanity may not be morally warranted. In this case, theological ethics would critique efforts to engineer humanity's genetic future. However, if one understands creation to be a process (*creatio continua*) that is not yet completed by the divine—a view that is shared by modern science—and if one understands the role of humans to be one of cooperation with the divine in bringing creation to its completion, then one might accord more responsibility and control to the human to intervene into the genetic pool, at least to correct defects. Curran adopts the latter view based on his dialogue with modern science and biotechnology. For him, however, the Christian mystery of mankind's fall might temper one's emphasis on human control over our genetic future, as would the mystery of eschatology (views of the final times). Each mystery would point to a limitation: the former mystery recognizes the limits on our abilities to do good; the latter recognizes a limit on the importance of science as good in relation to the total human good. Curran methodically develops each of his fivefold mysteries in dialogue with modern genetics and biotechnology and then systematically applies these mysteries back to the questions, developments, and applications of these sciences.

Two lasting contributions are found here. First, Curran's willingness to place modern science and technology in a critical dialogue with Christian ethics has encouraged others in the field to follow in a similar vein. Such a dialogue has surely been one of the forces that has resulted in a revised anthropology in Catholic ethics at least. Though Curran surely has not accomplished this alone, his writings are a model for how to carry on this dialogue. Second, his insistence that theological anthropology must be explicitly brought to bear on all questions of bioethics is important and instructive for others in the field. Some believe that much of the literature in bioethics today possesses little or no attention to this anthropological focus, and thus they argue that this lack leads to an impoverishment in the discussion of contemporary bioethical issues.[42]

The second area where Curran has made lasting contributions is concerned with various philosophical issues. The standard method for ethical analysis used in the Roman Catholic tradition, especially by the teaching authority of the church, has been the natural law. As a method of ethical analysis, it assumes that there is a range of basic goods or values that all pursue as part of their nature, and it assumes that knowledge of these goods is available to all people of goodwill. The theory of natural law found in the manuals of moral theology of the late-nineteenth through the mid-twentieth centuries seemed to too easily identify the physical action itself or the physical structure of its effects with the actual moral determination of the human action. In addition, the way this method was applied, especially to issues in bioethics and sexuality, was overly deductive and ahistorical. At the level of epistemology, the theory tended to search for certitude and did not trust human experience as a valid font of knowledge.

From both a methodological and an epistemological point of view, Curran sees multiple problems with the way the natural-law theory had been developed and then applied to questions in bioethics. From his vantage point, the received tradition on natural law is inadequate to deal with the contemporary issues in genetic medicine and biotechnology, and thus a dialogical conversation has to be opened to revise the theory. Much of Curran's early works in bioethics focuses on the revision of natural law, not its rejection.[43] He is committed to many of the presuppositions of natural-law theory—for example, its insistence on the ability of all to know the good—and thus his intent is to revise and reformulate the theory to deal with the bioethical issues facing his discipline. Curran's conception of natural law takes on many of the characteristics of modern consciousness: it is more historically minded, it gives a significant role to human experience as a valid font of moral wisdom, it is much more inductive in its approach, and it recognizes the limits of the certitude that we can have in our moral judgments. Many of these characteristics now regularly inform the analyses of Catholic bioethicists.

The final area of Curran's lasting contributions to the field is concerned with specifically ethical issues. Ethics is the systematic study of morality, and it involves the theoretical component to moral judgments. One of the components of ethics is called normative ethics or simply ethical theory. All ethical theories attempt both to articulate the objective criteria for judging actions and character to be right/wrong and good/bad and to discern the ways in which we might know these criteria to be fulfilled. Each relies in turn on various models of the moral life and human agency. Historically, the two standard ethical theories have been 1) teleological theories that focus on the goals of the moral life or on the ends and consequences of actions, and 2) deontological theories that focus on our duties and obligations or on the actions we perform.

Curran's contribution to this important discussion, and through it to issues in bioethics, is to offer an alternative to the existing ethical theories. Relying on the previous work of H. Richard Niebuhr,[44] Curran calls his theory a rationality-responsibility model, and he views it as distinct from the existing theories.[45] His model places much more emphasis on the relations between persons and the relations that exist between persons and the world. It also focuses centrally on the issue of responsibility that humans have toward themselves, others, and the world. Though Curran certainly needs to fill out more fully the exact criteria that must be used in judging actions, this model of the moral life has nonetheless attempted to meet the many complex challenges of contemporary biomedicine and technology.

Critical Assessment of Curran's Writings

Before beginning a brief critical assessment of Professor Curran's writings in bioethics, it might be helpful to remember two things. First, bioethics is not an area that he regularly worked in, and he never considered himself a bioethicist in the sense this term in used in current academic circles. Second, in many cases he is more interested in the dialogical conversation between contemporary medical genetics and biotechnology, on the one hand, and theological ethics, on the other. Thus, frequently Curran's writings in these areas focus more on the theological anthropological issues, philosophical presuppositions to ethical methodology, and on ethical theory than on the concrete bioethical issues themselves.

Briefly, there are three areas for critical assessment. First, because Curran is so deeply concerned with revising many of his own theological tradition's categories (e.g., natural law), some may view his analyses as somewhat parochial. Frequently, his dialogue with genetic science is less a deep ethical analysis of contemporary genetics than it is a deep analysis of the deficiencies that he sees in Roman Catholic ethics and the way the teaching authority of his church had used various anthropological, philosophical, and ethical concepts.

Second, the theory of compromise that he develops to deal with conflict situations that arise due to the existence of human sinfulness in the world[46] does not ultimately prove to be helpful.[47] He applies this theory to a few bioethical topics,[48] but Curran himself seems to abandon it in his later writings.

Finally, and possibly most importantly, Curran's corpus may need a more sustained, overarching theory or system that underlies his concrete ethical analyses of bioethical topics. His writings are probably best characterized as eclectic since he borrows from others inside and outside the field of Christian ethics. For example, he clearly borrows from some authors who have employed a personalist theory like Bernard Häring, but it may be inaccurate to type Curran's writings strictly as personalist. In addition, he borrows from H. Richard Niebuhr a phenomenology of human agency and applies these insights to the bioethical issues at hand, yet it would be inaccurate to type Curran's writings as phenomenological. Though one finds his essays on medical genetics and biotechnology to be very good and insightful, there still is lacking a general underlying system or theory that unifies his approach to these topics.

FUTURE AGENDA AND CHALLENGES

Medical genetics and biotechnology will continue to pose enormous challenges, and in fact the pace will only hasten as each of these areas develops and applies its newfound knowledge to human and nonhuman life. Thus a clear ethical agenda is necessary to confront these challenges. The list is not sacrosanct, but many in the field of bioethics would probably agree that there are seven or eight areas that need to be included. There is no necessary rank ordering of these priorities, but surely some are more important than others or the urgency of one will take priority over others.

First, there will be the need to put increasing pressure on the scientific community and biotechnology companies to protect the dignity of their research subjects. There is more and more evidence that harms are accruing to human subjects in various research protocols.[49] Part of this agenda must also deal with the protection of early embryos in research protocols and with their creation and use to benefit the health of others. Second, we will have to introduce new ethical and legal measures to protect the privacy of genetic information. We will need to sort through who should rightfully have access to this knowledge and who should be excluded. Since genes are inherited within families, do family members also have a right to this knowledge that could adversely affect their health? Genetic discrimination is a real possibility, especially in the workplace or in the clinic, but it is also a possibility in terms of securing health and life insurance.

Third, now that the human genome is basically mapped and sequenced and the scientific community is moving forward with not only identifying defective genes but also with the mapping of the proteins that cause disease, what will we do with this knowledge? Since our knowledge will outstrip our clinical abilities to cure many of these genetic diseases, how will we use this knowledge when counseling patients? Will we simply create the lifetime identity of a "sick person" when we tell an adolescent that she will get adult-onset Alzheimer's disease when she's eighty years old? Fourth, genetic screening of targeted populations must come under severe scrutiny. The chances for discrimination are enormous here, particularly if this type of screening is simply routine at birth or during a visit to the clinic. Fifth, human gene transfer, either with somatic cells or germline cells, for purposes of therapy or enhancement, will probably be introduced on a regular basis within the next twenty or thirty years at the clinical level. This technology could be combined with human cloning techniques and embryonic stem cell research, and thus different combinations of genetic medicine will develop over the next few decades. The agenda must sort out the differences between therapy and enhancement, and it must decide whether we should ever cross into the germline with any of these technologies.

Sixth, there are huge marketplace issues at stake, especially with the multinational pharmaceutical companies that stand to gain enormous profits. The fair pricing of the new drugs and therapies that will be developed must be constantly assessed. Ownership of the gene sequences must be decided at both the ethical and legal levels. Next, and very importantly, we must ensure that the development and use of these biotechnologies will not simply benefit the few who are rich enough to afford them. We will need to focus our attention on the equity of the delivery of health care in a way that we have not in the past. Not only are there millions in the United States who virtually go without any health care, there are millions and millions throughout the world who basically have no access to the wonders of modern medicine. Just social policies must be forged, not only in the scientific and medicine-rich West, but around the world.

Finally, for theological ethicists and their communities, there is the need to continue to develop methodologies and strategies for incorporating religious beliefs and traditions in the ethical assessment of these bioethical topics. The goal will be to establish a dialogue between religious traditions and science/technology while avoiding a reductionism. We are fortunate that Charles Curran has provided us with one very helpful example of how to carry on this dialogue.

ENDNOTES

1. Warren Thomas Reich, introduction, in *Encyclopedia of Bioethics*, rev. ed., vol. 1, edited by Warren T. Reich (New York: Simon & Schuster Macmillan, 1995), xxi. For Reich, the word "bioethics" was introduced in 1971 with the publication of Van Rensselaer Potter's book *Bioethics: Bridge to the Future* (Englewood Cliffs, N.J.: Prentice-Hall,

1971), but André Hellegers in Washington, D.C., first used the word in an institutional way to designate the focused area of inquiry. See Warren T. Reich, "The Word 'Bioethics': Its Birth and the Legacies of Those Who Shaped It," *Kennedy Institute of Ethics Journal* 4 (December 1994): 319–35. In either case, bioethics does not begin as a discipline until around this time.

2. Victor A. McKusick, *Human Genetics*, 2nd ed. (Englewood Cliffs, N.J.: Prentice-Hall, 1969), 181.

3. Lisa Sowle Cahill, "Genetics, Ethics and Social Policy: The State of the Question," in *Concilium: The Ethics of Genetic Engineering*, edited by Maureen Junker-Kenny and Lisa Sowle Cahill (London: SCM, 1998), vii.

4. Nanette Newell, "Biotechnology," in *Encyclopedia of Bioethics*, rev. ed., vol. 1, edited by Warren T. Reich (New York: Simon & Schuster Macmillan, 1995), 283.

5. Alison Taunton-Rigby, *Bioethics: The New Frontier* (Bentley College, Mass.: Center for Business Ethics, 2000), 6–8.

6. For the authoritative encyclopedia on this topic, see the *Encyclopedia of Ethical, Legal, and Policy Issues in Biotechnology*, 2 vols., edited by Thomas H. Murray and Maxwell J. Mehlman (New York: John Wiley & Sons, 2000).

7. For example, see the President's Commission for the Study of Ethical Problems in Medicine and Biomedical and Behavioral Research, *Splicing Life: The Social and Ethical Issues of Genetic Engineering with Human Beings* (Washington, D.C.: U.S. Government Printing Office, 1982).

8. Aaron Zitner, "Fields of Gene Factories," *Los Angeles Times*, June 4, 2001, A7.

9. For a helpful essay on the meaning of the phrase "playing God," see Allen Verhey, "'Playing God' and Invoking a Perspective," *Journal of Medicine and Philosophy* 20 (1995): 347–64.

10. For example, see Ronald Cole-Turner, *The New Genesis: Theology and the Genetic Revolution* (Louisville: Westminster/John Knox, 1993).

11. National Bioethics Advisory Board, *Cloning Human Beings*, 2 vols. (Rockville, Md.: U.S. Government Printing Office, 1997).

12. National Bioethics Advisory Board, *Ethical Issues in Human Stem Cell Research*, 3 vols. (Rockville, Md.: U.S. Government Printing Office, 2000).

13. At the end of his sabbatical Curran published his *Politics, Medicine, & Christian Ethics: A Dialogue with Paul Ramsey* (Philadelphia: Fortress, 1973).

14. Charles E. Curran, *The Prevention of Conception after Rape* (Rome: Pontifical Gregorian University, 1961).

15. Some of the other theologians, Protestant and Catholic, who belonged to this original group were Joseph Fletcher, Paul Ramsey, William F. May, James M. Gustafson, James F. Childress, Karen Lebacqz, Albert R. Jonsen, Bernard Häring, and Richard A. McCormick.

16. For example, see Charles E. Curran, ed., *Contraception: Authority and Dissent* (New York: Herder & Herder, 1969), especially 151–75.

17. Charles E. Curran, *New Perspectives in Moral Theology* (Notre Dame, Ind.: Fides, 1974), 163–93.

18. Charles E. Curran, *Moral Theology: A Continuing Journey* (Notre Dame, Ind.: University of Notre Dame, 1982), 112–40.

19. Charles E. Curran, *Issues in Sexual and Medical Ethics* (Notre Dame, Ind.: University of Notre Dame, 1978), 71–102.

20. Charles E. Curran, *Transition and Tradition in Moral Theology* (Notre Dame, Ind.: University of Notre Dame, 1979), 139–70.

21. Curran, *Politics, Medicine, & Christian Ethics*, especially 147–63.

22. Charles E. Curran, *Ongoing Revision: Studies in Moral Theology* (Notre Dame, Ind.: Fides, 1975), 144–72, especially 158–61.

23. Charles E. Curran, *Contemporary Problems in Moral Theology* (Notre Dame, Ind.: Fides, 1970), 189–224, especially 195.

24. Curran, *Contemporary Problems*, 192.

25. Curran, *Ongoing Revision*, 166.

26. Curran, *Ongoing Revision*, 193–94.

27. Curran, *Ongoing Revision*, 194–95.

28. Curran, *Ongoing Revision*, 216–17.

29. Curran, *Politics, Medicine, & Christian Ethics*, 218–19.

30. Charles E. Curran, *Moral Theology: A Continuing Journey* (Notre Dame, Ind.: University of Notre Dame, 1982), 130.

31. Charles E. Curran, *Critical Concerns in Moral Theology* (Notre Dame, Ind.: University of Notre Dame, 1984), 109.

32. Charles E. Curran, *Toward an American Catholic Moral Theology* (Notre Dame, Ind.: University of Notre Dame, 1987), 78.

33. Curran, *Critical Concerns in Moral Theology*, 99–100.

34. Curran, *Critical Concerns in Moral Theology*, 105–6.

35. Curran, *Critical Concerns in Moral Theology*, 107–10.

36. Curran, *Toward an American Catholic Moral Theology*, 77.

37. Curran, *Issues in Sexual and Medical Ethics*, 75–76.

38. Curran, *Politics, Medicine, & Christian Ethics*, 201.

39. Curran, *Contemporary Problems in Moral Theology*, 214.

40. Curran, *Toward an American Catholic Moral Theology*, 78.

41. For his essay on stance, see Curran, *New Perspectives in Moral Theology*, 47–86.

42. See Hubert Doucet, "How Theology Could Contribute to the Redemption of Bioethics from an Individualist Approach to an Anthropological Sensitivity," *Catholic Theological Society of America Proceedings of the Fifty-Third Annual Convention* 53 (1998): 53–66; and see my response, James J. Walter, "Response to Hubert Doucet," *Catholic Theological Society of America Proceedings of the Fifty-Third Annual Convention* 53 (1998): 67–71.

43. For example, see Charles E. Curran, *Medicine and Morals* (Washington, D.C.: Corpus Books, 1970).

44. H. Richard Niebuhr, *The Responsible Self* (New York: Harper & Row, 1963).

45. Charles E. Curran, *Directions in Fundamental Moral Theology* (Notre Dame, Ind.: University of Notre Dame, 1985), 173–96.

46. Curran, *Transition and Tradition in Moral Theology*, 59–80, especially 73–78.

47. For a thorough analysis and critique of Curran's theory of compromise, see Richard Grecco, *A Theology of Compromise: A Study of Method in the Ethics of Charles E. Curran* (New York: Peter Lang, 1991).

48. Curran, *New Perspectives in Moral Theology*, 163–93, especially 191–92.

49. As of this writing, the National Bioethics Advisory Commission has submitted a draft of its report on *Ethical and Policy Issues in Research Involving Human Participants* (December 2000).

11

Theological Perspectives on Cancer Genetics and Gene Therapy: The Roman Catholic Tradition

James J. Walter

Permit me to begin with a very general conclusion about the Roman Catholic perspective on cancer genetics and gene therapy. In principle, there is nothing in this tradition that theologically or morally prohibits interventions into the human genetic code, though in fact there may be circumstances in which a specific intervention might be immoral.[1] To prove this conclusion I focus my attention primarily on documents from the magisterium or teaching authority of the Catholic Church, that is, documents from recent popes, bishops, and the Second Vatican Council. I augment these teachings on occasion with various positions taken by Catholic theologians.

I proceed by analyzing three sets of issues that are stake for the Catholic tradition on this topic. These three sets are: 1) anthropological issues, 2) theological issues, and 3) moral issues. My analysis of each must necessarily be brief. I assume throughout that the types of genetic intervention are either somatic or germline and that the purposes of these interventions could be for either therapeutic or enhancement ends. Nonetheless, I limit most of my remarks to the area of the therapeutic. Though I realize there is an important dispute about what constitutes a "therapeutic" end and what constitutes an "enhancement" of the human genome,[2] I consider for our purposes that genetic interventions for either the cure or the prevention of cancer are therapeutic. These therapies could be used to elicit immune responses to cancer cells or to alter tumor tissue to enhance the effectiveness of chemotherapy.[3] I conclude with a brief summary of some definite positions taken by the Roman Catholic tradition on cancer genetics and gene therapy.

ANTHROPOLOGICAL ISSUES

There are several background beliefs about the human that function as starting points for a moral discussion of cancer genetics and gene therapy, but I will mention only two. First, the Roman Catholic tradition consistently argues not only that the nature of the human person is both body and spirit but also that there is a oneness among these distinguishable but inseparable aspects. As the "Pastoral Constitution on the Church in the Modern World" ("Gaudium et Spes") states the matter, "Though made of body and soul, man is one."[4] Pope John Paul II reiterated this belief in several of his statements on genetics. For example, in his 1982 address to the Pontifical Academy of Sciences, the pontiff claimed that "The human body is not independent of the spirit, just as the spirit is not independent of the body, because of the deep unity and mutual connection that exist between one and the other."[5] Thus, any genetic intervention into the human subject must recognize and respect this unity; any view that separates the two is dualistic and leads to a denigration of one or the other of the two aspects of the person.

Second, the Catholic tradition argues that there are various kinds of goods whose pursuit of and acquisition by persons will define their well-being and flourishing. Two of these goods are particularly important here: life and health. In their working report on genetic intervention, the British bishops argued that "to be fulfilled in our existence as human beings requires some degree of bodily well-being. Health is a good which is a dimension of the basic good of life."[6] Thus, if health is a basic good that all pursue, even though there are definite limits to this pursuit,[7] the nature of this good itself becomes the ground for the prima facie obligation on the part of both patients and physicians to seek remedies for cancer.[8] The role of medicine, then, is to serve health, and the technological means by which medicine realizes this good are ultimately subject to the objective standards of morality, which themselves are based on the nature of the human person in all its dimensions.[9]

THEOLOGICAL ISSUES

There are two distinctively theological issues that serve as interpretive frameworks for the morality of cancer genetics and gene therapy. The position one takes theologically on each of these issues will inform and shape how one reasons morally about genetic interventions.

The first issue concerns a question about whether or not we are "playing God" by intervening into the human genome in order to cure or prevent cancer.[10] This question obviously has definite anthropological implications, because at its core it is asking about the responsibility that we humans have over material reality, including the materiality (genes) of our own bodies. If the divine has not decided to share with us the dominion over our bodies but has reserved such dominion to itself, then it would seem that any act to change what God has given us in our bodies would be an improper exercise of human freedom and thus an act of "playing God." On the other hand, if one judges that God has indeed granted this responsibility to humans, then it would seem that we have at least a prima facie moral obligation to alter our genetic makeup for therapeutic ends. Such acts in this latter view, then, would not be improper acts of "playing God" but rather they represent the rightful taking up of our responsibility for the goods of life and health.

For the most part, Pope John Paul II[11] and much of the Catholic tradition[12] have argued rather strongly for the view that we humans, within certain moral limits, have been granted by the divine the responsibility over material nature, including our own genetic heritage. Consequently, as long as researchers respect the nature of the human person, a moral criterion that I develop below, therapeutic genetic interventions are theologically permitted in the Catholic community.

The second theological issue concerns whether or not a special sacred status should be conferred upon the human genome, for example, either because of its intimate connection to human reproduction and development or because of its participation in the image of God (*imago dei*) that resides in us.[13] If yes, then any intervention into our genetic code would constitute an improper act on the part of medical scientists. If no, then in principle our genes are like all other aspects of the created material world and thus possess no special sacred status. The Catholic tradition has understood the status of the human genome in terms of the latter view. For example, in their document on genetic intervention, the British bishops ask if the genome is morally untouchable by virtue of its special role in human development. Their answer: "We would argue not, in view of the fact that the genome is simply one highly influential part of our bodies: the part which directs the formation of other parts, both in ourselves and in our offspring. We believe that, like other parts of the body, the genome may *in principle* be altered, to cure some defect of the body."[14] Edmund Pellegrino and Joseph Cassidy have also argued for a similar position. They claim that human genetic material is a cause of great wonder, but in itself it does not deserve any special status such that interventions into our genome would per se constitute immoral acts.[15] Consequently, from a strictly theological perspective, the Catholic tradition would not prohibit interventions into the human genome for purposes of curing or preventing cancer.

MORAL ISSUES

Recent documents from the magisterium, especially those from John Paul II, reveal a remarkable positive thrust toward genetic intervention.[16] Many of these texts demonstrate an awareness of the difference between somatic cell and germline cell interventions, in which the latter is distinguished into gonadal cell and the cell line of the pre-embryo. The distinction between therapy and enhancement is acknowledged as well. In principle, none of these in itself is judged morally wrong, but each must be judged according to moral standards. Some of these standards are established moral principles; others serve as the foundation for the moral principles. In what follows, I list and briefly analyze four of these moral standards in relation to the various types of genetic intervention.

1. Do Good, Avoid Evil: The Fundamental Moral Imperative

Following Thomas Aquinas's discussion of the natural law in the thirteenth century,[17] this moral standard in the Catholic tradition has been considered the foundation for all moral principles. In the present discussion, the particular goods that we are to pursue are the goods of life and of health. The nature of these goods grounds the prima facie obligation to pursue them on behalf of ourselves and on behalf of others. However, we are only strictly obliged to avoid harm; we do not have a strict obligation to accomplish all good.[18] This understanding of our obligations clearly indicates that a good end does not justify a morally bad means and that a strict risk-benefit calculus is not the sole perspective from which to judge the moral appropriateness of genetic interventions.[19]

2. Genetic Interventions Must Respect the Dignity of the Human Person

This is clearly the most fundamental moral principle that applies to our discussion of genetic intervention, and it takes various forms in the documents under consideration.[20] In its most general terms, science and technology require *for their own intrinsic meaning* an unconditional respect for this principle.[21] Respect must be present from the very moment of conception,[22] and it requires that we not reduce life to a mere object.[23] Scientific interventions into the human genome respect the integrity of the person when they focus on benefits for the patient. Thus, genetic experimentation on human subjects, including embryos, can be justified morally as long as there is informed consent (by the patient or by proxy) and the experiments avoid harm and are directed to the well-being of the person.[24] Furthermore, experiments that are not strictly directed toward therapy but are aimed at improving the human biological condition (enhancement) can be justified, at least in part, on the grounds that the experiments respect the human person by safeguarding the identity of the person as one in body and soul (*corpore et anima unus*).[25] However, genetic experiments that are directed toward sex selection or other predetermined qualities[26] and those directed toward the creation of different groups of people[27] are forbidden morally because they violate the dignity of the person.

3. Genetic Interventions Must Promote the Well-Being of the Patient

I have already alluded to this standard, but it does have the status of a distinct moral principle in the Catholic tradition. John Paul II used it in part to justify morally the use of therapeutic genetic interventions to cure disease.[28] Likewise, the Science and Human Values Committee of the National Conference of Catholic Bishops has used this principle in permitting genetic testing for a cure or effective therapy of genetic diseases.[29]

4. Proportion between the Risks and Benefits

This is an important moral principle that applies to this topic, though most of the documents studied reject this as the sole principle that would apply to genetic interventions. The risks and benefits must be calculated in terms of their potential impact upon a patient's well-being and not in terms of their impact on existing others or future humanity.[30] In the end, if the benefits to the patient reasonably outweigh the risks, then this proportion can in part justify genetic interventions.

CONCLUSION

There are a substantial number of documents from the magisterium of the Catholic Church that have been produced on the topic of scientific and medical interventions into the human genome. For the most part, these teachings have been quite positive in their evaluation of these potential technologies. By way of conclusion, permit me to summarize the results of my analysis in relation to cancer genetics and gene therapy.

First, it seems clear that the Roman Catholic tradition would not only morally permit but would strongly encourage the development of somatic cell cancer therapies as long as these interventions do not violate any of the anthropological, theological, or moral issues discussed previously. In principle, these therapies raise no new moral problems that have not already been dealt with in other types of medical interventions to cure or prevent disease.[31] The goods of life and of health ground a prima facie moral obligation in the Catholic tradition to pursue research in this type of therapy.

Second, there seems to be an emerging, but not absolute, consensus that germline cancer therapy, if that were ever to become a possibility, would not be considered in principle unacceptable.[32] There are several qualifications that need to be made on this claim, though. It is important to note that this is an "in principle" argument; in practice, germline therapy is currently considered unacceptable for several reasons. For example, such therapy would be developed only after experimenting on embryos and exposing them to great harm.[33] In addition, even if one clearly distinguishes gonadal cell germline therapy from embryonic cell germline therapy, there are still problems. As the Catholic Health Association in the United States has noted, gonadal cell therapy would have to be justified on the grounds of possible beneficial results for future humanity, since this type of intervention does not alter the genetic makeup of the "patient."[34] This form of justification seems to violate, at least in a prima facie sense, the moral principle espoused by the Catholic tradition that any intervention should be for the benefit of the patient, not for some future humanity.

Finally, there is the possibility of genetic enhancement to improve the human. I have assumed throughout that the "enhancement" of our genes to resist cancer is not strictly a form of enhancement of our genetic code because it is aimed at the prevention of disease. Enhancement genetic interventions in this view are aimed per se at improving the human as such. Though there has not been much written on this specific type of genetic manipulation from the perspective of the magisterium, nonetheless at least John Paul II did not rule it out of hand by declaring it intrinsically immoral. Rather, he seemed to be open to such developments as long as they do not violate moral principles.[35]

ENDNOTES

1. One Catholic theologian who argued for this conclusion was Karl Rahner. For two of his most influential essays in this area of genetics, see "The Experiment with Man," in

his *Theological Investigations*, vol. 9, trans. Graham Harrison (New York: Herder and Herder, 1972), 205–24; and his "The Problem of Genetic Manipulation," *Theological Investigations*, vol. 9, trans. Graham Harrison (New York: Herder and Herder, 1972), 225–52.

2. For example, see Eric T. Juengst, "Can Enhancement Be Distinguished from Prevention in Genetic Medicine?" *Journal of Medicine and Philosophy* 22 (April 1997): 125–42.

3. Both forms of these therapies are cited by the British bishops' report: *Genetic Intervention on Human Subjects: The Report of a Working Party of the Catholic Bishops' Joint Committee on Bioethical Issues* (London: Linacre Centre, 1996), 4. Human gene therapy cancer trials have already been initiated for insertion of the tumor necrosis factor (TNF) gene into T-lymphocytes in order to enhance the ability of the T-lymphocytes to kill tumors. See K. Culver, "Current Status of Human Gene Therapy Research," *Genetic Resource* 7 (1993): 5–10.

4. "Gaudium et Spes," 14, in Walter M. Abbott, ed., *The Documents of Vatican II*, (New York: American Press), 212.

5. John Paul II, "Biological Research and Human Dignity," *Origins* 12 (October 22, 1982): 342–43. Also see his "The Ethics of Genetic Manipulation," *Origins* 13 (November 17, 1983): 385, 387–89, at 387.

6. British Catholic bishops, *Genetic Intervention on Human Subjects*, 17.

7. In the Roman Catholic theological tradition, to designate any potential medical intervention as "extraordinary" (i.e., that there is a disproportion between the benefits and burdens to a patient) would constitute a limit to the obligation that the patient would have to pursue that intervention. For a further discussion of the principle of proportionate versus disproportionate means (ordinary vs. extraordinary means), see the Congregation for the Doctrine of the Faith, "Declaration on Euthanasia," *Origins* 10 (August 14, 1980): 154–57, at 156.

8. The argument that the nature of a good itself grounds the prima facie moral obligation to pursue the good is based on a theory of natural law. For a helpful discussion of natural-law theory within the Roman Catholic tradition, see Richard M. Gula, *Reason Informed by Faith: Foundations of Catholic Morality* (New York: Paulist Press, 1989), chaps. 15 and 16.

9. John Paul II, *The Redeemer of Man* (*Redemptor Hominis*) (March 4, 1979), no. 16. The argument that the objective standards of morality are based on the nature of the human person originates from the "Pastoral Constitution on the Church in the Modern World" ("Gaudium et Spes"), 51. For a very helpful discussion of "the human person integrally and adequately considered," see Louis Janssens, "Artificial Insemination: Ethical Considerations," *Louvain Studies* 8 (Spring 1980): 3–29.

10. There are many different ways to understand the phrase "playing God." For some it functions as an actual moral judgment on scientific interventions, but for others it serves as a distinctively theological perspective from which to assess these interventions. For a very helpful discussion of these differences, see the Protestant theologian Allen Verhey, "'Playing God' and Invoking a Perspective," *Journal of Philosophy and Medicine* 20 (1995): 347–64. Also see James J. Walter, "'Playing God' or Properly Exercising Human Responsibility? Some Theological Reflections on Human Germ-Line Therapy," *New Theology Review* 10 (November 1997): 39–59; and James J. Walter, "Notes on Moral Theology: Theological Issues in Genetics," *Theological Studies* 60 (March 1999): 124–34.

11. For example, see John Paul II, *The Redeemer of Man* (*Redemptor Hominis*), no. 16.

12. For example, see the Congregation for the Doctrine of the Faith, "Instruction on Respect for Human Life in Its Origin and on the Dignity of Procreation" ("Donum Vitae"), in *Origins* 16 (March 19, 1987), introduction, 1, 699.

13. Though their focus was not on genetic interventions but on the patenting of genes, two Protestant theologians in the Southern Baptist community have recently argued for the special sacred status of genes based on the belief that the image of God (*imago dei*) pervades all aspects of human life, including one's genes. See Richard D. Land and C. Ben Mitchell, "Patenting Life: No," *First Things* 63 (May 1996): 20–23, at 21.

14. British Catholic bishops, *Genetic Intervention on Human Subjects*, 32. Emphasis in original.

15. Joseph D. Cassidy and Edmund Pellegrino, "A Catholic Perspective on Human Gene Therapy," *International Journal of Bioethics* 4 (1993): 11–18, at 12.

16. For example, see Pius XII's 1953 address on genetics, "Moral Aspects of Genetics," in *Medical Ethics: Sources of Catholic Teachings*, 2nd ed., edited by Kevin D. O'Rourke and Philip Boyle, 130–31 (Washington, D.C.: Georgetown University Press, 1993).

17. Thomas Aquinas, *Summa Theologiae*, trans. by the Fathers of the English Dominican Province (New York: Benzinger Brothers, 1947), I–II, q. 94, art. 2.

18. Bishops' Committee for Human Values, "Statement on Recombinant DNA Research," in *The Pastoral Letters of the United States Catholic Bishops*, vol. 4: 1975–1983, edited by Hugh J. Nolan, 200–204 (Washington, D.C.: USCC, 1984), 203; and John Paul II, "The Ethics of Genetic Manipulation," 388.

19. Bishops' Committee for Human Values, "Statement on Recombinant DNA Research," 203–4.

20. For example, see "Gaudium et Spes," 51; and the *Catechism of the Catholic Church* (New York: Paulist Press, 1994), 424.

21. Congregation for the Doctrine of the Faith, "Donum Vitae," introduction, 2, 699.

22. Bishop Friend/Pontifical Sciences Academy, "Frontiers of Genetic Research: Science and Religion," *Origins* 24 (January 19, 1995): 522–28, at 523.

23. See John Paul II, "The Ethics of Genetic Manipulation," 388; and the Catholic Health Association of the United States, *Human Genetics: Ethical Issues in Genetic Testing, Counseling, and Therapy* (St. Louis, Mo.: Catholic Health Association, 1990), 34.

24. "Donum Vitae," I, 4, 702; and Friend, "Frontiers of Genetic Research," 523.

25. John Paul II, "The Ethics of Genetic Manipulation," 388.

26. Catholic Health Association, *Human Genetics*, 26; and Friend, "Frontiers of Genetic Research," 524.

27. John Paul II, "The Ethics of Genetic Manipulation," 388.

28. John Paul II, "The Ethics of Genetic Manipulation," 388.

29. NCCB/Science and Human Values Committee, "Critical Decisions: Genetic Testing and Its Implications," *Origins* 25 (May 2, 1996): 769, 771–72, at 771.

30. Friend, "Frontiers of Genetic Research," 524.

31. For example, see the Catholic Health Association, *Human Genetics*, 19; British Catholic bishops, *Genetic Intervention on Human Subjects*, 28; and James F. Keenan, "What Is Morally New in Genetic Manipulation?" *Human Gene Therapy* 1 (1990): 289–98, at 292.

32. For example, see British Catholic bishops, *Genetic Intervention on Human Subjects*, 34.

33. British Catholic bishops, *Genetic Intervention on Human Subjects*, 42–43. For additional reasons, see the Catholic Health Association, *Human Genetics*, 20–21.

34. Catholic Health Association, *Human Genetics*, 21–22.

35. An earlier version of this chapter was published as "Catholic Reflections on the Human Genome," *National Catholic Bioethics Quarterly* 3 (Summer 2003): 275–83.

12

The Meaning and Validity of Quality of Life Judgments in Contemporary Roman Catholic Medical Ethics

James J. Walter

One of the most controversial and vexing issues in contemporary Catholic medical ethics concerns the validity of what are called "quality of life judgments" in deciding whether to forgo or withdraw treatment from patients. Scarcely a week goes by that we do not hear or read about cases of severely handicapped neonates or patients in a persistent vegetative state having all treatment, including nutrition and hydration, removed from them. Some Catholic ethicists and physicians view these judgments as just one more step toward an inevitable slide down the slippery slope toward the euthanasia of those who are the most vulnerable in society, namely, the dying, the comatose, the handicapped, and the incurably demented.[1] A growing number of theologians, on the other hand, argue that making quality of life judgments is fully consistent with the substance of the long-standing Catholic tradition on the distinction between ordinary and extraordinary means of preserving life.[2]

My intent is to locate and analyze a few of the definitional and ethical issues that are at stake in the discussion over the legitimacy of quality of life judgments. Though I cannot address the legal questions that the topic has raised, the seemingly intractable nature on this issue has been further complicated in the United States by the intervention of the courts[3] and some governmental agencies[4] during the past decade to decide patient treatment or nontreatment.

SOME PRELIMINARY DISTINCTIONS AND
THE GOALS OF MEDICINE

Statements about the "quality" or "qualities" of life can be descriptive, evaluative, or morally normative.[5] Descriptive statements about a quality of life are morally neutral in that they only make reference to the fact that a patient possesses a certain characteristic quality, for example, cognitive capacity. Evaluative statements, on the other hand, indicate that some value or worth is attached to a life that possesses the quality, and so evaluative statements assess that the quality (and thus the life) is desired, appreciated, or sacred. Finally, morally normative (prescriptive) statements about a quality of life always entail a moral judgment on the valued quality. These latter statements, then, presume that a quality is valued (e.g., cognitive capacity) but also involve judgments whether, and under which conditions, one *ought* to support or protect the life that possesses the quality or qualities (e.g., "Life that has cognitive capabilities always ought to be given all medical treatment"). Though descriptive and evaluative statements definitely come to bear on clinical and ethical decision making, all would agree that the key issue concerns the meaning and validity of morally normative claims about the quality of life.

When one makes either an evaluative or a normative claim about a quality of life, it is not altogether clear what the meaning of the word "life" is. Is one referring to life as mere physical or biological existence, or is one making a claim about life as personal existence (personhood)? At least part of the ambiguity or confusion in the discussion results from not clearly distinguishing life as mere biological existence from life understood as embodied personal existence. Anencephalic neonates and patients in a persistent vegetative state certainly have biological existence, but neither will ever experience personal existence as most of us understand that notion, that is, life with sapient consciousness and personal freedom.[6] By making this distinction we can become clearer about both what we value about physical life (evaluative claims) and what our duties and their limits are to preserve mere biological existence (morally normative claims).

Surely one of the key factors that has provoked this debate over quality of life has been the tremendous advancement of medical technology during the past several decades. Not to take this technology seriously in one's analysis is both to misread the "signs of the times" and to expect that traditional moral principles, which could not have anticipated these developments, can be equally applicable today as they were when they were conceived. We now have the capability of keeping patients biologically alive who would have certainly died only a few years ago.[7] These advancements in technology are well known and do not need to be detailed here. However, what this technology has done is to call into question the traditional goals of medicine. No doubt, medicine rightfully seeks to prevent death (especially an untimely death), to alleviate pain and physical suffering, and to promote health. Though these are important goals in the application of medical knowledge and skill, I would argue that they must be viewed as subordinate to the more encompassing goal of serving the purposefulness of personal existence.[8] Physicians promote health, prevent death, perform surgery, relieve pain, and so forth on behalf of others *in order that* we as patients might continue in some fashion to pursue values (material, moral, and spiritual) that transcend physical life. Pain, disease, general ill health, and death either frustrate our desires to pursue these values or make it impossible to pursue them at all. As a consequence, when medicine cannot any longer promote this goal for a patient at all, or when, by its interventions, medicine will place a patient in a condition that makes the pursuit of purposefulness too burdensome, then medicine has reached its limits *on the basis of its own principal reason for existence.*[9]

DEFINITION OF "QUALITY" OF LIFE

One of the more difficult problems in assessing the validity of quality of life judgments concerns the definition of the word "quality." Because this word is ambiguous, the entire phrase "quality of life" is subject to expansion to include just about anything, and so its use in medical decision making is open to serious abuse. Consequently, those who are entirely opposed to quality of life considerations in the medical environment have good reason to be concerned.[10] However, because there are ways to control the definition of the term and thus to restrict the range of its application, I argue that the issue is not *whether* we should employ this type of judgment but rather *how* do we circumscribe the limits of the judgment.

It is not infrequent in our consumerist society to link the word "quality" to the idea of excellence. So it is not unusual for us to talk about quality hotels, quality meals, and even quality medicine.[11] If "quality" is defined by reference to excellence, then the meaning of the term will be bounded only by the horizons of our imaginations and desires, and no doubt we will find it very difficult to find objective criteria by which to assess these judgments. One's worst fears about quality of life judgments will be realized because all patients who cannot live an excellent life, and they will surely include the handicapped and dying, will either not be given treatment or will be actively killed.

Another possibility is to define "quality" as a property or as an attribute.

The attribute or property at issue is an attribute or property of physical and/ or personal life. I find that most authors who argue against quality of life judgments, and even some who argue for their validity, will define the term in this way. There are a number of complex issues at stake once "quality" is so defined, but I only have space to analyze two of them: first, the evaluative status of physical life that does not possess the valued property and, second, the origin of and the limits to our obligations to preserve biological life (normative status).

The Evaluative Status of Life

When quality of life is defined by reference to an attribute or property of physical life, then basic questions are raised about the fundamental value of physical life (evaluative status) and the origin of this valuing. What is it that we value about physical life? Do we value physical life in and for the sake of itself, or do we value life because of some property that life possesses, for example, cognitive capacity? What philosophical or theological justifications can be offered for this valuing of life? Unfortunately, answers to these questions have led some to frame the contemporary debate in terms of a "quality of life ethic" versus a "sanctity of life ethic." I say unfortunately, because it is quite possible that this entire discussion about the evaluative status of human life may be misplaced.

Those who have argued for a sanctity of life ethic[12] over and against a quality of life ethic are aware that physical life is not an absolute value. On this point they are in total agreement with the proponents of the quality of life ethic. However, they maintain that those who support a quality of life ethic accord either no value or varying degrees of value to physical life contingent on the presence of some property that life possesses.[13] Such a view, they argue, is intolerable because 1) it denies the equality of physical life and the equality of persons, and thus it is a violation of justice; 2) it denies that all lives are inherently valuable, and so some lives can be truly "not worth living"; and 3) it denies the Christian (especially Roman Catholic) theological position that human life is valued holistically as body-spirit life by adopting a bilevel anthropology that is committed to sustaining physical life only as an instrumental value.[14] These authors conclude that a sanctity of life ethic is superior because it can affirm the equality of life on the grounds that physical life is truly a *bonum honestum* (a good or value in itself) and not a *bonum utile* (a useful or negotiable value that is dependent on some other intrinsically valuable property). Some argue the origin of this valuing philosophically by reference to a theory of goods that are incommensurable,[15] and others argue it theologically by reference to persons as created in the image of God.[16]

At first sight, these arguments against the so-called quality of life ethic seem formidable. In some ways, those who have supported the validity of quality of life judgments have not been as clear as they might be on the evaluative status of physical life, and in some instances they might have even poorly stated their own case. First, as I indicated above, it is necessary to distinguish clearly and consistently between physical or mere biological life and personal life (personhood). When this important distinction is not made, the opponents of quality of life judgments are prone to move back and forth between the value of biological life and the value of personhood.[17]

Second, those who support quality of life judgments should state explicitly and unequivocally that physical life is indeed a value that is not conditioned on any property. Some proponents, like Kevin O'Rourke and Dennis Brodeur, have stated, inappropriately in my mind, that "Mere physiological existence is *not* a value if no potential for mental-creative function exists."[18] Richard McCormick, who is one of the strongest supporters of quality of life judgments, has himself vacillated somewhat between claiming that physical life is a *bonum utile* and a *bonum honestum*.[19] David Thomasma et al. have also described physical life as a *conditional* value.[20] These ways of phrasing the issue of the evaluative status of physical life have led opponents of the position to the criticisms noted above. Unless I misunderstand what the proponents of quality of life judgments are driving at, I would suggest that it would be better to claim that physical life is a *bonum onticum*, that is, a true and real value, but by definition a created and therefore a limited good.[21] By so arguing, one can now affirm that all physical lives are of equal *ontic* value and that all persons are of equal *moral* value.

This leads me to my final suggestion, which I develop later. It is possible that the issue of the evaluative status of physical life is misplaced from the start. Despite some possible misstatements on the part of the proponents of quality of life judgments and misunderstandings on the part of the opponents, the word "quality" in the phrase "quality of life" does not and should not primarily refer to a property or attribute *of life*. Rather, the quality that is at issue is the quality *of the relationship* that exists between the medical condition of the patient, on the one hand, and the patient's ability to pursue life's goals and purposes (purposefulness) understood as the values that transcend physical life, on the other.[22] "Quality of life" may be an unfortunate phrase not only because it leaves the word "life" ambiguous (mere biological life as distinguished from personal life) but also because the word "quality" will tend to be construed as a property or an attribute that gives life its inherent meaning and value. Nonetheless, if we understand the phrase to refer to the quality of a relation and not to a quality of life itself, then the evaluative status of physical life is no longer a central issue in the debate. As a result, the formidable character of the arguments, if not the substance of the arguments, against the so-called quality of life ethic at this level loses its force.

The Normative Status of Life

Those who are opposed to the quality of life ethic believe that such an ethic logically entails a moral judgment on the valued qualities of life. Since morally normative judgments are statements about our moral duties and their limits toward supporting and protecting life, these authors fear that life and death decisions will be made solely on the presence or absence of certain qualities (properties) that a patient's life possesses. The result will be that our duties toward protecting life, especially those whose lives are most vulnerable, will be seriously eroded in society. The response to this erosion, and to the ethic that has precipitated it, is once again to argue for a sanctity of life ethic that refuses to ground our moral obligations on some valued quality (i.e., property or attribute) of life.

There are multiple issues involved in this discussion, but three particular questions clearly emerge at the heart of the matter. The first involves an attempt to define the normatively human, the second concerns the normative moral theory that underlies and grounds our moral obligations, and the third is concerned with how to establish limits and/or exceptions to our obligations and the justifications for such limits. Thus, the first issue is definitional in nature, though it also entails normative considerations; the second turns on the well-worn debate over the grounding of our moral obligations either deontologically or teleologically; and the last issue involves an assessment of the adequacy of the Catholic tradition's distinction between ordinary and extraordinary means of preserving life.

To define "quality" as a property of life (physical or personal) entails defining explicitly or implicitly what is called the normatively human. A number of years ago Joseph Fletcher attempted to isolate what he called the "indicators of humanhood."[23] He listed fifteen positive criteria (e.g., minimal intelligence, self-control, sense of futurity, concern for others, and curiosity) and five negative criteria (e.g., humans are not essentially parental, not essentially sexual, and not essentially worshipers) to define the normatively human. What he was doing in this essay was defining those qualities (positive and negative) that not only define who is human but also who is morally entitled to our care. The problem with Fletcher's position is that it falls into what William Aiken calls the "eudaimonistic" use of quality of life judgments, that is, it seeks to define the "good life" at its upper limits and then seeks to provide knowledge of both the necessary and sufficient conditions for its attainment.[24] The eudaimonistic use then becomes entrapped within what Aiken calls the "exclusionary" use of quality of life in which one cites the lack of certain qualities as a means of excluding potential patients from the normal standards of medical and moral treatment.[25] Thus, a judgment is made that, because a patient's quality of life is below the desirable level (i.e., it lacks a certain property), that patient's life is not worth living, and we are morally justified in treating him or her accordingly. The opponents of the quality of life ethic have rightfully perceived the problem of falling into the eudaimonistic and exclusionary uses of quality of life judgments, but, as I show below, the mistake they make is to attribute this problem to contemporary Catholic theologians who have argued for the legitimacy of quality of life judgments.

Normative moral theories are concerned with establishing standards for the moral evaluation of actions and a rationale for our moral obligations. To my knowledge, all the proponents of the so-called sanctity of life ethic subscribe to either a rights[26] or rule[27] deontology and accuse those who adopt a quality of life ethic of grounding moral obligations in some form of personal or social consequentialism.[28] In other words, in the sanctity of life ethic the duty to preserve physical life is grounded either in the patient's right to life or in the rules that require respect for life, justice, or care for another. This position contends that if our duties to preserve life are based on a prior judgment of whether a specific quality or property of physical life will result in benefits or good consequences to the patient himself or herself (personal consequentialism) or to society (social consequentialism), then our duties to preserve life are improperly grounded in what the patient earns through accomplishments to society or by means of the potentialities that the patient's life might possess.

This critique of a consequentialist grounding of our obligations to protect and preserve life is correct as far as it goes. It is true that the Christian tradition in general and the Roman Catholic tradition in particular have not based our duties simply on the presence of certain qualities or properties of physical life or on the contributions that a person has made or might make to society. Beyond any doubt, a critique should be leveled against any moral position that purports such a normative theory. The problem is that I remain unconvinced that this critique can really be applied to what many contemporary Catholic theologians have held on the validity of quality of life judgments. Though there might be some ambiguities in these theologians' positions on the evaluative and normative status of physical life, one could interpret their position as deriving our prima facie duties to preserve life from the ontic value of life and as deriving our actual *moral* obligations[29] from a teleological, but not *consequentialist*, assessment of the quality of the relationship that exists between the patient's medical condition and the ability to pursue life's goals and purposes.[30]

Because physical life is not an absolute value, those who argue for a sanctity of life ethic admit that there are definite limits to our obligations to preserve life. As a matter of fact, several authors admit that these limits and/or exceptions to our duties are controlled by "quality of life" considerations that are embodied in the traditional Catholic distinction between ordinary and extraordinary means of treatment. For example, John Connery,[31] Warren Reich,[32] and Brian Johnstone[33] all concede that "qualitative" factors or contingent qualities of life, such as the pain associated with using a certain medical treatment or the burden associated with the attainment of medical treatment, limit the duty to preserve life either on the part of the patient or on the part of health-care providers. Thus, they argue that the distinction between ordinary means (morally obligatory) and extraordinary means (optional and not morally obligatory) of treatment remains essentially valid and applicable today. The crucial point is not that the proponents of the sanctity of life ethic reject all quality of life factors; what they reject at the level of normative theory is the derivation of our duties from the presence of certain properties of physical or personal life, for example, the capacity for human relationships. In other words, quality of life judgments, which are judgments strictly circumscribed by an assessment of the benefits and burdens of medical treatment considered in itself and/or of those benefits and burdens that will accrue to the patient as a result of treatment, function appropriately in this ethic as ways of limiting or of making exceptions to our duties, which themselves are previously grounded on deontological considerations, for example, the right to life or respect for life. Thus, as long as the equality of both physical life and personhood is assured at the evaluative and normative levels, this ethic does in fact recognize the relative importance of quality of life judgments in medical decision making.

AN ARGUMENT FOR QUALITY
OF LIFE JUDGMENTS

The debate among contemporary Catholic theologians over the validity of quality of life judgments in the medical environment has reached an impasse as long as the terms of the debate continue to revolve around the opposition between two types of ethics, namely, sanctity of life ethic versus quality of life ethic. A successful negotiation of the impasse, but surely not the resolution of all the problems, will depend, at least in part, on the admission of the insights of the other's approach. Thus, in this final section I want to offer in broad strokes an outline to support the validity of quality of life judgments, while at the same time recognizing and admitting the insights of those who have opposed the use of such judgments.

One of the items that most often remains on a hidden agenda behind this debate concerns the goals and limits of medicine. In effect, a stalemate on almost all fronts—that is, moral, legal, and medical—exists because there is little or no agreement at this important level of discussion. I have already proposed above that the central and overarching end of medicine is to promote and enhance the purposefulness of physical and personal life. Such a proposal about the goal of medicine does not at all address the worth or value of physical or personal life. What the proposal does do is to state the raison d'être of medical interventions and its limits, on the one hand, and to give us some insight into what is meant *in a general way* by the terms "benefits," "burdens," and "best interests" of a patient, on the other hand.

As I have already noted, quality of life judgments should not be construed as judgments about the value of either physical or personal life. They are not concerned with assessing qualities or properties that, when present, make life itself valuable. Rather, these judgments are evaluative and normative claims or assessments about the relation between the patient's medical condition and the patient's ability to pursue material, moral, and spiritual values that transcend physical life but do not give that life its very meaning and worth. As such, they specify *concretely* the meaning of the terms "benefits," "burdens," and "best interests" of a patient as well as the limits of medical interventions within a given historical and cultural situation.

Whereas all physical life is of equal ontic worth and all personal life is of equal moral value, the quality of the relation between these lives and the pursuit of values is not equal. Due to multiple factors, a number of which have to do with genetic endowment and the ways in which we live our lives and a number of which are dependent on the nurturing and accessibility of values in culture, some people are fortunate enough to attain a high quality of life. Other individuals, regrettably, are not as fortunate, and they must live most of their lives pursuing life's purposes at a less than optimal level. But some have no discernible or such a minimal qualitative relation between their medical condition and the pursuit of values that a growing number of theologians have argued that those in this last category have no moral obligation to prolong their physical lives and thus that all treatment, including artificial nutrition and hydration, can be withdrawn from them. In the past, most, if not all, these lives in such conditions would have been mercifully ended by the underlying pathology, but the intervention of modern medical technology today has not been as merciful.

Two things are important to note here. First, none of the theologians proposing this view has accepted the active killing of patients. Second, this view
does not fall into either a eudaimonistic or an exclusionary use of quality of
life judgments. These theologians have not drawn a line at the upper limits of
pursuing life's purposes (eudaimonistic use), but they have sought to establish the lowest possible limits of what reasonable people would judge bearable and acceptable vis-à-vis the qualitative relation under consideration.[34]
Furthermore, this position does not employ the exclusionary use because it
does not exclude those who fall below these limits from our ordinary moral
obligations not to kill them or to care for them.

The duties and their limits to prolong life that bear on health-care professionals are correlative to the patient's obligations and their limits.[35] When it
is determined that a patient no longer has an obligation to prolong physical
or personal life—for example, when the pursuit of values is too burdensome
due to an underlying fatal pathology that cannot be removed—then medical
personnel do not exclude the patient from *their* obligations to offer treatment
but acquiesce to the limits of the *patient's* obligations. Thus, other things
being equal, when medicine can intervene to ameliorate the quality of the
relation between the patient's condition and the pursuit of life's goals, then
such an intervention can be considered a benefit to the patient and is in his or
her best interests. However, *because of the condition of the patient*, when a
proposed intervention cannot offer the patient any reasonable hope of pursuing life's purposes at all or can only offer the patient a condition where the
pursuit of life's purposes will be filled with profound frustration or with utter
neglect of these purposes because of the energy needed merely to sustain
physical life, then medical intervention 1) can only offer burden to the life
treated, 2) is contrary to the best interests of the patient, 3) is harmful to the
patient, and 4) medicine has reached its limits on the basis of its own reason
for existence and thus should not intervene except to palliate or to comfort
the patient.

What should be obvious is that quality of life judgments are concerned
with what the Vatican's "Declaration on Euthanasia"[36] called the assessment
of a due proportion between benefits and burdens. However, the proportionality referred to is not about the benefits and/or burdens of the treatments considered *in themselves* apart from the patient; rather, the assessment is
concerned with the proportionality of benefits/burdens (considered teleologically) that will affect the quality of the relation between the patient's medical
condition and his or her pursuit of values. By adopting this view of what
quality of life judgments are concerned with, it seems that the so-called "two
ethics of life" are not two but really one.

ENDNOTES

1. For example, see John R. Connery, "Quality of Life," *Linacre Quarterly* 53 (1986): 26–33; Daniel Callahan, "On Feeding the Dying," *Hastings Center Report* 13 (no. 5, 1983): 22; Eugene F. Diamond, "Nutrition, Hydration and Cost Containment," *Linacre Quarterly* 53 (1986): 24–34; and New Jersey State Catholic Conference, "Providing Food and Fluids to Severely Brain-Damaged Patients," *Origins* 16 (1987): 582–84.

2. For example, see Richard A. McCormick, *How Brave a New World? Dilemmas in Bioethics* (Washington, D.C.: Georgetown University Press, 1981), especially 339–51 and 393–411; Richard A. McCormick, "Notes on Moral Theology: 1980," *Theological Studies* 42 (1981): 100–110; John J. Paris and Richard A. McCormick, "The Catholic Tradition on the Use of Nutrition and Fluids," *America* 156 (1987): 356–61; Kevin O'Rourke, "The A.M.A. Statement on Tube Feeding: An Ethical Analysis," *America* 155 (1986): 321–23 and 331; and James J. Walter, "Food and Water: An Ethical Burden," *Commonweal* 113 (1986): 616–19. For a summary of these and other positions that have been taken recently, see Lisa S. Cahill, "Notes on Moral Theology: 1986," *Theological Studies* 48 (1987): 105–23.

3. The number of court cases during the past decade and a half is almost staggering. Some of the more publicized cases would include Karen Quinlan, Claire Conroy, Paul Brophy, Bro. Fox, Joseph Saikewicz, and Nancy Ellen Jobes.

4. The Department of Health and Human Services (DHHS) originally intervened after the Bloomington, Indiana, "Baby Doe" case (April, 1982). Since that time, DHHS has issued a number of regulations governing the treatment of neonates who are severely handicapped. The final regulations were published in the *Federal Register* 50 (1985): 14887–89.

5. Warren T. Reich, "Quality of Life," in *Encyclopedia of Bioethics*, vol. 2, edited by Warren T. Reich (New York: The Free Press, 1978), 830–31.

6. For a description of patients who are in a persistent vegetative state (PVS), see the President's Commission Report entitled *Deciding to Forego Life-Sustaining Treatment: A Report on the Ethical, Medical, and Legal Issues in Treatment Decisions* (Washington, D.C.: U.S. Government Printing Office, 1983), especially 171–81.

7. "Pastoral Constitution on the Church in the Modern World" ("Gaudium et Spes"), in *The Documents of Vatican II*, edited by Walter M. Abbott (New York: Association Press, 1966), no. 4; The longest case of coma on record is that of Elaine Esposito. She never recovered consciousness after receiving general anesthesia for surgery, and therefore she had to be fed and hydrated artificially. She remained in this condition for 37 years and 111 days before dying. See the President's Commission Report, *Deciding to Forego Life-Sustaining Treatment*, 177.

8. Albert R. Jonsen, "Purposefulness in Human Life," *Western Journal of Medicine* 125 (July 1976): 5–7.

9. For a similar view, see David Roy, "Issues in Health Care Meriting Particular Christian Concern—A Priority Issue: The Severely Defective Newborn," *Linacre Quarterly* 49 (1982): 60–80.

10. For example, see Mark Siegler and Alan J. Weisbard, "Against the Emerging Stream: Should Fluids and Nutritional Support be Continued?" *Archives of Internal Medicine* 145 (1985): 129–31; Patrick G. Derr, "Why Food and Fluids Can Never Be Denied,"

Hastings Center Report 16 (no. 1, 1986): 2830; and John R. Connery, "The Clarence Herbert Case: Was Withdrawal of Treatment Justified?" *Hospital Progress* 65 (February 1984): 32–35, 70.

11. Jonsen, "Purposefulness in Human Life," 5.

12. For example, see Warren T. Reich, "Quality of Life and Defective Newborn Children: An Ethical Analysis," in *Decision Making and the Defective Newborn: Proceedings of a Conference on Spina Bifida and Ethics*, edited by Chester A. Swinyard (Springfield, Ill.: Charles C. Thomas, 1978), 489–511; and Brian V. Johnstone, "The Sanctity of Life, the Quality of Life and the New 'Baby Doe' Law," *Linacre Quarterly* 52 (1985): 258–70.

13. Johnstone, "The Sanctity of Life," 263.

14. Reich, "Quality of Life and Defective Newborn Children," 504.

15. For example, see William E. May, *Human Existence, Medicine and Ethics* (Chicago: Franciscan Herald Press, 1977), 10.

16. Reich, "Quality of Life and Defective Newborn Children," 504.

17. For example, Warren Reich's theological position grounds both the value and the equality of "human life" on the belief that "all men are created as persons in the image of God"; Reich, "Quality of Life and Defective Newborn Children," 504. His use of the phrase "human life" is ambiguous here and therefore misleading. Though the context of his argument is a critique of what he believes to be McCormick's position on the inherent value of *physical* life, he completes his argument by referring to *persons* and their nature and value as images of God.

18. Kevin D. O'Rourke and Dennis Brodeur, *Medical Ethics: Common Ground for Understanding* (St. Louis, Mo.: Catholic Health Association of the U.S., 1986), 213 (emphasis added).

19. McCormick, *How Brave a New World?* 405–7; and Richard A. McCormick, *Health and Medicine in the Catholic Tradition: Tradition in Transition* (New York: Crossroad, 1984), 148.

20. David Thomasma et al., "Continuance of Nutritional Care in the Terminally Ill Patient," *Critical Care Clinics* 2 (1986): 66.

21. For two important articles on the distinction between the ontic and the moral levels in moral analysis, see Louis Janssens, "Ontic Evil and Moral Evil," *Louvain Studies* 4 (1972): 115–56; and Louis Janssens, "Ontic Good and Evil-Premoral Values and Disvalues," *Louvain Studies* 12 (1987): 62–82.

22. Richard McCormick has proposed that the minimal potential for human relationships is one of the central criteria in quality of life judgments. It is probably the case that McCormick intended "potential for human relationships" to mean a property or attribute *of life* in his quality of life criterion. (See his *How Brave a New World?* 339–51, 393–411.) Whereas this may be true, I think that the basic thrust of McCormick's position is to assess the quality *of the relation* between the patient's medical condition and the pursuit of life's purposes. For McCormick, the fact that a patient does not possess any capacity for relationality means that the patient will not have any qualitative relation between his or her medical condition and the pursuit of life's values. Indications of my interpretation can be found throughout his more recent writings. For example, see his "The Best Interests of the Baby," *Second Opinion* 2 (1986): especially 23. For my earlier interpretation and evaluation of McCormick's position, see James J. Walter, "A Public Policy Option on the Treatment of Severely Handicapped Newborns," *Laval Théologique et Philosophique* 41 (1985): 239–50.

23. Joseph Fletcher, "Indicators of Humanhood: A Tentative Profile of Man," *Hastings Center Report* 2 (November 1972): 1–4.

24. William Aiken, "The Quality of Life," *Applied Philosophy* 1 (1982): 27.

25. Aiken, "The Quality of Life," 30.

26. For example, see Reich, "Quality of Life and Defective Newborn Children," 491–92.

27. For example, see Connery, "Quality of Life," 31–32; Johnstone, "The Sanctity of Life," 264–65; and Paul Ramsey, *Ethics at the Edges of Life: Medical and Legal Intersections* (New Haven, Conn.: Yale University Press, 1978), especially 153–88.

28. Reich, "Quality of Life," 833; and Reich, "Quality of Life and Defective Newborns," 503–4.

29. For the distinction between prima facie and actual moral obligations, see W. D. Ross, *The Right and the Good* (Oxford: Clarendon, 1930).

30. McCormick himself argues that we have a prima facie obligation to preserve *physical* life. To my knowledge, none of his critics has pointed out this fact about his position. See McCormick, "The Best Interests of the Baby," 21.

31. Connery, "Quality of Life," 31.

32. Reich, "Quality of Life and Defective Newborns," 506–9.

33. Johnstone, "The Sanctity of Life," 265–69.

34. For McCormick's formulation of his "reasonable person" standard, see his *How Brave A New World?* 383–401.

35. The substance of my position is based on Pius XII's allocution "The Prolongation of Life," *Pope Speaks* 4 (1958): 393- 98.

36. "Declaration on Euthanasia," *Origins* 10 (1980): 156. It seems to me that the Pontifical Academy of Sciences departs from the essential substance of the "Declaration on Euthanasia" when it requires that food and water must always be given (regardless of the proportionality between the benefits and burdens) to patients who are in a persistent vegetative state. See "The Artificial Prolongation of Life," *Origins* 15 (1985): 415.

IV

ISSUES AT THE END OF LIFE

13

Terminal Sedation: A Catholic Perspective

James J. Walter

There is no official Roman Catholic teaching on terminal sedation. What follows is one theologian's view of how the tradition might think on this topic. I start with a couple of introductory comments and distinctions as well as the background to this discussion. This is concerned with the nature of suffering and the duty, within the Catholic tradition, to alleviate suffering. Then I turn my attention to the two moral issues that are at stake in either terminal or palliative sedation. Before one places the patient into a coma, one must have already made the decision not to artificially deliver nutrition and hydration, thus allowing or permitting the patient to die of dehydration. The other moral issue follows once the patient is in a coma. I discuss the ethical dimensions of these two issues and their distinctions. Finally, I finish with when I think it is morally permissible or not permissible to perform this procedure, according to the Catholic tradition.

First, I want to make two careful distinctions. The first involves intentions. Terminal sedation generally refers to the intent to end the life of the patient. In my mind it is very similar to physician-assisted suicide and euthanasia. Palliative sedation, on the other hand, refers to the intent from the perspective of the caregiver to relieve refractory pain. Only recently has this distinction between the two kinds of sedation entered into the literature.

The second distinction revolves around suffering. There are two types. One is neurophysiological suffering that originates from actual physical pain. Then there is one I call "agent narrative suffering." It originates within the alienation of the patient, within the hopelessness the patient experiences, and the burden the patient may feel he or she will impose on his or her family. How does the Catholic tradition view suffering? And does the tradition argue within itself a duty on the part of the health-care community to alleviate suffering when possible? These are important questions. Pope John Paul II, in a speech titled "The Christian Meaning of Human Suffering" (1984), made a distinction between physical and moral suffering. He said that this distinction was based on the double dimension of the human being and indicated the bodily and the spiritual element as the immediate or direct subject of suffering.

Physical suffering relates to the body. Moral suffering relates to the soul. In one way what the pope called moral suffering is what I call "agent narrative suffering." Physical suffering from the pope's perspective can have meaning. It is possible to find meaning and value within suffering when it is experienced in close connection with love received and love given. It can also have redemptive meaning in identifying one's own suffering with the suffering of Jesus Christ on the cross.

Is there a duty to alleviate pain and suffering? When physical suffering originates out of pain, it ought to be relieved, if possible. When patients seek relief, physicians have a duty to offer painkillers to alleviate the pain. This is not just an option; it is a duty for the physician within the Roman Catholic community. A document was written in 1980, titled "Declaration on Euthanasia," and it states that

> human and Christian prudence suggest for the majority of sick people the use of medicines capable of alleviating or suppressing pain, even though these may cause as a secondary effect semiconsciousness and reduced lucidity. As for those who are not in a state to express themselves, one can reasonably presume that they wish to take these painkillers and have them administered according to the doctor's advice. (www.cin.org/vatcong/euthanas.html)

This now sets the stage for the two moral issues needing to be addressed as palliative sedation.

The first ethical issue is whether to put the patient into a coma. How would one approach this particular issue morally? Two Catholic principles may be used to address these issues. One could use the principle of double effect as it applies to a specific case. The case is that this is an instance in which one action produces two results: one good and one evil. From the Catholic tradition, one must consider the motive, intention, and means of the individual. The intention arises from the will. The will targets a specific end that it wants to achieve. The means are the ways to bring about the desired end. However, in every action there are always further consequences: some I foresee and want; some I foresee, but don't want; and some I don't foresee and, of course, don't want.

Henry Ford didn't invent the internal combustion engine. What he did was to mass-produce automobiles. And we can assume that what he intended to do, what he wanted and targeted, was in fact to bring about a machine in a mass-produced way so people could move easily and quickly about their lives. He created factories in order to produce this. What moved him to do that? Probably profitability, among other things. There were a number of consequences or results of Mr. Ford's actions, some of which he was aware of and foresaw and wanted. He certainly foresaw that people driving automobiles would be able to get where they wanted quickly. There are other things that he foresaw, but didn't want. He surely foresaw that people were going to kill one another with this machine; presumably, Mr. Ford did not want that. There are other things he did not even foresee with the mass-production of automobiles, and he obviously did not want them, such as the amount of pollution that would occur with this machine. Are we going to hold him responsible for everything that occurs as a consequence?

What types of consequences am I responsible for, even if I don't foresee them? Even when I don't want them, can I attribute them morally to the person doing the action? One of the problems that can occur within this kind of schema is the reduction of all of the consequences and the end of the act into a single category. This category is called "results."

This is what the circuit court of appeals did that preceded the *Vacco* v. *Quill* Supreme Court's decision (supct.law.cornell.edu/supct/html/95–1858.ZS.html). The Second Circuit Court of Appeals said, "A patient has the right, under Cruzan, to refuse any treatment even if that results in death. So, what's the difference if a physician gives the patient something that would take their life? The result is the same." Here, the court simply combines the end and consequences into "results." By doing that, one does not know what the agent intends and what the consequences are.

If one reduces intention/end and consequence into a single category of "results," then the Second Circuit Court is absolutely correct. However, if the distinction between intention/end and consequences within palliative sedation is maintained, the intention of the physician, the target of the will, is to palliate the patient and free the patient from neurophysiological pain. The physician uses drugs to accomplish that, with the end of alleviating the patient's pain and with the further foreseen, but unwanted consequence, of the unconsciousness and possible death of the patient. That seems to be morally legitimate as long as it can be shown that the physician has titrated the dosage of the drug, not walked in and simply given the patient 100 mg. of morphine. As long as the dosage is given over a period of time to control the

pain of the patient, it seems to be an entirely different scenario from physician-assisted suicide or terminal sedation. Although the motive is the same—
namely, compassion—the intention is different. In physician-assisted suicide,
the consequence category is the alleviation of pain, and the death of the
patient is the intention/end. These two categories get switched between terminal sedation and palliative sedation.

In the Roman Catholic tradition, these categories are kept distinct. There
is the refusal to elide "end" and "consequence," what are called effects: one
good and one evil. One of those effects will become the end. The other one
will become the consequence.

What does one do once the patient is placed in the coma? The physician,
with the patient's or surrogate's consent, has already made the moral decision
that he or she will not medically deliver nutrition and hydration. It makes no
moral sense to place the patient into a permanent coma and then insert a feeding tube in this case. The Roman Catholic tradition here would use the distinction between ordinary and extraordinary means. Ordinary and
extraordinary are not defined by the references used in clinical practice, that
is, by reference to what is customary versus unusual or experimental. Rather,
these are carefully defined moral terms that relate to a proportion between
benefit and burden to the patient. Ordinary means are all of those potential
treatments, surgeries, medications, and anything else that could offer the
patient a reasonable hope of benefit *and* that can be offered without excessive
expense, pain, or inconvenience. What is expensive, painful, and inconvenient for me may not be for someone else. This is patient centered. There are
no abstract standards to determine what is excessively painful, excessively
expensive, or excessively inconvenient. Notice two conditions have to be met.
The treatment has to offer reasonable hope of benefit *and* it must be attained
without excessive burden. On the other hand, extraordinary means are all of
those potential treatments, surgeries, medications, and anything else that
could not offer a reasonable hope of benefit *or* could not be obtained without
excessive pain, expense, or other inconvenience. This is always a patient or
family determination after calculating benefit and burden. The claim might
be made that the delivery of nutrition and hydration could be considered
extraordinary for a patient in that it would offer no reasonable hope of benefit
or that it would simply be too burdensome for that patient to accept treatment,
given their condition of unrelieved neurophysiological pain.

Given those two, I think it is possible to justify limited cases of palliative
sedation, but not terminal sedation. Cases that are not morally permissible
within the Roman Catholic tradition are as follows: placing patients into a
coma that involves "agent narrative suffering" that results from hopelessness,
alienation, and so on; and/or when the intention is to end the life of the

patient. Neither of these instances is permissible and each is an instance of "terminal sedation." Cases that might be morally permissible within the Roman Catholic tradition involve neurophysiological suffering only that give rise to truly refractory pain. Evidently, under the most optimal conditions, approximately 5 percent of dying patients experience refractory, unrelieved, and excruciating pain. The principle of double effect, along with the distinction between ordinary and extraordinary means, in fact, might justify limited cases of palliative sedation.

14

The PVS Patient and the Forgoing/Withdrawing of Medical Nutrition and Hydration

Thomas A. Shannon and James J. Walter

Over the past several decades, modern medicine has progressed at a rate that has astonished even its practitioners. Developments in drugs, vaccines, and various technologies have given physicians an incredible amount of success over disease and morbidity as well as allowing them to make dramatic interventions into the body to repair or replace a problematic system or organ. Yet there are limits we are coming to recognize slowly and only reluctantly, for even many of our best technologies are only halfway technologies, that is, the technology or intervention compensates for a function but cannot cure the underlying pathology or correct the damaged organ. The respirator is probably the most frequently encountered example of this phenomenon.

Another intervention is our capacity to provide nutrition and hydration to those in a persistent vegetative state (PVS). For long-term feeding of such individuals, a gastrostomy tube is inserted directly into the stomach and the liquid protein diet is delivered in a controlled fashion by a pump. If the individual is reasonably healthy and other reflexes are intact, the life expectancy may be several decades.[1] The PVS will not be cured, and the liquid protein serves to maintain the status quo. The question of how to treat these patients medically is now heavily debated nationally and internationally.

In this chapter, we examine the issue in several ways: 1) report on a survey of the U.S. hierarchy on bioethics committees in general and on forgoing or withdrawing nutrition and hydration in particular; 2) propose a structured argument that includes a reconceptualization of quality of life judgments; and 3) offer suggestions for the future conduct of this debate.

A SURVEY OF THE U.S. HIERARCHY

General Analysis

In January 1988, one of the authors (TAS) developed a brief questionnaire that sought information on two broad areas: 1) Were there diocesan bioethics committees and, if so, what was their composition; and 2) did dioceses have specific policies on the issue of nutrition and hydration.[2]

A total of 167 questionnaires were sent to the ordinaries of the U.S. dioceses, and seventy-eight ordinaries responded. Of these, sixty-two indicated that there was no diocesan bioethics committee, sixteen indicated the existence of such a committee, and of these, seven sent in detailed information, which is evaluated separately below.

Of those indicating no diocesan committee, eight said that there were committees at local Catholic hospitals. Another eight identified a specific individual within the diocese to whom the ordinary turned for assistance. Another three indicated the formation of such a committee, either on a diocesan or state level. Finally, one respondent stated there was an inoperative committee.

The survey then asked for a description of the membership of the committee, frequency of meetings, its role, whether or not there were guidelines, and how it functioned within the diocese.

Committee size ranged from nine to twenty-three members, which allowed for a good representation of professions, typically including hospital administrators, physicians, nurses, chaplains, ethicists, lawyers, and other theologians. Six of the committees met monthly, two met bimonthly, and one as needed. Three respondents said their role was to set policy, two were to be advisory, and one was to be primarily educational. Two respondents had no guidelines, and nine indicated some form of guidelines ranging from church teachings on medical issues to specific pronouncements of the hierarchy over the past decade.

Part 2 of the survey focused specifically on the moral evaluation of feeding tubes. Of the seventy-eight answering, seventeen made no comment on part 2, thirty-seven made some comments, and twenty-two respondents reported no cases of PVS patients in their diocese.

Nine respondents reported knowledge of PVS patients within their dioceses. Of those nine, eight reported figures ranging from one to four or five per year, and one respondent indicated ten cases in the past year. Eight committees were asked to consider cases and eleven had not been asked. Additionally, four respondents reported that they have specific guidelines they follow in such instances and eight indicated that they have none.

The survey asked if the committee considered feeding tubes to be a medical technology. Six said yes, four said no, eight gave no answer, and one said "it depends." The respondents were then asked if they considered the use of such feeding tubes to be routine care. Six said yes, four said no, eight gave no answer, and one said "it depends." The next question was whether the removal of a feeding tube from a PVS patient was ordinary or extraordinary care, or if they had no position. Four responded the care was ordinary, four that it was extraordinary, one had no position, nine gave no answer, and nine said "it depends." The final question asked whether removal was an act of involuntary euthanasia, which is direct and forbidden, or indirect and permitted, or no position. Four responded that removal was direct, five that it was indirect, two had no position, four said "it depends," and eight had no answer.

Before turning to an analysis of the seven detailed responses (Documents A–G), we would like to make a few general observations about the data so far.

Given the seriousness of contemporary bioethical questions and their pervasiveness within society, it is surprising so few dioceses have these committees or that so few local Catholic hospitals were indicated as having one. While neither seeking to bureaucratize all life nor to reject appropriate patient and family autonomy, nonetheless such committees on a diocesan or state level serve a useful function, minimally by providing workshops or other resources to hospitals or other groups in the diocese. Of those that are in place, the composition is well represented from a disciplinary perspective, and the committees meet with appropriate regularity. The committees appear to be accessible and, while maintaining patient privacy and confidentiality, there is some degree of openness in the committees.

Part 2 of the questionnaire provides more interesting data. Nine committees had cases brought to them and, taken together, they had a moderately large number of cases—about forty-five. Six committees considered feeding tubes to be a medical technology and also routine care, four thought they were not a medical technology, and one did not consider them routine care. One committee was uncertain in each case. Yet of these committees, only four thought that feeding tubes were ordinary means whose removal constituted active euthanasia.

Four committees considered the technology ordinary and four judged it to be extraordinary. Four thought their removal to be direct euthanasia, while five considered it passive euthanasia. But even more interesting is that nine committees thought that the placing of the technology into the ordinary/

extraordinary categories depended on the individual circumstances of the case, and eight thought the same thing about the determination of active or passive euthanasia. This suggests substantial ambiguity about the moral status of feeding technologies for PVS patients.

First, there is a difference over whether the procedure is a medical technology. If a technology, its moral evaluation fits conceptually more easily into the traditional format of ordinary/extraordinary means. If not, one might have to structure the argument differently. Most interesting are the differences in perception between whether the therapy is considered ordinary or extraordinary means, on the one hand, and whether its forgoing/withdrawal is morally evaluated as direct or indirect euthanasia, on the other. This interest is compounded when combined with the additional judgment—on the part of nine and eight respondents respectively—that such a determination "depends" on the circumstances. Such evaluations suggest room for various analyses of the problem and the possible moral acceptability of several resolutions.

Analysis of Specific Guidelines

Seven respondents sent more detailed information about committee makeup and the bylaws governing these committees. We discuss each document in some detail, but, to maintain a promised confidentiality, we will simply refer to these documents as A–G.

Document A suggests that the primary locus for decision making is the local hospital, with the diocesan or proposed statewide committee serving as a resource. Yet part of the task of the proposed statewide committee will be to develop guidelines for the local committee. At present, discussions are ongoing among committees but no consensus has been reached.

Document A affirms a presumption in favor of the use of feeding tubes but states that each case must be examined on its own merits. On the other hand, in very exceptional and extraordinary cases, the withdrawal of feeding tubes might be passive and, therefore, permissible euthanasia. Thus, while removal of these tubes is exceptional, their removal is not prohibited either. As the document states it, "each case must be considered on its own merits."

Document B represents the responses from three diocesan hospitals since this diocese has no diocesan committee. B1 indicated that, while there have been cases, the committee did not meet as a committee on them. Rather, individual members of the committee served as resources to the medical staff and the families. This document stated that there is no consensus within the hospital about the issue, and so each case is to be examined on its own merits. The committee understands the practice as passive euthanasia, and thus permissible, but also recognizes that there is no consistent position in the hospital.

We detect a problematic area in this document. B1 argues feeding tubes might be withdrawn on the basis "that continued treatment *will result in* prolonged total dependence, persistent pain, or discomfort, or in a *persistent vegetative state*" (emphasis added). However, one wonders how the withdrawal of feeding tubes causes PVS? This technology is used to *support* patients in this condition; its administration does not *result* in PVS.

Document B2 states that their consultation has been on the placement of such technologies rather than on their withdrawal. Since it has no fixed policy, each case must be dealt with individually. Additionally, this committee considers tube feeding to be a medical technology and can become an extraordinary means in specific cases "which must be individually assessed and reassessed." The decisions are to be considered in "light of the effect of this nutrition and/or the burden to the patient which would be experienced." Again, these decisions cannot be based on a broad application of a policy but must be made according to "case specific evaluations."

Document B3 comes from an ethicist at a medical center that has no committee. The respondent indicates that conversations about this problem show that many individuals at the medical center have concerns about the issue.

Tube feeding, in this individual's judgment, is a technology, but its moral significance resides in "its function in the ongoing treatment of the patient." Thus, the central issue is: Does the treatment contribute to restoring life and health, or does it prolong the patient's dying? "If the former I think it [is] routinely required. If the latter, I judge it foregoable, permissibly not obligatorily foregoable. . . . Tube feeding is some cases is proportionate, hence required, in others, disproportionate, hence not required."

Two other relevant comments were made by this hospital ethicist. First, can feeding tubes ever be withdrawn? If one can

> admit that sometimes tubal feeding need not be *instituted*, then you are already describing conditions which might eventuate *within a case* which justify discontinuing tubal feeding. Put another way, a patient on tubal feeding might become the sort of patient you don't want to begin on tubal feeding. Since you need not start the intervention on the latter patient, why must you stay with it for the former one? (emphasis in the original)

Second, never starting or, once begun, removing the tubes is not an intending of death; rather, these decisions indicate that families "recognize and consent to [accept] a dying process which is judged irreversible and imminent."

The two common themes in these three documents from diocesan hospitals are a recognition of the ambiguities in the issue and a strong affirmation of a case-by-case evaluation. The more crucial moral elements are case specific and determining the usefulness of the technology in relation to the condition of the patient. In addition, the suggestion to use the same criteria for not instituting the therapy as the criteria for withdrawing it is a helpful one and could aid in resolving several problems.

Document C is testimony to a state legislature on a natural death act. At issue is the inclusion of a proviso for withholding feeding tubes in a living will. After a strong affirmation of the dignity, sanctity, and value of all human life, this document states: "The concern to affirm life, however, does not require the maintenance of physiological life by all means. It is recognized that aggressive overtreatment is as ethically unacceptable as is undertreatment. Both lack respect for the dignity and welfare of each person."

This testimony makes four points that lay out several issues very clearly.

1. A clear presumption in favor of life should be established. People who are able to eat, but only with assistance, cannot be discriminated against or be refused appropriate treatment.
2. The law should recognize the right of individuals to be allowed to die in circumstances where medical treatments, including nutrition and hydration, are ineffective or too burdensome for the patient.
3. The law must carefully define useless or ineffective treatment to clearly identify those treatments that offer no benefit of recovery or no relief of pain. The burdens associated with continued medical treatment should be defined in terms of the burdens that an individual experiences in pursuing the goals or ends of life and not defined by a level of invasiveness that may or may not be associated with forced feeding.
4. The clinical setting distinguishes between nutrition and hydration. Although both terms are used as though they are identical, it should be recognized that individuals may not require forced nutrition while still requiring hydration to alleviate thirst, provide comfort, relieve pain, or provide an open channel for IV medications.

Document C is very nuanced and makes careful distinctions. In particular, the document emphasizes the distinction between basic nutrition and hydration that requires time and effort on the part of medical personnel to feed the patient orally and the medical procedures that require total parenteral nutritional support (TPN) or invasive medical techniques to provide nutrition and hydration, for example, insertion of gastrostomy tubes.

Document D comes from a research center whose writings and contributions were mentioned by many respondents as a source of guidance for their committees. Two major points are made. First, forgoing or withdrawing foods and fluids on the rationale of the "assumption that life itself can be useless or an excessive burden" is morally wrong because it is euthanasia by omission. This carries out the "proposal, adopted by choice, to end someone's life because that life itself is judged by others to be valueless or excessively burdensome." The crucial issues here are the moral intention of those who would withdraw the means of providing nutrition, on the one hand, and the justification for the argument adduced to support such a withdrawal, on the other. For this document, the intention is to end life, and the justification for so acting is that the life is burdensome or useless. This constitutes direct euthanasia.

Second, the forgoing or withdrawing of medically provided nutrition and hydration "do not necessarily carry out a proposal to end life." When certain conditions are met—"if the means employed is (sic) judged either useless or excessively burdensome"—one may forgo or withdraw treatment.

> Nonetheless, *if it is really useless or excessively burdensome* to provide someone with nutrition and hydration, then these means may rightly be withheld or withdrawn, *provided* that this omission does not carry out a proposal to end the person's life, but rather is chosen to avoid the useless effort or the excessive burden of continuing to provide the food and fluids. (emphasis in the original)

Two applications follow. If a person is imminently dying, nutrition may become useless and burdensome, whether administered by tube or otherwise. On the other hand, if the patients are not dying, feeding provides a great benefit: "the preservation of their lives and the prevention of their death through malnutrition and dehydration." Yet even in this instance, this treatment could become useless or futile: "(a) if the person in question is imminently dying, so that any effort to sustain life is futile or (b) the person is no longer able to assimilate the nourishment or fluids thus provided."

On the basis of this analysis, Document D states:

> We thus conclude that, in the ordinary circumstances of life in our society today, it is not morally right, nor ought it to be legally permissible, to withhold or withdraw nutrition and hydration provided by artificial means to the permanently unconscious or other categories of seriously debilitated but non terminal persons. Food and fluids are universally needed for the preservation of life, and can generally be provided without the burdens and expense of more aggressive means of supporting life.

This document makes a strong argument in favor of such feeding based on the value of human life, the fact that such feeding can provide benefits to the patient and is not generally burdensome, and that the withdrawal of such technology many times includes the intention to end a person's life. Only when the individual is actually dying and/or cannot assimilate nourishment could the feeding be considered an extraordinary means.

Document E represents an advisory opinion of an archdiocese. This opinion bases its position on Pius XII's teaching on ordinary and extraordinary means, the Congregation for the Doctrine of the Faith's (CDF) "Declaration on Euthanasia" and documents from the National Conference of Catholic Bishops (NCCB) Committee for Pro-Life Activities. Document E uses the standards of reasonable hope of success and a determination of excessive burdens as the criteria for decision making. In addition, it recognizes and accepts the presumption of the use of medically providing nutrition and hydration for individuals.

The advisory opinion makes two statements of importance. The first concerns the decision to forgo or withdraw.

> It can hardly be denied that in certain circumstances artificial hydration and nutrition can be just as burdensome and useless as other means and under these circumstances would not be obligatory. A Catholic in good conscience can come to the conclusion that in a particular set of circumstances such treatment need not be initiated or continued, because it holds no hope that it will be successful in prolonging life or is unduly burdensome for oneself or another.

The second point concerns the intention involved in ending treatment. Document E argues that "even though the omission may shorten life, the intention is not to bring on death but to spare the patient a very burdensome treatment." These actions could constitute direct euthanasia if the intention is to end the life, but if omitted because they are too burdensome or useless in preserving life, "they do not constitute killing any more than any other such omission."

Document E uses the categories of ordinary and extraordinary means and then draws the conclusions that a decision to forgo or withdraw nutrition can be made in good conscience and that people should not be prevented from doing what is morally permissible. While the document does not encourage forgoing or withdrawal, neither does it prohibit such actions.

Document F supports the removal of nutrition and hydration within the context of the Catholic moral tradition that permits withdrawal of all medical technologies either on the basis that a patient has entered the dying phase or that the technologies are nonbeneficial or burdensome. These evaluations are moral as well as medical: "not what will the treatment do . . . but will the treatment promote human activities and values."

> Merely maintaining biological life is not evaluated as being in and of itself humanly beneficial. Life is something more than biological existence. Life is a conditional

value which couples biological existence with social, spiritual and human activities such as loving, praying, remembering, forgiving and experiencing. Life is all these things.

Consequently, when these activities can no longer be realized, there is no moral obligation to continue medical treatment, unless to relieve suffering. The conclusion that treatment can stop "does not mean that the person is worthless, but that the person has activated all human potential." Thus, there is "no moral requirement to administer artificial nutrition and hydration. In fact it might be violating the person." Document F concludes on the interesting note that "people feel intuitively that it is wrong and want to find ways to escape imprisonment by technology."

Finally, Document G discusses this issue within the context of policies of life-sustaining treatment. The general context for thinking about this issue is "Prolonging physiological function by itself is not of value if it seems all potential for cognitive functions—mental creativity, the capacity to know and to love—if all that is irreversibly destroyed. Respect for life is at the heart of medicine, and a person in such a condition must not be put to death, but may be allowed to die." The document then considers various forms of supportive care following the decision to allow to die. First, when medical procedures that prolong life are to be withheld or withdrawn, other medical procedures not directed to supportive care may also be omitted. These include lab work, diagnostic procedures, dialysis, nutritional support by mouth or vein, or transfer to an ICU, for example. Measures not to be omitted are "basic nursing care, including patient hygiene, adequate analgesia, oxygen for comfort, positioning, intake for comfort including intravenous hydration, and nutritional support as tolerated." The document then notes that there may be exceptions to hydration and nutritional support.

Exceptions to the last two care elements do exist, especially when they offer no benefit or comfort to the patient. Intravenous hydration may not be appropriate when it prolongs or increases discomfort. With careful deliberation, nutritional support may be withheld when all three of the following conditions are present, namely:

[1] The patient has a terminal condition that is irreversible in the final stages.
[2] The patient is comatose and shows no clinical evidence of experiencing hunger or thirst.
[3] The patient (or substitute decision-maker) has requested no further treatment.

Other situations not meeting the above criteria for withdrawal or nutritional support care will be decided on a case-by-case basis.

Document G concludes that any treatments during this time of dying should aim at maintaining the dignity of the individual and providing compassion and comfort. The guidelines wisely state that the dying are more in need of comfort and company than treatment and diagnostic procedures.

These documents represent a range of opinions, arguments, and conclusions. All are carefully stated, clearly argued, and located squarely within the Catholic tradition—yet different conclusions are drawn from this common heritage, which indicates that the debate is far from finished. There is strong preference for a case-by-case consideration of the issues and a reluctance to have fixed rules to decide cases. On the other hand, there is a recognition that some consensus needs to be developed. Finally, there is no enthusiasm or joy about the conclusion that forgoing or withdrawing is morally permissible. While the arguments are sound, the conclusion is reached with sadness and reluctance.

In the second part of this chapter we turn to our own contribution to the development of a moral consensus by arguing for the permissibility of forgoing or withdrawing medical procedures that provide nutrition and hydration to PVS patients.

AN ARGUMENT IN SUPPORT OF FORGOING/ WITHDRAWING MEDICAL NUTRITION AND HYDRATION

The results of this survey demonstrate to us that the question of forgoing or withdrawing medical procedures for supplying nutrition and hydration[3] is far from settled. In this section we make our contribution to the debate by proposing arguments supporting the forgoing of this procedure.

The Medical Situation

An important fact about a PVS patient is that he or she is not dying. In these patients the brain stem is intact with the major damage to the brain occurring in the neocortex and cortex. Thus, these patients breathe spontaneously, have their eyes open, have a sleep-wake cycle, their pupils respond to light, and they typically have a normal gag and cough reflex.[4]

With respect to the diagnosis of PVS patients, there is "no set of specific medical criteria with as much clinical detail and certainty as the brain death criteria. Furthermore, even the generally accepted criteria, when properly applied, are not infallible."[5] Furthermore, "It is not uncommon for patients to survive in this condition for five, ten, and twenty years."[6] Survival is contingent on age, economic, familial, and institutional factors, the natural resistance of the body to disease and infection, and changing moral and social views of this condition.

Of critical importance is knowing whether these patients experience pain and/or suffering. Cranford, following the amicus curiae brief of the American Academy of Neurology in the Paul Brophy case, argues that PVS patients "may 'react' to painful and other noxious stimuli, but they do not 'feel' (experience) pain in the sense of conscious discomfort"[7] because the centers of the brain required for these experiences are too compromised to be functional. Thus, PVS patients are not clinically dying and, if they are otherwise in good health and receive appropriate care, they can have a rather long life expectancy. We obviously have the medical capacity to provide nutrition and hydration for these individuals, but the ethical difficulty, of course, is must we do everything we can to sustain their existence in this clinical condition?

The Value of Life

Clearly, the preservation of life is an important goal of the human community in general and of the profession of medicine in particular. Intuitively we know life is valuable and sacred; for were it not, then nothing else would be. Yet when all is said and done, especially in the Christian framework, life—even human life—is not of ultimate value. Philosophically and politically, we affirm a variety of values that transcend human life: justice, freedom, charity, the good of the neighbor, and so forth. On the basis of these values or for their sake, we can qualify our protection of individual human lives. Theologically, only God is of ultimate value; all else, no matter how good or valuable, must take second place. Though heresy trials are one, perhaps unfortunate, example of this priority, we also have the celebrated examples of martyrdom and individual self-sacrifice.

This perspective reminds us, particularly in the health-care context, that while preserving life is a good—and even a great good—biological life is neither the highest value nor a value that holds ultimate claim on us. To make biological life the ultimate value is to forget our real priorities and to create an idol by making a lesser good our ultimate reality.

The Quality of Life

The meaning and validity of quality of life judgments have been debated in the literature for quite some time.[8] One example in recent decades is Joseph Fletcher's criteria of humanhood.[9] Though his criteria establish standards for being human, they also implicitly argues that life without a certain level of rationality is not human and, consequently, not worth living. Most recently,

Robert Jay Lifton's examination of Nazi doctors emphasizes the role of the concept of *lebenunvertes Leben*: life unworthy of life.[10] Such unworthiness consists primarily in being Jewish, but also extends to mental illness and retardation, as well as to severe physical handicaps.[11]

Quality of life judgments can serve as a code for a life judged to be worthless or useless. This orientation comes partially from our consumerist society in which quality is linked with individuals' norms of excellence and is limited only by the horizons of their imagination and desires.[12] This perspective realizes one's worst fears about quality of life judgments because the removal of any transcendent significance or value to human lives gives the state, institutions, or other individuals final control over a person's fate.

The two most crucial levels in the quality of life debate are the evaluative and the normative. At the evaluative level, three points need to be made. First, it is necessary to distinguish clearly and consistently between physical or biological life and personal life (personhood). When this important distinction is not made, quality of life judgments can equivocate between the value of biological life and the value of personhood.[13] This possibility must be removed. Second, physical life is indeed a value that is not conditioned on any property or characteristic of the person. Here, we disagree with Documents F and G, which appear to imply such a conditional value of physical life, for example, its rationality.[14] In our view, physical life is a *bonum onticum*, a true and real value, although created and, therefore, limited. By arguing that physical life as such is a *bonum onticum* and not a conditional value (i.e., a *bonum utile*), we can affirm that all physical lives are of equal *ontic* value and that all persons are of equal *moral* worth. Third, the issue of the evaluative status of physical life may be misplaced from the start. The word "quality" does not and should not refer to a property or attribute *of life*. Rather, the quality that is at issue is the quality *of the relationship* that exists between the medical condition of the patient, on the one hand, and the patient's ability to pursue life's goals and purposes, understood as the values that transcend physical life, on the other.[15] We maintain that this reconceptualization of quality of life judgments is entirely congruent with the substance of the Catholic tradition.

Normatively, those who oppose quality of life judgments fear that life and death decisions will be made solely on the presence or absence of certain qualities or properties that a patient's life possesses. This erodes our duties to protect innocent lives, especially of those most vulnerable in our society.

If one contends that our duties to preserve life are based on a prior judgment of whether a specific quality or property of physical life will result in benefits or good consequences to the patient (personal consequentialism) or to society (social consequentialism), then in our judgment those duties to preserve life are improperly grounded in what the patient earns through social accomplishments or potentialities that the patient's life might possess. We reject such a normative position because it denies, at least implicitly, the equal ontic value of all physical lives.

We argue that one derives the prima facie duty to preserve physical life from the ontic value of life and the actual moral obligation to preserve life from a teleological, but not consequentialist, assessment of the relationship between the patient's overall condition and his or her ability to pursue life's goals and purposes. The structure of the actual moral obligation is teleological in that the patient's condition is always viewed in relation to the pursuit of life's purposes, and the grounding of the obligation always involves an evaluative assessment of the qualitative relation that exists between these two components. Because physical life is not an absolute value, even those arguing for the sanctity of life position recognize definite limits to the obligation to support life.[16] We should not reject quality of life judgments, but we should rightly reject any normative deriving of our moral duties from the presence of certain properties of physical or personal life.

"Quality of life" judgments, which are judgments strictly circumscribed by an assessment of the benefits and burdens of medical treatment considered in itself and/or of those benefits and burdens that will accrue to the patient as a result of treatment, function appropriately as ways of qualifying our duties to preserve life. Thus, as long as the value of both physical life and personhood is assured at the evaluative and normative levels, we not only support the role of "quality of life" judgments in medicine but also judge them to be indispensable in proper decision making. In our view, then, quality of life judgments properly supplement and enhance the Christian emphasis on the sanctity of life.[17]

The Technological Imperative

We cannot discuss this debate without including a reference to the technological imperative—"if we can do it, we should (or must) do it"—which infers a moral obligation either from a capacity or from the mere existence of a technology.

In the context of high-tech medicine, such an imperative, even if not explicitly subscribed to, is difficult to resist. The same is true even for low-tech or simple technologies. Some medical technologies that administer nutrition and hydration are relatively simple, for example, parenteral methods of delivering nutrients. Other methods are more invasive (e.g., gastrostomy tubes) and they carry with them potential iatrogenic dangers, such as infection resulting from the surgical creation of the stoma. Yet they are much less invasive than other procedures and are more risk-free if properly cared for. Furthermore, their use provides a clear and demonstrable benefit: the prolongation of physical life. Indeed, feeding tubes may be unique among all medical technologies in that they almost exceptionlessly deliver on their claims. The technological imperative is augmented by simplicity and predictability of outcome and consequently presents an apparently unassailable case for use. But this very simplicity, ease of use, and ready availability disguise the moral dimension of the technology's use.

One must consider the use with respect to outcome. The outcome, of course, is the preservation of physical life. Prima facie, such an outcome is valuable, but it must be considered with respect to other values and/or goods, for physical life is not the only or absolute good. Thus, other goods, such as human dignity, ought to be considered. Our point is that, in and of itself, the presence of a technology and the capacity to use it constitute at most a prima facie case for its use. One cannot automatically or necessarily infer an actual moral obligation from the mere existence or presence of a technology.[18]

The Ordinary/Extraordinary Means Distinction

This well-used distinction can be dated as early as the seventeenth century and has been used by popes and theologians in arguments to determine one's moral obligation to preserve human life.[19] Some maintain that the key element in the traditional use of the distinction is the *classification* of technologies, medicines, or procedures. Consequently, they are considered apart from the patient on whom they are used. Once classified, the moral question is then essentially resolved. In the feeding tube example, the late John Connery argued that since nutrition and hydration kept individuals alive, the technology fit the classic definition of ordinary treatment and, therefore, was morally mandatory.[20]

If one shifts the perspective from an abstract classification of technologies to a *patient-centered* approach,[21] which gives moral weight to the autonomy of the patient and looks to the impact of these technologies on the patient's medical and nonmedical condition as a whole, one can establish a different moral argument. Here, the expressed wishes of the patient have a legitimate moral claim based on our valuing the dignity of the individual and on our respecting the sacredness of his or her conscience. Second, it is the proportionality or disproportionality of benefits and burdens *to the patient* that makes any medical treatment or procedure, including the medical provision of nutrition and hydration, obligatory or optional. Because the technology can neither ameliorate a PVS patient's general clinical condition nor restore this individual to any state of health where the patient might pursue the values of life, the means are extraordinary and not morally required. Therefore, ordinary and extraordinary are determined not by classifying the technology but by considering its impact on the patient and his or her overall condition. Additionally, and following directly from the above, the distinction must adopt a patient-centered perspective to avoid the technological imperative.

The Burdensomeness of Life

The specific issue here is whether the burdensomeness of the life preserved by the offering of nutrition/hydration can or should be part of the overall assessment of burden in the determination of ordinary/extraordinary as we have just outlined it. Considered only *in itself*, the medical provision of nutrition and hydration would most often be considered ordinary. Thus, for some people any considerations beyond the technology itself would lead to an improper questioning of the value of the patient's life.

We think the concepts of burden and quality of life should be linked. Burden can accrue to the patient precisely through the administration of modern technology and can be a consequence of a life lived merely at the biological level with no hope of restoration or further pursuit of temporal or even eternal goals. In this sense, the burden is iatrogenic. For the PVS patient, medicine has reached its limit in bringing this individual to any level of health and wholeness. Again, this patient-centered approach focuses on the conditions under which this valued life is to be lived and seeks to identify what interests of the patient can be achieved. Thus, we argue that burden is to be assessed not only from the perspective of the burdensome effects of the technology itself but, like Document C, also from the perspective "of the burdens that an individual experiences in pursuing the goals or ends of life" as a result of the intervention of the medical technology. Though it is doubtful that the PVS patient would experience this burden personally, the burden is real, even if experienced secondhand by the family and/or by those professionals who must care for the patient.[22]

Fear of Being "Trapped"

The expected benefit of tube feeding is the preservation of life post-trauma or post-treatment so that other important work can go on, for example, treatment or diagnosis. But there comes a time—sometimes sooner and sometimes later—when one knows that all has been tried and cure is not possible. What was formerly appropriate to do—that is, trying to cure—is now inappropriate, and our efforts must shift to accompanying the patient on his or her final journey.

We agree with Document F that it is precisely here that a family may feel or actually be trapped. Having appropriately initiated medical feeding to preserve life while other tests, procedures, and medications were tried, the family may now be frustrated in its desire to remove the feeding tube. Though such feeding only preserves biological life, attempts to withdraw the feeding may be challenged by medical personnel or by others.

Our fear is that individuals or families may inappropriately refuse to initiate medical procedures for delivering nutrients because of the fear of not being able to withdraw these procedures when that becomes appropriate. Thus, individuals who may genuinely benefit from this type of procedure could be deprived of its goods. Such a situation would be tragic beyond belief. But because of the technological imperative, our near absolutizing of biological life, and the fear of taking personal responsibility in medical decision making, this outcome is almost guaranteed. However, recognizing patient autonomy and shifting to a patient-centered calculation of benefits and burdens in the fashion we have described will counter this unfortunate situation.

Summary

In our judgment, the cumulative effect of our arguments supports the legitimate forgoing or withdrawing of nutrition and hydration to PVS patients. This judgment can properly be reached without supporting any efforts or claims for euthanasia and without making any improper judgments about the worth of a particular life. After carefully considering both the patient's known wishes and the qualitative relation between the patient's medical condition and the pursuit of life's purposes, one may appropriately judge that such a therapy is disproportionate and morally optional. This conclusion seems to be very close to, if not the same as, the judgment contained in Document E.

SUGGESTIONS FOR FUTURE DISCUSSION

Having reviewed the results of the survey, the points raised in the various documents submitted to us, and identified several ethical arguments supporting the removal of medical feeding tubes, we wish to make some suggestions for the future conducting of this debate.

Nomenclature

The Misuse of "Euthanasia" in the Debate

In our survey, ordinaries were asked whether the diocesan committee considered the removal of feeding tubes from PVS patients to be an act of involuntary euthanasia. The responses are very interesting. Most answered that they considered the withdrawal of these tubes to be "passive or indirect and therefore permitted." A significant number responded that "it depends," and only four respondents answered that this action was "active or direct and therefore forbidden."

The response from the research center, Document D, states that the withdrawal of feeding tubes from PVS patients, except in very limited cases, is an act of "euthanasia by omission," and in most cases anyone who does this has the moral intention to end a life that is considered valueless or excessively burdensome. Two assumptions, frequently cited among those who consider such actions as euthanasia, seem to underlie this conclusion. The first is that the medical provision of nutrients offers a benefit by preserving the life of the patient. The second is that this nourishment should be considered as ordinary *care*, similar to all other types of care.

The moral characterization of the intention of the one authorizing withdrawal as "ending a life" forces this discussion into the context of euthanasia. In its brief to the New Jersey Supreme Court on the case of Nancy Ellen Jobes, the New Jersey Catholic Conference argued that the withdrawal of feeding tubes is "intentional euthanasia."[23] Because we disagree both with the two basic assumptions that underlie this argument and with the description of the moral intention of these acts of withdrawal as killing, we argue that the use of the term euthanasia should be avoided in the debate.

A moral analysis of euthanasia necessarily involves an assessment of the intention. Though they may be motivated by humane reasons, morally, all acts of euthanasia intend the death of the patient, either by commission or by omission, and thus by definition these acts constitute the unjustified killing of a patient. However, we argue that in withdrawing nutrition and hydration the intent is either to end a procedure that no longer benefits the patient or to prevent the person from being entrapped in technology. The patient's death, while foreseen, results from the justified discontinuance of a technology that itself can neither correct the underlying fatal pathology—that is, the permanent inability to ingest food and fluids orally—nor offer the patient any reasonable hope for what we have defined as quality of life. In our judgment, then, it is inappropriate to characterize the withdrawal of medical nutrition and hydration from PVS patients as euthanasia.

The Use of "Forgo," not "Withhold"

We suggest that in any future discussion of this issue the word "forgo" should be used rather than "withhold." The reason is that "withhold" connotes that something is denied to someone who has some entitlement to it. When family members appropriately decide that a medical treatment will not truly benefit the PVS patient, their decision is to refrain from pursuing what is not useful to the loved one, not to deny something to which the patient has a need or a right. Our intent is twofold: to avoid a begging of the question and to suggest a terminology that allows the argument to come forward and be evaluated on its own merits. The terminology of forgoing and withdrawing, we think, will prevent the argument from becoming confused linguistically and prejudged methodologically.

Description of Nutrition and Hydration

What to call the nourishment administered to a patient introduces a variety of problems, descriptive as well as symbolic. The terms "food and water" conjure up, among other things, a variety of images depending on taste and ethnic background. They also connote a meal in which one actively participates or, if with others, shares. The symbolism associated with food and water is deep, and rightly so. They symbolize membership and participation in a community, and to deny these common but significant realities to someone is more than depriving that individual of nourishment; it is cutting him or her off from the community.

The symbolic level of food and water is what inclines several individuals to argue against the removal of nourishment from the PVS patient.[24] The forgoing or the removal of nutrition says that the individual has been marked and put outside the community, outside society. This further signifies the valuelessness of the person and his or her uselessness to the community. Therefore, one must continue to provide this nourishment precisely as a symbol of inclusion.

However, one must also recognize the limits of this symbolism, particularly in the case of PVS patients. First, we have a situation in which the patient is fed and does not eat; the experience is entirely passive. Orderlies or nurses do not deny trays of food to patients nor do they forcibly remove these from the hands of patients. Nutrition and hydration are administered to the patient and the body absorbs them; the feeding process is completely involuntary. Second, the symbolism of the meal is utterly absent, even if others are there. There is no meal, but a medical feeding. Though nourishing, it is difficult to consider such a liquid protein diet as food. For food, in addition to having a certain biological reality, is also a human construct and is more than the sum of its nutritional value. It is the color, texture, aroma, taste, and company in which it is shared. For the PVS patient, all of this is absent. To call this nourishment *food* is to invest it with more meaning than the reality of the situation can bear.

Also, these patients do not consciously experience hunger or thirst. But even if these states were experienced, medical procedures for supplying nutrition and hydration might not relieve the feelings.[25] "Medical nutrition and hydration" seems an appropriate phrase for this form of nourishment because it captures in a nonjudgmental fashion the medical provision of the nourishment as well as the passivity of the experience. The patient is fed and, consequently, the body is nourished, but he or she certainly does not participate in a meal and clearly does not share table fellowship. This terminology also describes the procedure without begging the moral question of whether one ought to provide it, and it avoids the intrusion of inappropriate symbolism. This terminology will keep us from making more of the situation than is there, but it will also keep us from making less of it.

Ordinary and Extraordinary Treatment

Change in the Use of the Terms

As we noted above, there is a difference in how these traditional terms can be used. For some, the terms are the basis on which the procedure or technology is classified. Once classified, the correct action is relatively clear. If ordinary, the procedure or technology is morally obligatory; if extraordinary, it is morally optional. This schema encounters significant problems when the pace of technological change increases. In addition, the term *ordinary* in its moral or normative sense has been used to declare a certain technology routine or customary in a medical or descriptive sense. The descriptive use of ordinary generally refers to what *is* usually done, but this involves little or no moral analysis of what *ought* to be done.

These equivocations have precipitated a rethinking of the terminology that now aims at the evaluation of the benefit-burden ratio for the patient.[26] Consequently, a procedure is judged ordinary in a normative sense if its effects on the patient provide proportionately more benefits than burdens. On the other hand, a treatment is extraordinary in a moral sense if the evaluation produces the contrary conclusion. Thus, these terms are now seen as the *conclusion* of a process of evaluation rather than as a *classification* of a procedure. It is not unusual that a Jehovah's Witness would judge a clinically routine blood transfusion morally extraordinary because of the disproportionate consequences for his or her eternal salvation. Similarly, a person on long-term dialysis might conclude in some circumstances that use of this technology is extraordinary because of its impact on diet and lifestyle.

Understanding ordinary and extraordinary as conclusions of an evaluative process rather than as a classification schema permits a much more appropriate use of the terms in the practice of contemporary medicine. Furthermore, the danger of equivocation is now removed, and the meaning of the terms is moral, not descriptive.

Autonomy

Though the concept of autonomy has undergone some criticism in the last few years because it has been taken to an extreme by functioning independently of or to the exclusion of other values, nonetheless, we might do well to remember the old adage that abuse does not take away its use. Autonomy is an important value, and the proper starting point for these discussions is the expressed wishes of the competent patient. To begin at this point is to respect the dignity of patients and their conscientious decisions. Statements that individuals make about their death or the circumstances of their dying are extremely important. Minimally, they form the foundation of any and all discussions about the initiation or withdrawal of therapy. These statements, which need to be discussed and evaluated in light of the clinical situation and other relevant moral values, always constitute a core element in the final decision about treatment.

Quality of Life Considerations and the Goal of Medicine

As we have noted, quality of life judgments should not be construed as judgments about the worth of either physical or personal life. They are not concerned with assessing qualities or properties that, when present, make life itself valuable. Rather, these judgments are evaluative and normative claims or assessments about the relation between the patient's overall condition and his or her ability to pursue material, moral, and spiritual values that transcend physical life but do not give that life its very meaning and worth. Consequently, quality of life judgments help specify concretely the meaning of the terms "benefits," "burdens," and "best interests" of a patient as well as the limits of medical interventions within a given historical and cultural situation.

Whereas all physical life is of equal ontic worth and all personal life is of equal moral value, the quality of the relation between these lives and the pursuit of values is not equal. Due to multiple factors, some of which have to do with individual genetic endowment and the ways in which we live our lives and some of which are dependent on the nurturing and accessibility of values in a given culture, a large portion of the population is fortunate enough to attain a high quality of life. Other individuals, regrettably, are not as fortunate, and they must live most of their lives pursuing life's purposes at a less than optimal level. But some have no discernible or such a minimal qualitative relation between their overall condition and the pursuit of values that we would argue that those in this last category have no moral obligation to prolong their physical lives. In these cases, all treatment can be withdrawn from them. Not long ago, all PVS patients' lives would have been mercifully ended by their inability to ingest food orally, but the intervention of modern technology today has not been as merciful.

No doubt, one of the principal factors that has provoked this debate has been the ambiguity about the central goal of medicine itself. Medicine rightfully seeks to prevent death (especially an untimely death), to alleviate pain and physical suffering, and to promote health as far as possible. Indeed, these are important goals. However, we argue that all these goals are really subordinate to the more encompassing goal of serving the purposefulness of personal existence.[27] In other words, the central and overarching goal of clinical medicine is to enhance the qualitative relation between the patient's condition and the pursuit of life's goods. Thus, other things being equal, when medicine can intervene to ameliorate the quality of the relation between the patient's condition and the pursuit of life's goals, then such an intervention can be considered a benefit to the patient and is in his or her best interests. On the other hand, because of the overall condition of the patient, when a proposed intervention cannot offer the patient any reasonable hope of pursuing life's purposes at all or can only offer the patient a condition where the pursuit of life's purposes will be filled with profound frustration or with utter neglect of these purposes because of the energy needed merely to sustain physical life, then any medical intervention 1) can only offer burden to the life treated, 2) is contrary to the best interests of the patient, 3) can cause iatrogenic harm or the risk of such harm, and 4) has reached its limit based on medicine's own principal reason for existence, and thus treatment should not be given except to palliate or to comfort.[28]

Responsibility in Decision Making

Playing God: People or Technology?

When the biotechnological revolution began in earnest and humans discovered new powers and capacities, one of the first slogans to describe this new state of affairs was "playing God." This phrase denoted the power humans now wielded over previously untamed and uncontrolled natural realities. But we detect a shift emerging. Rather than humans "playing God," it is now technology that is "playing God." Our machines seem to have developed a life and power of their own. How, for example, does someone with an artificial heart die? How does someone on a respirator stop breathing? How does someone with a feeding tube refuse to be nourished? Very often, once in place, there seems to be no way—short of a cosmic power failure—to end the domination of the machine. We are, clearly, much better about removing machines now than we were initially, but many are still very reluctant to intervene in the activities of the machinery. Often enough, court intervention is the only recourse the family or guardian has to stop a machine.[29]

Have we surrendered our decision-making powers to machines? Do they "play God" by exercising their untiring, endless vigilance over us and our loved ones? We have not improved our situation much if, indeed, we have turned our appropriate decision-making responsibilities over to machines. Although such decisions are dangerous and difficult at times, humans have a legitimate level of responsibility for deciding about the forgoing or withdrawing of treatment. Surrendering that responsibility because a machine is in place is truly the worship of a false god.

Role of the Family

The family typically plays an important role in these decisions because often enough the individual most affected by a decision cannot participate directly. Such involvement is proper because generally the family has a relationship with the patient and knows his or her wishes. The family is normally in the best position to discern the patient's wishes or desires. Thus, they can either relate what the patient actually wanted or, failing that, relate their best judgment of what the patient would have wanted. If the family has no direct knowledge of the patient's wishes, they are still the appropriate decision maker. They have a socially recognized relation to the patient and can be presumed to have the best interests of the patient in mind.

Should conflicts arise that simply cannot be resolved at the local level with the assistance of the physicians, an ethics committee, a patient's rights advocate, the clergy, or other resources, then—and only then in our judgment—is it appropriate to think of turning to the courts for a resolution of the issue. The family, even without knowledge of the patient's wishes, has at least a relation with the patient and is a more appropriate locus for decision making. However, when they cannot resolve the issues and a decision is necessary, then the courts are an appropriate avenue for seeking a decision.

CONCLUSION

On both practical and theoretical levels, the question of forgoing or withdrawing medical nutrition and hydration from PVS patients appears to have reached no clear consensus inside or outside the Catholic community, although our sense is that many, if not most, people are uncomfortable with continuing this technology when there is no reasonable hope of an improvement in the patient's prognosis. This is not to say that there is an atmosphere of joy about the situation or a zeal to begin a withdrawal procedure. Rather, there is a sense of reluctance, a very great sense of caution and care, and a most careful focusing on the moral arguments.

Finally, we wish to highlight two aspects of the debate that we think are particularly crucial. First, the moral intention to forgo or withdraw medical nutrition and hydration is not identical with the intention in euthanasia. This conclusion is confirmed by our own work and in most of the literature. People who advocate the forgoing or the withdrawal of feeding tubes are not advocating any kind of euthanasia policy. The clear intent is to end a procedure that is not proportionately benefiting the person or to release the person from entrapment in technology. Thus, while forgoing or withdrawing feeding tubes is not "medical killing" as some have claimed, it may well be "involuntary medical living." Second, forgoing or withdrawing this technology is argued as a moral option, not as a mandatory practice. Therefore, the conclusion that we share with most authors is either that forgoing or withdrawal is not prohibited or it is within the permitted range of moral activities. We also agree with Document E that individuals who conclude that such a practice is morally appropriate should not to be prohibited from acting on that conclusion.

We expect that the debate will continue and that different aspects of it will be further examined. Our hope is that this report and presentation of an argument will help structure that process and assist in its resolution.[30]

ENDNOTES

Support for the survey was provided by the Research Development Council of Worcester Polytechnic Institute, and the authors acknowledge their gratitude for this assistance.

1. The longest case of coma is that of Elaine Esposito, who died 37 years and 111 days after falling into coma. See the President's Commission for the Study of Ethical Problems in Medicine and Biomedical and Behavioral Research, *Deciding to Forego Life-Sustaining Treatment: A Report on the Ethical, Medical, and Legal Issues in Treatment Decisions* (Washington, D.C.: U.S. Government Printing Office, 1983), 177, n. 16.

2. Some dioceses may not have received a survey either because the see was vacant or because of error on TAS's part. Additionally, not every respondent answered every

question. Thus, in terms of data analysis there is no constant "n"; yet, an overall impression can be gained from the data.

3. Throughout the remainder of this chapter we have adopted the terminology used by the Hastings Center in describing the technique by which nutrition and hydration are provided to the PVS patient. As defined by the Hastings Center, "medical procedures for supplying nutrition and hydration are medical enteral procedures and parenteral nutritional procedures." "Medical enteral procedures are procedures in which nutritional formulas and water are introduced into the patient's stomach or intestine by means of a tube, such as a gastrostomy tube or nasogastric tube." "Parenteral nutritional procedures are procedures in which nutritional formulas and water are introduced into the patient's body by means other than the gastrointestinal tract. Such procedures include total parenteral nutritional support (TPN), in which a formula capable of maintaining the patient for prolonged periods is infused into a vein—usually a large, central vein in the patient's chest—and intravenous procedures in which water and/or a formula supplying limited nutritional support is introduced into a peripheral vein." The Hastings Center, *Guidelines on the Termination of Life-Sustaining Treatment and the Care of the Dying* (Briarcliff Manor, N.Y.: Hastings Center, 1987), 140–41.

4. For a more detailed discussion of the condition of a patient in persistent vegetative state, see Ronald E. Cranford, "The Persistent Vegetative State: The Medical Reality (Getting the Facts Straight)," *Hastings Center Report* 18 (February/March 1988): 27–32. Also, see the President's Report, *Deciding to Forego Life-Sustaining Treatment*, 174–81.

5. Cranford, "The Persistent Vegetative State," 29.

6. Cranford, "The Persistent Vegetative State," 31.

7. Cranford, "The Persistent Vegetative State," 31. In addition, see the recent "Position of the American Academy of Neurology on Certain Aspects of the Care and Management of the Persistent Vegetative State Patient," reprinted in *Medical Ethics Advisor* 4 (August 1988): 111–13.

8. For example, see George J. Annas, "Quality of Life in the Courts: Earle Spring in Fantasyland," *Hastings Center Report* 10 (August, 1980): 9–10; Daniel Callahan, *Setting Limits* (New York: Simon & Schuster, 1988), 187–93; John R. Connery, "Quality of Life," *Linacre Quarterly* 53 (February, 1986): 26–33; Brian V. Johnstone, "The Sanctity of Life, the Quality of Life and the New 'Baby Doe' Law," *Linacre Quarterly* 52 (August, 1985): 258–70; Edward W. Keyserlingk, *Sanctity of Life or Quality of Life in the Context of Ethics, Medicine and Law* [A study written for The Law Reform Commission of Canada] (Ottawa: Minister of Supply and Services Canada, 1979), 49–72, 75–105, 185–90; Richard A. McCormick, "A Proposal for 'Quality of Life' Criteria for Sustaining Life," *Hospital Progress* 59(1975): 76–79; Richard A. McCormick, "The Quality of Life, the Sanctity of Life," *Hastings Center Report* 8 (February, 1978): 30–36; Warren T. Reich, "Quality of Life," in *Encyclopedia of Bioethics*, vol. 2, edited by Warren T. Reich (New York: Free Press, 1978), 829–40; and Warren T. Reich, "Quality of Life and Defective Newborn Children: An Ethical Analysis," in *Decision Making and the Defective Newborn: Proceedings of a Conference on Spina Bifida and Ethics*, edited by Chester A. Swinyard (Springfield, Ill.: Charles C. Thomas, 1978), 489–511.

9. Joseph Fletcher, "Indicators of Humanhood: A Tentative Profile of Man," *Hastings Center Report* 2 (November 1972): 1–4.

10. Robert Jay Lifton, *The Nazi Doctors: Medical Killing and the Psychology of Genocide* (New York: Basic Books, 1986), 21.

11. For an interesting contrast between the Nazi interpretation of "quality of life" and what contemporary authors tend to mean by this criterion, see Cynthia B. Cohen, "'Quality of Life' and the Analogy with the Nazis," *Journal of Medicine and Philosophy* 8 (1983): 113–35.

12. Albert R. Jonsen, "Purposefulness in Human Life," *Western Journal of Medicine* 125 (July, 1976): 5.

13. For example, Warren Reich's theological position grounds both the value and the equality of "human life" in the belief that "all men are created as persons in the image of God" (Reich, "Quality of Life and Defective Newborn Children," 504). His use of the phrase "human life" is ambiguous here and therefore misleading. The context of his argument is a critique of what he believes to be Richard A. McCormick's position on the value of *physical life*, yet Reich completes his argument by referring to *persons* and their nature and value as images of God.

14. In fact, several contemporary Catholics have given the impression that the value of physical life is dependent on some inherent property or attribute that, when present, gives physical life its value. It is possible that this way of phrasing the value of physical life is due to the lack of a terminology in the contemporary discussion that can mediate between the two traditional categories of value, namely, *bonum honestum* and *bonum utile*. For example, see Kevin D. O'Rourke and Dennis Brodeur, *Medical Ethics: Common Ground for Understanding* (St. Louis, Mo.: Catholic Health Association of the U.S., 1986), 213; Richard A. McCormick, *How Brave a New World? Dilemmas in Bioethics* (Washington, D.C.: Georgetown University Press, 1981), 405–7; and David Thomasma et al., "Continuance of Nutritional Care in the Terminally Ill Patient," *Critical Care Clinics* 2 (January 1986): 66.

15. See James J. Walter, "The Meaning and Validity of Quality of Life Judgments in Contemporary Roman Catholic Medical Ethics," *Louvain Studies* 13 (Fall 1988): 195–208, especially 201.

16. For example, see John R. Connery, "Prolonging Life: The Duty and Its Limits," *Linacre Quarterly* 47 (May 1980): 151–65; Johnstone, "The Sanctity of Life, The Quality of Life," especially 265–69; and Reich, "Quality of Life and Defective Newborn Children," especially 505–9.

17. Keyserlingk also argues a similar position in his report for the Law Reform Commission of Canada. See his *Sanctity of Life or Quality of Life*, especially 49–72.

18. We agree with the report from the Hastings Center that "All invasive procedures for supplying nutrition and hydration—all enteral and parenteral techniques—should be considered procedures that require the patient's or surrogate's consent." Hastings Center, *Guidelines on the Termination of Life-Sustaining Treatment and the Care of the Dying*, 61.

19. See Gerald Kelly, *Medico-Moral Problems* (St. Louis, Mo.: Catholic Hospital Association, 1958), 128–41.

20. John R. Connery, "The Clarence Herbert Case: Was Withdrawal of Treatment Justified?" *Hospital Progress* 65 (February 1984): 32–35, 70.

21. Recently, several authors have argued for a patient-centered approach in clinical decision making. For example, see Robert M. Veatch, *Death, Dying, and the Biological Revolution: Our Last Quest for Responsibility* (New Haven, Conn.: Yale University Press, 1976); and James J. Walter, "Food & Water: An Ethical Burden," *Commonweal* 113 (November 21, 1986): 616–19.

22. Though we have refrained from making any judgment about the financial burden either on society or on insurance companies in providing funds for PVS patients, the fact that there are approximately 10,000 of these patients in the United States strongly inclines us to agree with Daniel Callahan that "It is hard to see how a debate on that reimbursement issue can be forestalled much longer." See Callahan's "Vital Distinctions, Mortal Questions: Debating Euthanasia & Health-Care Costs," *Commonweal* 115 (July 15, 1988): 404. It is important to note here that the *Declaration on Euthanasia* and Document E, both following Pius XII, do permit one to assess the burden on the family or on the community in judging whether a treatment is disproportionate. See the *Declaration on Euthanasia* in *Origins* 10 (August 10, 1980): 16.

23. New Jersey State Catholic Conference Brief, "Providing Food and Fluids to Severely Brain Damaged Patients," in *Origins* 16 (January 22, 1987): 583. The conference was following the Lutheran theologian Gilbert Meilaender in his "On Removing Food and Water: Against the Stream," *Hastings Center Report* 14 (December 1984): 11–13. An opposing position was taken by Bishop Gelineau of Providence, Rhode Island, in the Marcia Gray court case. See his statement in *Origins* 17(January 21, 1988): 546–57.

24. For example, see Daniel Callahan, "On Feeding the Dying," *Hastings Center Report* 13 (October 1983): 22.

25. Hastings Center, *Guidelines on the Termination of Life-Sustaining Treatment and the Care of the Dying*, 59.

26. See the *Declaration on Euthanasia* where the terminology has shifted to a discussion of proportionality between the benefits and the burdens.

27. Jonsen, "Purposefulness in Human Life," 6.

28. Walter, "The Meaning and Validity of Quality of Life Judgments," 207.

29. There have been several court cases recently involving patients in a persistent vegetative state. Two of the more notable cases are Paul Brophy and Nancy Ellen Jobes.

15

Artificial Nutrition and Hydration: Assessing the Papal Statement

Thomas A. Shannon and James J. Walter

In addressing an international congress on Life-Sustaining Treatments and Vegetative State: Scientific Advances and Ethical Dilemmas that was sponsored by the World Federation of Catholic Medical Associations and the Pontifical Academy for Life, Pope John Paul II argued, according to a statement from the Vatican Information Service on March 22, 2004, that the administration of artificial nutrition and hydration (ANH) through feeding tubes is "a natural means of preserving life, not a medical procedure." At one point, the pontiff claims that ANH for patients in a persistent vegetative state (PVS) is not a medical treatment (*non un atto medico*), yet later he claims that its use must be considered ordinary and proportionate (*ordinario e proporzionato*), which seems to imply that this kind of intervention is indeed a type of treatment, though an ordinary and morally required one. Additionally, people in a persistent vegetative state will always remain human, maintain their dignity, and have "the right to basic health care (nutrition, hydration, hygiene, warmth, etc)." Furthermore, according to the pope, the "moral principle according to which even the slightest doubt of being in the presence of a person who is alive requires full respect and prohibits any action that would anticipate his or her death." Additionally, the pope stated that "it is necessary to promote positive activities to counteract pressure for the suspension of food and hydration, as a means to putting an end to the lives of these patients." Finally, the pope noted that "Death by starvation or dehydration is, in fact, the only possible outcome as a result of their withdrawal. In this sense it ends up becoming, if done knowingly and willingly, true and proper euthanasia by omission."

This analysis and the conclusions drawn from it appear to represent a major reversal of the moral tradition of the Catholic Church in assessing whether a particular medical or other intervention is morally obligatory, particularly in the determination of whether this intervention is ordinary or extraordinary treatment. Also whether an intervention is a medical treatment or some other intervention is not the primary determinant of whether the intervention is morally ordinary or extraordinary. Whether some intervention is considered a "natural means" (*un mezzo naturale*), as the pope did, also does not determine the moral or obligatory status of the intervention. A few remarks are therefore in order.

First, the Catholic moral tradition determines whether an intervention is ordinary or extraordinary based on a proportionate-disproportionate means test, according to the 1980 CDF "Declaration on Euthanasia." "In any case, it will be possible to make a correct judgment as to the means by studying the type of treatment to be used, its degree of complexity or risk, its cost and the possibilities of using it, and comparing these elements with the result that can be expected, taking into account the state of the sick person and his or her physical and moral resources" (para. 4). The "Declaration" then gives four examples. The patient can choose to use the most advanced medical means available; such participation in research may also be a service to the rest of humanity. Second, the patient is permitted to stop interventions when the results fall short of expectations. Third, the refusal of a technique in use but that carries a risk or is burdensome is not the equivalent of suicide. Finally, "When inevitable death is imminent in spite of the means used, it is permitted in conscience to take the decision to refuse forms of treatment that would only secure a precarious and burdensome prolongation of life, so long as the normal care due to the sick person in similar cases is not interrupted" (para. 4).

The basic point here is that ordinary and extraordinary forms of treatment are not determined by classifying an intervention according to whether or not it is routinely used by physicians. This empirical definition of ordinary-extraordinary is not helpful in this context, and it is not what the Catholic tradition had in mind when the distinction was developed. Whether a medical intervention is *morally* ordinary has historically been determined by its effect on the patient or on those who have the responsibility to care for the patient. To argue that what is *medically* ordinary as determined by its routine usage by physicians is also *morally* ordinary equivocates on the term ordinary and misrepresents the core of the medical ethical tradition of the Catholic Church, a tradition in place since at least the sixteenth century. Early moral theologians, for example, taught that cloistered nuns who might be embarrassed by a medical examination were under no obligation to have such an examination. It was an extraordinary procedure because of the burden it placed on them.

Second, to determine that an intervention is morally extraordinary and therefore should either not be initiated or withdrawn is not to deny the personhood of the patient or to devalue the person's dignity. Likewise, such forgoing or withdrawal does not necessarily imply that the intention of the physician or family is to end the life of the patient. It might simply be to recognize that either the proposed intervention is not useful in helping to restore the patient to health or that the patient is dying or in a condition that will lead to death and that the moral obligation is to accompany this person on his or her final journey. The intention might also be to respect the patient's considered wishes when competent not to have such interventions put in place when the patient falls into a PVS state. Mandating useless or unwanted interventions might well be the violation of the person's dignity, and therefore we should be deeply worried about this in a clinical setting.

Third, when people begin dying, they frequently stop eating and drinking. This is a part of the dying process, and interfering with it may in fact interfere with this process and actually harm the patient. Such interventions are morally contraindicated as both harmful and extraordinary. A person in a persistent vegetative state, assuming a correct diagnosis (and such a diagnosis will and should take some time), is incapable of orally eating or drinking by his or her self. To the best medical knowledge when properly diagnosed, such a condition is irreversible. It cannot be cured. The damage to the brain is so severe that nothing can be done to reverse that condition, and the patient will not return to any level of sapient or sentient existence. There is a whole medical literature about the medical condition of such patients that is most relevant for the discussion of this question.

What can be done is to intervene with artificial nutrition and hydration to maintain the physiological process and to prevent death. All the artificial feeding does is maintain the biological processes of the person. It does not directly contribute to the person's recovery or maintain the person in a stable condition as part of an ongoing therapeutic process. Artificial nutrition and hydration cannot make such contributions because recovery is not an option for a person in a persistent vegetative state or for one in the dying process. Such interventions can, in some instances, harm the person because of the possibility of known harmful side effects, such as infections at the site of the insertion of the tube, nausea, vomiting and the possibility of the vomitus choking the patient, abdominal swelling, cramping, and perhaps diarrhea. Some patients occasionally tear them out. And whether this is done consciously or unconsciously, the tube needs to be reinserted, and this exposes the patient to more risks. There is a well-established medical literature on the harms and burdens associated with tube feeding. It might be helpful to consult such literature before claiming that such interventions are not a medical treatment.

There has been a strong moral argument, grounded in the history of Catholic medical ethics, that the use of feeding tubes for nutrition and hydration can be judged in some circumstances as extraordinary, and thus not morally obligatory. This argument has been based on the view that no intervention in the abstract can be judged either ordinary or extraordinary. Such a prudential judgment always requires knowledge of a specific patient and his or her own evaluation of the proposed intervention. Not only the means (proposed intervention) but the ends toward which the intervention is aimed are important in the moral analysis. In the concrete medical setting, it would be improper to say that there are never any burdens connected to feeding tubes. There are physical burdens and harms that can be associated with ANH. The treatments can be expensive, especially the placing of the feeding tube by medical personnel. According to the CDF's "Declaration," one may refuse an intervention from a desire "not to impose excessive expense on the family or the community." This statement recognizes that there is no moral obligation to spend either one's own or the community's money on treatments that do not bring benefit to a patient's overall condition or that might be judged burdensome or psychologically repulsive.

Fourth, this address by John Paul II seems to represent to us an elevation of biological or physical life to an almost absolute value. The statement comes close to saying that life must be preserved for its own sake. Yet in his encyclical "Evangelium Vitae," he clearly stated, "Certainly the life of the body in its earthly state is *not an absolute good* for the believer, especially as he may be asked to give up his life for a greater good" (sec. 47). The Catholic medical ethics tradition has not required that a person actually be dying before interventions could be terminated, as the pope implied in this statement and in "Evangelium Vitae." In the latter document he states, "In such situations, when *death is clearly imminent and inevitable*, one can in conscience 'refuse forms of treatment that would only secure a precarious and burdensome prolongation of life'" ("Declaration on Euthanasia," IV, sec. 65). In the broader Catholic tradition, interventions can be removed when they are defined as morally extraordinary because of their burdens or because they are no longer useful in securing a medical benefit for the patient. If such interventions can no longer be forgone or withdrawn, then we are in severe danger of making biological life an absolute value and an end in itself. Human life, of course, has not been so evaluated in the Catholic medical ethics tradition, nor in the Catholic theological tradition.

Finally, though this papal statement sought to prevent the practice of euthanasia, whether by commission or by omission, this way of stating the matter may in fact have the reverse outcome. If people are told that removing useless and burdensome interventions is morally prohibited and that they are morally obligated to provide such interventions right up to the point of natural death, many people may conclude that this moral advice contradicts their deepest moral instincts and will simply ignore it. And if the most pastorally sensitive part of Catholic medical ethics—the recognition that once an intervention is judged either useless or burdensome, it can be rejected—is jettisoned, many people will conclude, rightly or wrongly, that one might just as well go directly to euthanasia since there is no relevant moral analysis for considering the appropriate medical and moral treatment of the sick or the permanently unconscious.

Many other important questions remain. Why is this statement not framed within a broader theological reflection on the meaning of life? One thinks of Pope Pius XII's allocution on "The Prolongation of Life" in 1957 that placed these decisions about forgoing and withdrawing of medical interventions in the theological context of the spiritual ends of life. He stated, "Life, health, all temporal activities are in fact subordinated to spiritual ends." Furthermore, what is the level of magisterial authority with which this statement is proclaimed? Is it an application of the pope's positions enunciated in "Evangelium Vitae" on end-of-life questions? Does this statement apply only to patients in PVS, or does it also extend to other categories of patients who need permanent feeding tubes inserted but are not in PVS? If the traditional distinction between ordinary and extraordinary means applies to other categories of patients on this issue, then on what grounds do we argue that it is always required of patients in PVS? Surely, the reason cannot be that these patients might not have made their wishes known ahead of time and thus are vulnerable to others' interpretations of their informed judgment. We know that many Catholics have already signed "living wills" while competent and in good faith that they do not want such interventions used if they fall into a PVS state. Therefore, families that refer to these documents are attempting to be faithful to the wishes of the patient and not attempting to end the life of the patient because the patient is a burden on them. Many more questions remain, but we are left with a sense that the pope's rightful purpose to protect PVS patients and to curb the movement toward euthanasia has not achieved its goal in this statement.

16

Implications of the Papal Allocution on Feeding Tubes

Thomas A. Shannon and James J. Walter

The papal allocution to the international congress on Life-Sustaining Treatment and Vegetative State: Scientific Advances and Ethical Dilemmas on March 20, 2004, has been the occasion for significant discussion concerning the use of artificial feeding tubes for nutrition and hydration. Briefly, the pope stated that such tubes were "not a medical act" and their use "always represents a natural means of preserving life" and is part of "normal care." Therefore, their use is to be morally evaluated as ordinary and obligatory. "If done knowingly and willingly" the removal of such feeding tubes is "euthanasia by omission." The person's medical condition is not relevant in making a determination about the use of feeding tubes because the food and water delivered through such tubes is ordinary care and provides a benefit—"nourishment to the patient and alleviation of his suffering."[1]

What is interesting about this papal allocution is that it seems to represent a significant departure from the Roman Catholic bioethical tradition with respect to both the method and the basis upon which such decisions are made. Historically the method for making a determination about the use of a medical intervention was the proportion between the benefits of the intervention and its harms to the individual, family, and community. The method is a teleological balancing of the impact of the intervention. This has been the central teaching of the tradition from the mid-1600s through Pope Pius XII and the 1980 "Declaration on Euthanasia" by the Congregation for the Doctrine of the Faith.[2] The method announced by Pope John Paul II seems to be deontological. The use of feeding tubes to deliver artificial nutrition and hydration is declared ordinary, and such an intervention apparently ought not be forgone or withdrawn.

The traditional method is a balancing of benefit and burden. The basis of such determinations is the impact principally on the patient. The history of the Roman Catholic tradition is filled with examples of impacts that are considered disproportionate, ranging from the use of expensive medications, food beyond the budget of the individual, interventions that are painful in both the short and long term, and even the refusal of a physical examination if that will cause excessive embarrassment to the individual. Included in such a listing and specifically noted in the "Declaration on Euthanasia" is the financial impact on both the patient and family. Interventions that will provide a significant financial hardship need not be used.

The question of the use of artificial feeding tubes has been much debated in Roman Catholic bioethics, especially when used for patients in persistent vegetative state.[3] One early statement was from the revered Jesuit moral theologian Gerald Kelly.

> I see no reason why even the most delicate professional standard should call for their [oxygen and intravenous for a patient in a terminal coma] use. In fact, it seems to me that, apart from very special circumstances, the artificial means not only need not but also should not be used, once the coma is reasonably diagnosed as terminal. Their use creates expense and nervous strain without conferring any real benefit.[4]

There were further arguments made on both sides of the issue by theologians, bishops, and bishop conferences. Over time, a consensus developed that seemed to be that the forgoing or withdrawal of artificial feeding tubes could be judged morally optional in some circumstances.

The reason the papal statement is so startling to many is because it came out of the blue. It seems to depart from the tradition of Roman Catholic bioethics on how to analyze such questions and substitutes a deontological principle for the traditional proportion of benefits to burdens. Thus, the statement raises a number of very practical questions for patients, theologians, medical personnel, and Catholic hospital administrators.

One set of questions relates to the degree of authority of the statement itself. Traditionally allocutions are given to a variety of groups that meet in Rome, but they have not always been seen as the locus for making a major policy shift. Such statements have been used by popes for discussing particular issues, as Pius XII was wont to do. He used allocutions to discuss the use of analgesics to relieve pain at the end of life[5] and organ transplantation.[6] Many of these allocutions at that time were understood to be made in relation to the state of the question in moral theology, and it was well understood that the statements were subject to interpretation by moral theologians. So a first question is, what is the authority of the text?

A second question is, should the text be read broadly or narrowly? That is, should the text be understood to apply to all instances in which a feeding tube is involved or should it be restricted to the specific case of the patient in persistent vegetative state? Profound personal and institutional implications follow from one's reading of the application of the text.

A third question concerns how the allocution will be implemented. That is, what will the U.S. bishops do with this text? Will they consider it a directive that must be implemented in all Catholic health-care institutions, will they need to study what it means in terms of its implications for Catholic health care, or will they leave its meaning up to individual health-care institutions? Part of this implementation issue is how the right-to-life movement in the Catholic Church will enter this debate. It is clear that questions related to the beginning of life are to be resolved deontologically with little or no attention given to circumstances. What may now be the case is that end-of-life questions are to be resolved in a similar way. The political and religious power of the right-to-life movement was clearly manifest in the Terri Schiavo case in Florida. Additionally, it must be noted that Pope John Paul II appointed almost every single bishop in the United States, and it is clear that primary criteria for such appointments are fidelity to church teaching and loyalty to the pope.

Although these questions are of direct concern to Roman Catholics, their resolution will have implications beyond the church. Furthermore, there is another set of questions that will impact persons and institutions. We will now briefly discuss these.

For the past several decades in the United States, persons have been encouraged to make some sort of advance directive. The purpose of this directive, of course, is to help the individual clarify what his or her wishes with respect to health care are in the event that he or she becomes incompetent. Such directives ensure the implementation of the person's wishes, can also be the means by which a decision maker is designated for health-care purposes, and can serve to reassure the family that the patient's wishes are being carried out. In addition, such advance directives might also have the consequence of easing the responsibilities of the family at a time of great stress. If there is an advance directive, the family will know that they are doing what the patient wanted—and this may be a great comfort for many families.

Are Catholics no longer to be encouraged to make advance directives? Or are they to be directed to include no statement about the use of artificial feeding tubes? But suppose that the individual has already directed that he or she does not want a feeding tube, or, should it no longer prove beneficial, have it removed. Will family members be torn between the wishes of the patient and what they understand to be the teaching of the Catholic Church? Practically speaking, the bedside of a dying patient is not the place to have a crisis of faith or morals. By following what the family thinks is church teaching, they will violate the wishes of the patient, and they may in fact cause harm to the patient by the continuation of his or her life with the use of feeding tubes. Yet if they do not follow what they think is church teaching, they might think they are sinning or at least not being good Catholics.

What is a Catholic hospital, nursing home, or palliative care facility to do? If the bishop of the diocese in which these facilities are located mandates a literal implementation of this directive, one would assume that such facilities would be under some obligation to develop policies that prohibit the forgoing or removal of feeding tubes regardless of whether the patient directly asks for such forgoing or removal, regardless of whether his or her advance directive states the same, or regardless of whether the family makes such a request. As a matter of practical fact, most Catholics probably will not know what, if any, instructions the local bishop has given, and they certainly will not know what policies the local Catholic hospital has. Thus, the time they will find out what such policies are is when they are confronted with the reality of the policy at a time of critical decision making, the absolutely worst time for such a discovery.

Several difficult situations might present themselves here. One can envision patients or families insisting on either forgoing or removing a feeding tube and one can then see hospitals refusing such a request.

The medical staff is then caught in the middle, and in the United States, one will consequently have a lawsuit with major implications for church-state relations—one that will make the mandating of the provision of contraceptives in the California Supreme Court ruling in March 2004 against Catholic Charities of Sacramento pale in comparison. One solution that has been proposed is for the patient to be transferred to another hospital—as if one's insurance plan would facilitate that or that another hospital would take such a patient under those circumstances.

Another solution would be not to have oneself admitted to such a facility to begin with. It is the case now that upon admission to a hospital, patients are informed about advance directives and given the opportunity to fill one out. This practice could now be complemented with an additional statement that because this is a Catholic health facility, any instructions concerning the forgoing or removal of feeding tubes will be disregarded. The patient could then determine whether he or she wished to be admitted. The problems with this solution are almost infinite: this is where the physician sent the patient, this is the facility that performs this particular procedure, this is the hospital covered by the insurance plan, and so on and so forth. And this solution does nothing for people admitted to the facility through the emergency room.

There may be any number of administrators of Catholic health-care facilities or physicians, nurses, or other health-care providers who will conscientiously object to a strict interpretation and unilateral application of this teaching. This will present a problem for the hospital at least with respect to the sort of privileges that it grants to physicians. What should the facility do with administrators and staff, the ethics committee, the various chaplains, and other people involved in the daily working of the facility who might conscientiously disagree with the allocution?

What if the patient in the facility is not a Catholic and demands either the forgoing or removal of a feeding tube? Will there be exemptions for non-Catholics? On what basis would these be granted, since the papal allocution states that such a practice would be euthanasia by omission? One would assume that a Catholic facility instructed by the bishop to implement the pope's allocution strictly would mean that it would do this across the board, lest it participate in euthanasia by omission.

The fact that this allocution is understood by many Catholic moral theologians to sit uneasily with the dominant method and basis for determining when a treatment is ordinary or extraordinary pales in comparison with the myriad of personal and institutional issues that the allocution raises. If there were institutional policies in the United States that prohibit the forgoing or withdrawing of artificial feeding tubes, there could be a lawsuit with monumental implications for understanding church-state relations. Also, what would be the implications, financial and otherwise, for Catholic hospitals that are in cooperative relations with non-Catholic health-care facilities?

The decision-making process at the end of life is difficult enough as it is. It is a time fraught with tension, pain, suffering, sorrow, guilt, and grieving. The strict implementation of a policy such as that in the pope's allocution seems to us simply to prolong such agony by prohibiting a responsible medical and moral evaluation of the patient's condition and acting in accordance with the Catholic tradition of medical ethics. Such a policy also has the potential to cause enormous difficulties for Catholic health-care facilities and their staffs. While we certainly support every effort to prevent acts of euthanasia, we do not support policies that require medical staff to provide unwanted medical treatments. Such policies, in fact, may drive people to euthanasia because they feel that they have lost a traditional and sympathetic ally in their final journey with their loved one.

ENDNOTES

1. The allocution "Care for Patients in a 'Permanent' Vegetative State" can be found on the Vatican website, www.vatican.va/holy_father/john_paul_ii/speeches/2004/march/documents/hf_jp-ii_spe_20040320_congress-fiamc_en.html or in *Origins* 33(April 8, 2004): 737, 739–40.

2. Congregation for the Doctrine of the Faith, "Declaration on Euthanasia," in *Origins* 10 (August 14, 1980): 154–57.

3. For example, see Thomas A. Shannon and James J. Walter, "The PVS Patient and the Forgoing/Withdrawing of Medical Nutrition and Hydration," *Theological Studies* 49 (December 1988): 623–47; Joseph Torchia, "Artificial Hydration and Nutrition for the PVS Patient," *National Catholic Bioethics Quarterly* 3 (Winter 2003): 719–30; Gerald D. Coleman, "Take and Eat: Morality and Medically Assisted Feeding," *America* 190 (April 5, 2004): 16–20; Thomas A. Shannon and James J. Walter, "Artificial Nutrition, Hydration: Assessing Papal Statement," *National Catholic Reporter*, April 16, 2004 (http://nat-cath.org/NCR_Online/archives2/2004b/041604/041604i.php); Ron Hamel and Michael Panicola, "Must We Preserve Life?" *America* 190 (April 19, 2004): 6–8.

4. Gerald Kelly, "The Duty of Using Artificial Means of Preserving Life," *Theological Studies* 11 (June 1950): 203–20.

5. Pope Pius XII, "Christian Principles and the Medical Profession," *The Human Body: Papal Teachings* (November 12, 1944): 56–58.

6. Pope Pius XII, "Tissue Transplantation," *The Human Body: Papal Teachings* (May 14, 1956): 380–83.

17

Assisted Nutrition and Hydration and the Catholic Tradition: The Case of Terri Schiavo

Thomas A. Shannon and James J. Walter

The Terri Schiavo case in Florida focused attention on a variety of issues related to the end of life: who is the decision maker, the status of advance directives, the role of family members with respect to married adult children, and issues related to the removal of life support systems, particularly assisted nutrition and hydration. Terri Schiavo is now linked to two other young women who played a critical role in thinking through ethical issues at the end of life. Karen Ann Quinlan and her family helped us think through the removal of a ventilator. The physicians in her case were reluctant to do this because they feared legal repercussions. The legal and ethical analysis concurred that such removal was justified because it constituted extraordinary means of treatment. Nancy Cruzan and her family focused attention on the removal of artificial nutrition and hydration (ANH). Again, law and ethics concurred that such removal was justified, particularly because people testified that being maintained in such circumstances was not her wish.

On February 25, 1990, Terri Schiavo suffered a heart attack, possibly brought on as a result of chemical imbalances from an eating disorder. She suffered loss of oxygen to her brain and was eventually diagnosed as being in a persistent vegetative state. A decade later, in February 2000, her husband, Michael Schiavo, requested that her feeding tube be removed. The circuit court judge agreed, and this set off a lengthy appeal and counterappeal process, including attempted legislative initiatives from the state of Florida and the U.S. Congress and thirty-seven court reviews, that was complicated by increasing family acrimony and public commentary from a variety of sources, religious, political, ethical, and legal. After a five-year legal battle, the feeding tube was removed, and Terri Schiavo died on March 31, 2005, at the age of forty-one.

A critical element in the debate was the ethics of the use of feeding tubes for patients in a persistent vegetative state. Several bishops, particularly in light of the papal allocution in March 2004 on feeding tubes, argued that their use was morally obligatory. Thus Bishop Vaga of Baker, Oregon, stated, "She may well die in the future from an inability to digest food but it would be murder to cause her death by denying her the food she still has the ability to digest and which continues to provide for her a definite benefit—life itself."[1] That sentiment was echoed by Rep. Thomas DeLay of Texas who said, "That act of barbarism can be and must be prevented."[2] A comment on the ethical issue underlying the provision of ANH was offered by Bishop Loverde of Arlington, Virginia, who said: "If Mrs. Schiavo were facing imminent death, or were unable to receive food and water without harm, then removing nutrition and hydration would be morally permissible. It is however never permissible to remove food and water to *cause* death. Food and water are basic human needs, and therefore basic human rights."[3] And Richard Doerflinger of the USCCB (United States Conference of Catholic Bishops) was reported to have articulated the normative nature of this position in an interview with the *Washington Post*:

> Before the pope made his statement about feeding-tube cases at a conference last year there was enough uncertainty about the church's position that Catholics could remove feeding tubes without fear of committing a sin. No one could fairly have said to you that you were dissenting from clear Catholic teaching. Now you would have to say, "Yes, you are."[4]

The issue to be focused in this note is the state of the question in the Catholic tradition regarding the use of assisted nutrition and hydration, an issue that became central to the medical and public debate.

Our position is that there have been four unacknowledged shifts within the last twenty-five years from the traditional method of analyzing our moral obligations during illness and the dying process. The first of these is a shift in the very method itself: from proportionate reasoning as in the "Declaration on Euthanasia" from the Congregation for the Doctrine of the Faith (CDF) in 1980 to a deontological reasoning as in the March 2004 papal allocution "Care for Patients in a 'Permanent' Vegetative State." Second, there is a shift in applying the ordinary-extraordinary distinction from the general context of obligations to oneself while ill to restricting the application to the context of imminent dying. Third, there has been a shift from making a determination of whether or not to use an intervention such as chemotherapy or assisted nutrition and hydration to a presumption in favor of using such interventions. Finally, following John Paul II's allocution, there is a shift from a presumption to use to an obligation to use. Thus, in a series of statements from various ecclesial commissions and magisterial authorities, the tradition has been moved recently from both a patient-centered focus and obligations determined through the use of proportionate reason to a technology and intervention-centered focus with obligations being determined by deontological principles. We call this more recent position the revisionist position.

THE DEVELOPMENT OF THE REVISIONIST POSITION

Methodological Shift

Many moral theologians argue that there are two different ethical methodologies in operation in Roman Catholicism. The first is deontological or a principle-based ethic and is used primarily in the areas of sexual morality and in medical morality where sexual morality is the content, for example, assisted reproduction. The resolutions of ethical issues are deducted from the principles, and there are no exceptions to the principles and no parvity of matter in sexual issues. The principles bind absolutely and are not qualified by circumstances. The other method is the one used in the area of social justice, for example, in the analysis of the morality of war or economic policy. This method, used in the two pastoral letters of the American bishops, "The Challenge of Peace" in 1983 and "Economic Justice for All" in 1986, includes scriptural and philosophical perspectives, empirical analysis, expert testimony, and an examination of a variety of contexts and circumstances. The conclusions drawn are recognized to be provisional in that new data can reshape the conclusion, and there is a recognition that one can come to different conclusions that are in harmony with one's starting principles.

Historically, the method of analysis of issues related to end-of-life issues has mostly uses the second method. This ethic has traditionally been patient-centered and focused on an evaluation of benefits and burdens or on whether the intervention was proportionate or disproportionate. This is the method of, for example, the 1980 "Declaration on Euthanasia" from the Congregation for the Doctrine of the Faith.

First, the congregation notes in section IV that it "pertains to the conscience either of the sick person, or of those qualified to speak in the sick person's name, or of the doctors, to decide, in the light of moral obligation and of the various aspects of the case." The "Declaration" says that the patient can make a correct decision about whether a treatment is proportionate or disproportionate by "studying the type of treatment to be used, its degree of complexity or risk, its cost and the possibilities of using it, and comparing these elements with the result that can be expected, taking into account the state of the sick person and his or her physical and moral resources." Finally, the "Declaration" notes that one can refuse treatments based on a "desire not to impose excessive expense on the family or the community."

This position is essentially supported by the Pontifical Council *Cor Unum* when it says:

> The fundamental point is that the decision should be made according to rational arguments that have taken well into account the many and various aspects of the situation, including what effect will be had upon the family. The principle to follow is, therefore, that no moral obligation to have recourse to extraordinary measures exists; and that, incidentally, a doctor must follow the wishes of a sick person who refuses such measures.[5]

The "Declaration on Euthanasia" is a clear and articulate summary of the moral teaching of the Catholic Church on end-of-life issues from about the sixteenth century to the present. Many of these teaching are summarized in the doctoral dissertation by now-Bishop Cronin.[6] The constant theme of the moralists is that the patient needs to determine what is extraordinary in light of his or her medical circumstances, financial situation, and values. If the effects of the intervention are disproportionate to the desired outcome, they need not be used.

However, a shift seems to be occurring in this tradition and in the method over the past two and a half decades. When one reads the 2004 allocution by John Paul II on assisted nutrition and hydration, there is a methodological shift to deontology and determination of principles by definition or stipulation. Briefly, the pope stated that such tubes were "not a medical act" and their use "always represents a natural means of preserving life" and is part of "normal care." Therefore, their use is to be considered in principle ordinary and obligatory. "If done knowingly and willingly," the removal of such feeding tubes is "euthanasia by omission." The person's medical condition is not really relevant in making a determination about the use of feeding tubes because the food and water delivered through such tubes is ordinary care and provides a benefit—"nourishment to the patient and alleviation of his suffering."[7]

What is interesting about this papal allocution is that it seems to represent a significant departure from the Roman Catholic bioethical tradition with respect to both the method and the basis upon which such decisions are made. Historically, the method for making a determination about the use of a medical intervention was the proportion between the benefits of the intervention and its harms or burdens to the individual, family, and community. The method is a teleological balancing of the impact of the intervention. This has been the central teaching of the tradition from the mid-1600s through Pope Pius XII and the 1980 "Declaration on Euthanasia" by the Congregation for the Doctrine of the Faith.[8] The method announced by Pope John Paul II appears to be deontological in nature. The use of feeding tubes to deliver artificial nutrition and hydration is stipulated as in principle ordinary, and such an intervention apparently must not be forgone or withdrawn unless or until the body cannot assimilate the nutrients or they do not alleviate the suffering of the patient.[9]

The Shift from Illness to Imminent Dying

When one reads the manualist tradition on this question, the general framing of the question is in terms of preserving one's life during an illness. Historically, particularly up to about 1950, there was a coincidence of becoming ill and dying, but that was because of the general lack of any genuinely useful medical interventions. Typically when one got seriously ill, one died. However, the moralists did not cast the teaching as applicable only in the context of dying. For example, when Francisco de Vitoria in the sixteenth century spoke of "protecting his life," of "employing all the means to conserve his life," he believed that "one is not held to lengthen his life."[10] Thomas Sanchez, in the same century, says that "it is inferred that one is not obliged to use medicines to prolong life even where there would be the probable danger of death, such as taking a drug for many years to avoid fevers."[11] Thus the obligation is cast in terms of the general context of illness and the prolongation of life.

Pius XII, in his 1957 address on "The Prolongation of Life," discusses the possibility of terminating attempts at resuscitation by not placing a patient on a mechanical ventilator. In this address the discussion of termination of life support occurs within the context of deep unconsciousness and hopelessness but not within the context of dying or of terminal illness. Additionally, Pius does not posit a presumption to resuscitate but rather uses the traditional burden-benefit method to determine whether or not there is an obligation to resuscitate.[12]

Finally, the "Declaration on Euthanasia" speaks in this vein, as well. Section IV, as noted above, discusses the issue under the rubric of caring for one's health and how to determine what remedies to use. The last six sentences of section IV refer to the dying process but only in that one can refuse "means of treatment that would only secure a precarious and burdensome prolongation of life." The condition of dying or being terminally ill is not the general context for the application of the decision-making process, but rather one more situation in which one can apply the method of analysis.

A shift in analysis seems to stem from "Evangelium Vitae" (EV) in which John Paul II, in talking about aggressive medical therapies that are disproportionate or too burdensome, says "in such situations, when death is clearly imminent and inevitable, one can in conscience"[13] refuse treatments. The footnote for this section is to the CDF "Declaration on Euthanasia," but this seems to misrepresent what the document says. The "Declaration" does talk about imminent death in section IV, but it does not do it in the manner that EV suggests. EV restricts the application of the criteria of proportionality and burden to the situation of imminent and inevitable death. But this is not what the CDF document says. Rather, the analysis of section IV is to identify the method of decision making and what is to be included in it as the patient makes decisions about his or her treatment. The context of dying is yet another time when this method can be brought to bear on the situations. The restriction of the application of the ordinary-extraordinary distinction to imminent death is new and has not been part of the general moral tradition nor of the CDF document.

The Shift from an Argument about the Appropriateness of a Therapy to the Presumption of Its Use

Imbedded in the distinction between ordinary and extraordinary means of medical technology is the possibility of an equivocation on the term "ordinary." When we discuss medical interventions, we frequently discuss some of them as routine, standard, the treatment of choice, standard of care, or ordinary. What is meant in this discussion is that for this particular situation, this is what is usually or ordinarily done. Such interventions can range from a blood transfusion to chemotherapy to cardiac bypass surgery to dialysis to the insertion of a feeding tube, and so on and so forth. However, no determination has yet been made on the effect of such an intervention on the patient or on others. From the perspective of the tradition, this is where the moral evaluation begins. What is the impact on the patient? What benefits or burdens will it bring him or her? What is the likely outcome of the intervention? What is the cost, both psychological and economic for the patient and his or her family? The patient must determine whether there is a proportion between what is done ordinarily in medicine and the expected benefits, both short term and long term. What may be *medically* ordinary or routine may not in fact be *morally* ordinary because of a disproportion of the benefit-burden ratio for the patient. We must avoid the common equivocation on the word *ordinary*.

Another version of this equivocation concerns the distinction as a means of categorizing interventions. When one categorizes medical interventions in the abstract apart from the concrete circumstances of the patient, the basis of the classification itself determines the moral status of the intervention, not the effects of the intervention on the patient. Thus we look at the intervention and ask if this is routinely done. If the answer is yes, then we must use it. Again the assumption is that, because an intervention is customarily used, it must be morally obligatory. And again the moral analysis is short-circuited because of the equivocation, and one attempts to draw an "ought" or moral obligation directly from an "is" or what is routinely done.

Another problem this equivocation sets up is that the terms *ordinary* and *extraordinary* are used as methods of classification or categorizations of interventions. If an intervention is categorized as ordinary—based on the observation that this is customary or ordinary medical practice—then it is morally obligatory. Unfortunately, the tradition does not use the terms *ordinary* and *extraordinary* as a means of abstract classification but as the conclusion of an argument about the proportion or disproportion of benefits and burdens, as the CDF phrases it. This point was also nicely made by the founder of American Catholic bioethics, Gerald Kelly, who noted in 1950 that sometimes even "ordinary artificial means are not obligatory when relatively useless."[14] This conclusion led him to revise the definitions of the terms even more carefully, away from any sense of using them as means to categorize the intervention in the abstract to an evaluation of the impact on the patient.

The equivocation on the term *ordinary* and the use of the terms as means of categorizing interventions set the context for the presumption of use of assisted nutrition and hydration. For example, in 1986, the Committee for Pro-Life Activities of the then NCCB noted that food and water are necessities of life. And since they can be provided without risks and burdens associated with more aggressive life-supporting interventions, there should be a presumption in favor of their use. This idea of a presumption in favor of ANH was reiterated by the New Jersey Catholic Conference in 1987 when it argued against the removal of ANH in the case of Nancy Jobes. The bishops noted a positive duty to prolong human life and, since food and water are basic to human life, they should always be provided.[15] This position was repeated in the *Ethical and Religious Directives for Catholic Health Care Services* issued in 1994 by the NCCB/USCC. After repeating the traditional means of determining burden and benefit, the document states, "There should be a presumption in favor of providing nutrition and hydration to all patients, including patients who require medically assisted nutrition and hydration, as long as this is of sufficient benefit to outweigh the burdens involved to the patient."[16]

What is interesting is the structure of the sentence. The tradition would usually begin with an analysis of whether there is burden or benefit and then determine whether ANH is required or not. The revisionist position begins with a presumption and then moves to disprove the presumption. The problem with this comes from either an equivocation on the term *ordinary* or from using the term as a method of classification. The position of the long-standing tradition has been to evaluate the proposed intervention and then come to a moral conclusion.

A final difficulty with this shift concerns determining to what we have presumptive or prima facie obligations. In the tradition, one had a presumptive obligation to preserve one's life, not a presumptive obligation to accept or take any particular medical technology, for example, mechanical ventilators, heart transplants, or assisted nutrition and hydration. In recent statements, however, patients have a presumptive obligation to take artificial nutrition and hydration. This presumptive obligation can be overridden if and when it can be shown from the circumstances—for example, the body cannot assimilate the nutrients or the patient is imminently dying or they do not alleviate the suffering of the patient—that this obligation is not one's actual moral obligation.

The Shift from Presumption of Use to the Necessity of Use of Assisted Nutrition and Hydration

The first note of a shift away from considering the context of the sick person as morally relevant to decision making at any stage of the illness is in the previously cited *Cor Unum* document of 1981. This document states:

> There remains the strict obligation to apply under all circumstances those *therapeutic measures* which are called "minimal": that is, those which are normally and customarily used for the maintenance of life (*alimentation*, blood transfusions, injections, etc.). To interrupt these minimal measure would in practice, be equivalent to wishing to put an end to the patient's life.[17]

Note here that feeding is defined as a medical intervention and that there is the presumption of benefit of this intervention.

The Pontifical Academy of Sciences in 1985 noted, "If the patient is in a permanent irreversible coma, as far as can be foreseen, treatment is not required, but all *care* should be lavished on him, *including feeding*."[18] Note here that "feeding" is not placed within the category of "medical treatment" but is defined as "care," which indicates that such interventions are not subject to the normal moral criterion of proportionality between benefits and burdens.

This position is repeated in John Paul II's allocution on assisted nutrition and hydration in which the pope stated in March 2004 that such tubes were "not a medical act" and their use "always represents a natural means of preserving life" and is part of "normal care." Therefore, their use is to be morally considered in principle as ordinary and obligatory. "If done knowingly and willingly," the removal of such feeding tubes is "euthanasia by omission." Other than the inability of the body to absorb the nutrients or that the patient is imminently dying or that the patient's suffering cannot be alleviated, the person's medical condition is not relevant in making a determination about the use of feeding tubes because the food and water delivered through such tubes is ordinary care and provides a benefit—"nourishment to the patient and alleviation of his suffering."[19] Such a shift to the requirement that assisted nutrition and hydration must be used essentially takes the decision about this intervention out of the patient-centered approach that has so characterized the historical tradition of the past.

CONCLUSIONS

The Terri Schiavo case provides an interesting insight into a major change in the methodology to determine whether or not an intervention is a benefit or a burden, whether or not it is proportionate or disproportionate. To our knowledge, no one in any of the discussions has argued that there is no moral obligation to provide cures or care for those who are ill or in medically compromised positions. At issue is how one determines that obligation. Our observation is that the tradition from at least the sixteenth century through Pius XII, the Congregation for the Doctrine of the Faith in 1980, and the vast majority of moral theologians has determined this obligation by having the patient consider the benefits and burdens of the intervention to determine if they were proportionate or disproportionate. The tradition did not start with assumptions about interventions, nor did it categorize interventions.

Since the early to mid-1980s, though, a revisionist position has been emerging in the statements from the pontifical academies, commissions, and committees that radically change the methodology. These statements categorize interventions and stipulate obligations. The method shifts from proportionality of effects on the patient (teleology) to deontology.

The shift seems to be motivated by two moves: one ethical and the other political. The ethical move seems to emerge out of an eliding of two distinct but related elements that make up a moral judgment. The axiological element, which is concerned with the determination of value, affirms the value or sanctity of life of the patient. This assessment opposes, correctly, efforts to devalue life lived under difficult circumstances or problematic medical conditions, such as permanent coma. Thus, the axiological element of the moral judgment in the Catholic tradition opposes any use of the phrase "quality of life" as a shorthand way of arguing that a patient's life is not worth preserving. The second and distinct element, the normative, is a determination of what obligations one has in the concrete to maintaining this *valued* life. This normative element has traditionally been resolved by determining the burden-benefit ratio of the proposed intervention. Failure to make this important and traditional ethical distinction between axiology and normativity leads one to affirm wrongly that the affirmation of the value or sanctity of life of the patient in and of itself imposes normative obligations with respect to medical interventions. In addition to being the fallacy of deriving an "ought" from an "is," the failure also implicitly may signify a form of vitalism that affirms that biological life is the only or most important value. Finally, the failure to make the distinction leads to a form of a "medical indications policy" as the moral criterion that mandates that particular interventions necessarily must follow from the diagnosis.

The political move both incorporates the failure to make the distinction between the axiological and the normative and incorporates this into the rhetoric of the right-to-life movement. Thus the rhetoric of the right-to-life movement focuses on the obligation to maintain biological life under virtually any and all conditions and in the more excessive strands of the movement comes close to committing idolatry by making biological life the only value to be considered. This is certainly not the traditional Catholic "sanctity of life" position, and, in fact, it begins to move this rhetoric into materialism in that biological life is the only or most important value under consideration. There is no doubt that recent magisterial attempts to protect the dignity of unconscious patients are important and utterly necessary, but the movement to require the use of technologies that sustain biological life may in fact have the opposite effect on a society that is prone to devaluing life.[20]

In an earlier article we developed the following position, and we continue to argue that it will serve as an appropriate basis on which to make decisions about the morality of the use of assisted nutrition and hydration.

When a proposed intervention cannot offer the patient any reasonable hope of pursuing life's purposes at all or can offer the patient a condition where the pursuit of life's purposes will be filled with profound frustration or with utter neglect of these purposes because of the energy needed merely to sustain physical life, then any medical intervention (1) can only offer burden to the life treated, (2) is contrary to the best interests of the patient, (3) can cause iatrogenic harm or risk of such harm, and (4) has reached its limit based on medicine's own principal reason for existence, and thus treatment should not be given except to palliate or to comfort.[21]

The more recent revisionist perspective approaches end-of-life judgments by defining and categorizing particular interventions in the abstract as ordinary, and, on the basis of this maneuver, mandating these interventions. This method, which appears to have entered magisterial statements by stipulation, undercuts the traditional benefit-burden method and risks imposing great hardship on patients and families at a time of great crisis. We can think of no greater burden to impose on people at this time than to have them feel abandoned by the church when they are in greatest need of its benefits. Bluntly stated, the Catholic tradition on end-of-life issues has never mandated doing useless or inane things to people in the name of morality. We should not start doing this now.

ENDNOTES

1. www.catholicmediacoalition.org/bishops%20on%20terri.htm#BishopVasa

2. www.cnsnews.com/ViewPolitics.asp?Page=%5CPolitics%5Carchive%5C2005 03%5CPOL20050318c.html

3. www.catholicmediacoalition.org/bishops%20on%20terri.htm. Emphasis in the original.

4. Manuel Roig-Franzia, "Catholic Stance on Tube-Feeding Is Evolving," *Washington Post*, March 27, 2005.

5. Pontifical Council *Cor Unum*, *Questions of Ethics Regarding the Fatally Ill and the Dying*. (Rome: Vatican Press, 1981), 8–9.

6. This dissertation is now included as part I of the book *Conserving Human Life*, edited by Russell E. Smith (Braintree, Mass.: Pope John XXIII Medical-Moral Research and Educational Center, 1989).

7. John Paul II, "Care for Patients in a 'Permanent' Vegetative State." This allocution can be found on the Vatican website, www.vatican.va/holy_father/john_paul_ii/speeches/2004/march/documents /hf _jp-ii_spe_20040320_congress-fiamc_en.html, or in *Origins* 33 (April 8, 2004): 737, 739–40.

8. Congregation for the Doctrine of the Faith, "Declaration on Euthanasia," in *Origins* 10 (August 14, 1980): 154–57.

9. John Paul II, "Care for Patients in a 'Permanent' Vegetative State," 739. Though the pope made an "in principled" argument here, some have not carefully articulated this in their remarks about the allocution. For example, see the published interview noted above with Richard Doerflinger in the *Washington Post*, March 27, 2005.

10. Cronin, *Conserving Human Life*, 34–37.

11. Cronin, *Conserving Human Life*, 43.

12. Pius XII, "The Prolongation of Life" (November 24, 1957), *The Pope Speaks* 4 (1958): 395–98.

13. John Paul II, "Evangelium Vitae," 65.

14. Gerald Kelly, "The Duty of Using Artificial Means of Preserving Life," *Theological Studies* 11 (1950): 220. See also "Notes," *Theological Studies* 12 (1951): 550–56 for the revised definitions of ordinary and extraordinary.

15. New Jersey Catholic Conference, "Providing Food and Fluids to Severely Brain Damaged Patients," *Origins* 16 (January 22, 1987): 582–84.

16. USCC, *Ethical and Religious Directives for Catholic Health Care Services* (Washington, DC: USCC, 1994), Directive No. 58. Interestingly, in the latest version of the ERDs (2001), the introduction to part V, in which directive 58 is found, states, "These statements agree that hydration and nutrition are not morally obligatory either when they bring no comfort to a person who is imminently dying or when they cannot be assimilated by the person's body." Note here that a proportion between benefit and burden is not the criterion used.

17. Pontifical Council *Cor Unum, Questions of Ethics*, 8–9. Emphases added.

18. The Pontifical Academy of Sciences, "The Artificial Prolongation of Life," *Origins* 15 (December 5, 1985): 415. Emphases added.

19. John Paul II, "Care for Patients in a 'Permanent' Vegetative State," 739.

20. See Thomas A. Shannon and James J. Walter, "Implications of the Papal Allocution on Feeding Tubes," *Hastings Center Report* 34 (July–August 2004): 18–20.

21. Thomas A. Shannon and James J. Walter, "The PVS Patient and the Forgoing/ Withdrawing of Medical Nutrition and Hydration," *Theological Studies* 49 (December 1988): 645.

Index

abortion: anthropological parameter concerning, 152–57; Catholic moral teachings on, 148–51; dignity and sanctity of human life, 153–54; ethical parameter concerning, 157–62; Hebrew scriptures and, 172n10; individualism and, 156; legal parameter concerning, 166–69; modern concepts of the pre-embryo and, 85; notions of ensoulment and, 78; for reasons other than birth control, 164; value parameter concerning, 162–65; women's freedom to choose and, 164

abortion debate: complexity of Catholic position in, 169–70; in public life, 145–46; values and, 170

abortion laws, 51

acrosome reaction, 70

active conception, 79

adoption, 138

adult protective services, 50–51, 54–55

Advanced Cell Technology, 94

advanced directives, 265–66

advertising, in vitro fertilization and, 128–129

affectio commodi, 115–16

affectio justitiae, 116–17

agape, 41

"agent narrative suffering," 225–26, 228

Aiken, William, 214

allocution(s): on artificial nutrition and hydration, 272–73, 277; degree of authority of, 264–65; on feeding tubes, implications of, 263–68

aloneness, 14

Altizer, Thomas J. J., 38

American Academy of Neurology, 241

analogue models. *See* disclosure models

Andrews, Lori, 30, 51

angels, 104

Anselm of Canterbury, 80, 89n59, 146

anthropology, theological, 190–92

applied philosophy, 4–6

Aquinas, Thomas. *See* Thomas Aquinas

Aristotle, 109, 112

artificial conception: "Humanae Vitae" on, 129–30; *See also* assisted reproduction

artificial nutrition and hydration: argument in support of forgoing/withdrawing, 240–46; described, 248–49; moral option of forgoing/withdrawing, 253; papal allocution on, 272–73, 277; papal statement on analyzed, 257–61; persistent vegetative state patients and, 231–40; potential burdens and harms from, 259–60; Terri Schiavo case, 269–79; *See also* feeding tubes

281

About the Authors

James J. Walter is the Austin and Ann O'Malley Professor of Bioethics and the Chairperson of The Bioethics Institute at Loyola Marymount University in Los Angeles, California. He has published four other books, most recently *The New Genetic Medicine: Theological and Ethical Reflections* with Thomas A. Shannon, and he has published in many scholarly journals on bioethical topics.

Thomas A. Shannon is Professor Emeritus in the Department of Humanities and Arts at Worcester Polytechnic Institute. He is the author of many essays in bioethics and the editor of four Sheed & Ward readers in bioethics.